T0329133

Thresholds of Genotoxic Carcinogens

Thresholds of Genotoxic Carcinogens

From Mechanisms to Regulation

Edited by

Takehiko Nohmi
Biological Safety Research Center,
National Institute of Health Sciences,
Setagaya-ku, Tokyo, Japan

Shoji Fukushima
Japan Bioassay Research Center,
Japan Industrial Safety & Health Association,
Hadano, Kanagawa, Japan

AMSTERDAM • BOSTON • HEIDELBERG • LONDON
NEW YORK • OXFORD • PARIS • SAN DIEGO
SAN FRANCISCO • SINGAPORE • SYDNEY • TOKYO
Academic Press is an imprint of Elsevier

British Library Cataloguing-in-Publication Data
A catalogue record for this book is available from the British Library.

Library of Congress Cataloging-in-Publication Data
A catalog record for this book is available from the Library of Congress.

ISBN: 978-0-12-801663-3

For Information on all Academic Press publications
visit our website at http://www.elsevier.com/

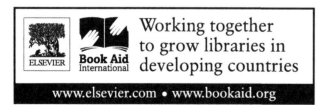

Working together
to grow libraries in
developing countries

www.elsevier.com • www.bookaid.org

Publisher: Mica Haley
Acquisition Editor: Erin Hill-Parks
Editorial Project Manager: Molly McLaughlin
Production Project Manager: Chris Wortley
Designer: Maria Inês Cruz

Typeset by MPS Limited, Chennai, India

Contents

List of Contributors.. *xi*

Preface .... *xiii*

Chapter 1: Qualitative and Quantitative Assessments on Low-Dose Carcinogenicity of Genotoxic Hepatocarcinogens: Dose–Response for Key Events in Rat Hepatocarcinogenesis *1*

Shoji Fukushima, Min Gi, Anna Kakehashi and Hideki Wanibuchi

Introduction 1
Qualitative and Quantitative Analyses on Low-Dose Carcinogenicity of
    2-Amino-3,8-dimethylimidazo[4,5-*f*]quinoxaline in the Rat Liver 3
Qualitative and Quantitative Analyses on Low-Dose Hepatocarcinogenicity of
    2-Amino-3-methylimidazo[4,5-*f*]quinoline in the Rat Liver 7
Qualitative and Quantitative Analysis on Low-Dose Hepatocarcinogenicity
    of *N*-nitrosodiethylamine in the Rat Liver 9
Discussion...9
References...15

Chapter 2: Thresholds for Hepatocarcinogenicity of DNA-Reactive Compounds *19*

T. Kobets and G.M. Williams

Introduction 19
Dose–Effect Studies of Initiation of Liver Carcinogenesis 22
Conclusions 28
Relevance to Humans 30
References...32

Chapter 3: Interaction of Low-Dose Radiation and Chemicals in Cancer Risk...........*37*

Shizuko Kakinuma, Benjamin J. Blyth and Yoshiya Shimada

Epidemiological Analysis of Cancer Risk 38
    Solid Cancer..38
    Leukemia...40
Interaction of Radiation and Other Carcinogens 41
Data From Animal Experiments 42
    Skin Tumors 42
    Thymic Lymphoma 43

Conclusion 46
Acknowledgments 46
References..46

Chapter 4: Possible Mechanisms Underlying Genotoxic Thresholds: DNA Repair and Translesion DNA Synthesis 49

Takehiko Nohmi and Teruhisa Tsuzuki

Introduction 49
Challenges in Identification of Genotoxicity of Chemicals......................52
Possible Mechanisms Underlying Genotoxic Thresholds 54
Significance of DNA Repair Mechanisms in the Suppression of Mutagenesis
    and Tumorigenesis in Mammals..55
TLS as a Critical Factor for Mutagenesis 58
Future Perspectives 62
Acknowledgments 63
References..63

Chapter 5: DNA Repair and Its Influence on Points of Departure for Alkylating Agent Genotoxicity 67

Adam D. Thomas and George E. Johnson

Introduction 67
The Paradigm Shift in Response to Low Doses of Alkylating Agents 69
Alkylating Agent Mechanism of Action 70
DNA Repair of Alkyl Adducts: Potential Influences on PoDs 71
Mechanistic Evidence Supporting a PoD for EMS 74
Mechanistic Evidence Supporting a PoD for ENU 75
Mechanistic Evidence Supporting a PoD for MMS 76
Mechanistic Evidence Supporting a PoD for MNU 76
Concluding Remarks 77
References..77

Chapter 6: The Role of Endogenous Versus Exogenous DNA Damage in Risk Assessment 83

*James Swenberg, Yongquan Lai, Rui Yu, Vyom Sharma, Benjamin C. Moeller,
Hadley Hartwell, Jacqueline Gibson and Jun Nakamura*

Introduction 83
Aldehydes 84
Alkylating Agents 88
Oxidative Stress 90
Ionizing Radiation 92

Quantifying Complex Dose–Response Relationships to Support
  Risk Assessments...92
    Approach 1: Threshold Models..93
    Approach 2: Bottom-Up Method..93
    Approach 3: Distributional Method..94
    Approach 4: Bayesian Belief Networks...95
  Conclusion..98
  References..98

Chapter 7: Thresholds of Toxicological Concern for Genotoxic Impurities in
Pharmaceuticals *103*
  Masamitsu Honma

  Introduction 103
  Genotoxic and Nongenotoxic Carcinogens 104
  Thresholds of Chemical Genotoxicity..105
  Risk Management for Genotoxic Carcinogens..107
  Risk Assessment and Control of Genotoxic Impurities in Pharmaceuticals............109
    Principles for Assessment and Control of Genotoxic Impurities in
      Pharmaceuticals... 109
    Less-Than-Lifetime TTC 112
    Compound-Specific TTC 112
  Conclusion..114
  References..114

Chapter 8: Practical Thresholds in the Derivation of Occupational Exposure
Limits (OELs) for Carcinogens *117*
  Hermann M. Bolt

  Introduction 117
  Derivation of Occupational Exposure Limits for Carcinogenic Substances 118
  Concept of the German DFG (MAK (Maximale Arbeitsstoffkonzentration)
    Commission)..118
  Discourse and Further Development in Europe..120
  The Concept of SCOEL...121
  Recent Examples of Carcinogens With a Practical Threshold Assigned
    by SCOEL..122
    Propylene Oxide 122
    Naphthalene...123
    Nickel...124
    Cadmium 125
  Conclusions 126
  Abbreviations..126
  References..126

Chapter 9: Experimental Design and Statistical Analysis of Threshold Studies 129
David P. Lovell

Introduction 129
    Definitions of Thresholds 131
    Dose–Response Modeling in Radiation (The No Safe Dose of
        Radiation Concept) 132
    Linear and Nonlinear 132
    Experimental Designs for Dose–Response Modeling 133
No-Observed Genotoxic Effect Level 138
Dose–Response Modeling 139
Interpolation and Extrapolations 143
Goodness of Fit Issues: Acceptance and Rejection of Models 143
BMD Approach 145
Mathematical Modeling for the BMD 146
Software 146
    BMDS 147
    PROAST 147
    Drsmooth 147
    Other R Packages 148
    GraphPad PRISM 148
Conclusions 149
Acronyms 149
References 150

**Chapter 10: Nrf2 as a Possible Determinant of the Threshold for
Carcinogenesis 155**

Yasunobu Aoki

Introduction 155
The Regulation of Gene Expression by Nrf2 158
The Susceptibility of Nrf2 Knockout Mice to Xenobiotics 159
The Carcinogenicity and Mutagenicity of Xenobiotics in Nrf2 Knockout Mice 160
Human Carcinogenesis in Regard to Nrf2 Activity 163
Do Nrf2 and Nrf2-Regulating Genes Contribute to the Creation of a
    Threshold to Carcinogenesis? 164
Conclusion 164
Abbreviations 165
References 165

**Chapter 11: Assessment of Nongenotoxic Mechanisms in Carcinogenicity
Test of Chemicals; Quinone, Quinone Imine, and Quinone Methide as Examples 171**
Yasushi Yamazoe and Kunitoshi Mitsumori

Quercetin 172
    Genotoxicity 173
    Pharmacokinetics 173
    Carcinogenicity 174
    Toxicology 175

Eugenol and Methyleugenol 175
    Genotoxicity 175
    Pharmacokinetics 176
    Carcinogenicity 177
Phenacetin and Acetaminophen 178
    Genotoxicity 178
    Pharmacokinetics 179
    Carcinogenicity 180
Menadione 180
    Genotoxicity 181
    Pharmacokinetics 181
    Carcinogenicity 182
    Toxicology 182
Ethoxyquin 183
    Genotoxicity 183
    Pharmacokinetics 184
    Carcinogenicity 184
    Mechanism of Carcinogenicity of Ethoxyquin 185
General Discussion for All the Chemicals Shown 185
References 188

Chapter 12: Mode of Action and Assessment of Human Relevance for Chemical-Induced Animal Tumors 193

Masahiko Kushida, Tomoya Yamada and Yasuyoshi Okuno

Introduction 193
Importance of Mode of Action (MOA) Analyses for Chemical-Induced Animal
    Tumors and Assessment of Human Relevance Based on MOA 194
Human Relevance of the Constitutive Androstane Receptor (CAR)
    Activator-Induced Liver Tumors in Rodents Based on MOA 195
    Hepatic Tumor Induction by CAR Activators in Rodents 195
    MOA for Rodent Liver Tumor Formation via CAR 195
    Human Relevance of a Rodent CAR-Activator Liver Tumor MOA 196
Human Relevance of the Mutagen-Induced Tumors in Rodents
    Based on Threshold 197
Future Prospects of the Mechanistic Research in Genotoxic and
    Nongenotoxic Tumor Inducers 199
References 200

Index 205

List of Contributors

Yasunobu Aoki   Center for Health and Environmental Risk Research, National Institute for Environmental Studies, Tsukuba, Japan

Benjamin J. Blyth   Radiobiology for Children's Health Program, Research Center for Radiation Protection, National Institute of Radiological Sciences, Chiba, Japan

Hermann M. Bolt   Leibniz Research Centre for Working Environment and Human Factors, TU Dortmund, Dortmund, Germany

Shoji Fukushima   Japan Bioassay Research Center, Japan Industrial Safety & Health Association, Hadano, Kanagawa, Japan

Min Gi   Department of Molecular Pathology, Osaka City University Graduate School of Medicine, Abeno, Osaka, Japan

Jacqueline Gibson   Department of Environmental Sciences and Engineering, University of North Carolina, Chapel Hill, NC, United States

Hadley Hartwell   Department of Environmental Sciences and Engineering, University of North Carolina, Chapel Hill, NC, United States

Masamitsu Honma   Division of Genetics and Mutagenesis, National Institute of Health Sciences, Tokyo, Japan

George E. Johnson   DNA Damage Research Group, Institute of Life Science, College of Medicine, Swansea University, Swansea, United Kingdom

Anna Kakehashi   Department of Molecular Pathology, Osaka City University Graduate School of Medicine, Abeno, Osaka, Japan

Shizuko Kakinuma   Radiobiology for Children's Health Program, Research Center for Radiation Protection, National Institute of Radiological Sciences, Chiba, Japan

T. Kobets   Chemical Safety Program, Department of Pathology, New York Medical College, Valhalla, NY, United States

Masahiko Kushida   Environmental Health Science Laboratory, Sumitomo Chemical Co. Ltd., Osaka, Japan

Yongquan Lai   Department of Environmental Sciences and Engineering, University of North Carolina, Chapel Hill, NC, United States

David P. Lovell   Institute of Medical and Biomedical Education (IMBE), St George's, University of London, London, United Kingdom

Kunitoshi Mitsumori   Food Safety Commission, Government of Japan, Akasaka Minato-ku, Tokyo, Japan

Benjamin C. Moeller   Department of Environmental Sciences and Engineering, University of North Carolina, Chapel Hill, NC, United States; Lovelace Respiratory Research Institute, Albuquerque, NM, United States

Jun Nakamura   Department of Environmental Sciences and Engineering, University of North Carolina, Chapel Hill, NC, United States

Takehiko Nohmi   Biological Safety Research Center, National Institute of Health Sciences, Setagaya-ku, Tokyo, Japan

Yasuyoshi Okuno   Sumika Technical Information Service, Inc., Osaka, Japan

Vyom Sharma   Department of Environmental Sciences and Engineering, University of North Carolina, Chapel Hill, NC, United States

Yoshiya Shimada   Radiobiology for Children's Health Program, Research Center for Radiation Protection, National Institute of Radiological Sciences, Chiba, Japan

James Swenberg   Department of Environmental Sciences and Engineering, University of North Carolina, Chapel Hill, NC, United States

Adam D. Thomas   DNA Damage Research Group, Institute of Life Science, College of Medicine, Swansea University, Swansea, United Kingdom

Teruhisa Tsuzuki   Department of Medical Biophysics and Radiation Biology, Faculty of Medical Sciences, Kyushu University, Higashi-ku, Fukuoka, Japan

Hideki Wanibuchi   Department of Molecular Pathology, Osaka City University Graduate School of Medicine, Abeno, Osaka, Japan

G.M. Williams   Chemical Safety Program, Department of Pathology, New York Medical College, Valhalla, NY, United States

Tomoya Yamada   Environmental Health Science Laboratory, Sumitomo Chemical Co. Ltd., Osaka, Japan

Yasushi Yamazoe   Food Safety Commission, Government of Japan, Akasaka Minato-ku, Tokyo, Japan

Rui Yu   Department of Environmental Sciences and Engineering, University of North Carolina, Chapel Hill, NC, United States

Preface

In the modern world, people are inevitably exposed to many chemical agents. These chemicals are mostly man-made and are essential to maintain and improve the quality of life. However, these chemicals sometimes exhibit unexpected adverse effects on humans. In particular, carcinogenicity of chemicals is a major public concern because cancer is the leading fatal disease in many countries. To protect human health from chemical carcinogens, international communities have set up several guidelines for their regulation. In general, chemical carcinogens are regulated under two distinct disciplines. If the chemicals induce tumors via genotoxic mechanisms such as mutations, they are referred to as "genotoxic carcinogens" and under this discipline regulates that there are no thresholds or safe levels, even at very low doses. In other words, genotoxic carcinogens are thought to impose cancer risk on humans even at quite low doses. In contrast, if the chemicals induce tumors via nongenotoxic mechanisms such as cell proliferation, inflammation, cell toxicity, or hormonal effects, they are referred to as "nongenotoxic carcinogens" and this discipline regulates that there are thresholds or safe levels at low doses. Nongenotoxic carcinogens can be used in society when the doses used are below the threshold levels.

Recently, however, the nonthreshold discipline for genotoxic carcinogens has been challenged by experimental and theoretical approaches. In fact, this discipline is counterintuitive because humans possess many defense systems against genotoxic chemicals. The defense mechanisms include antioxidants, detoxication metabolisms, DNA repair, error-free translesion DNA synthesis, apoptosis, and so on. These mechanisms may reduce the mutagenic effects of chemicals at low doses below the spontaneous levels. In addition, the doses usually used for cancer bioassay with rodents are much higher than the doses where humans are actually exposed to the chemicals in everyday life. Experiments with large number of rodents at doses close to the actual human exposed levels reveal that there are doses where no increase in number of tumors is observed. Therefore, it is questionable whether cancer risk at high doses can be linearly extrapolated to low doses.

This book *Thresholds of Genotoxic Carcinogens: From Mechanisms to Regulation* was designed to cover current scientific activities regarding the risk assessment of genotoxic carcinogens at low doses. As is written in the subtitle, the scientific contents of the book are diverse, that is, from mechanisms to regulatory practices. Therefore, the authors' expert areas are diverse, including experimental pathology, analytical chemistry, DNA repair, radiation biology, food safety, pharmaceuticals, occupational health, and statistics. Thus, this book includes scientific opinions in different expert areas. We hope that the book will provide insights into the basis of the regulatory policy of chemical carcinogens and also that it will be informative not only for scientists but also for regulators of chemical agents.

Finally, we acknowledge all the contributors of this book and Ms Molly M. McLaughlin (Elsevier) for her guidance and assistance.

Takehiko Nohmi PhD and
Shoji Fukushima MD, PhD

Qualitative and Quantitative Assessments on Low-Dose Carcinogenicity of Genotoxic Hepatocarcinogens: Dose–Response for Key Events in Rat Hepatocarcinogenesis

Shoji Fukushima[1], Min Gi[2], Anna Kakehashi[2] and Hideki Wanibuchi[2]

[1]Japan Bioassay Research Center, Japan Industrial Safety & Health Association, Hadano, Kanagawa, Japan [2]Department of Molecular Pathology, Osaka City University Graduate School of Medicine, Abeno, Osaka, Japan

Chapter Outline

Introduction   1
Qualitative and Quantitative Analyses on Low-Dose Carcinogenicity of 2-Amino-3, 8-dimethylimidazo[4,5-f]quinoxaline in the Rat Liver   3
Qualitative and Quantitative Analyses on Low-Dose Hepatocarcinogenicity of 2-Amino-3-methylimidazo[4,5-f]quinoline in the Rat Liver   7
Qualitative and Quantitative Analysis on Low-Dose Hepatocarcinogenicity of N-nitrosodiethylamine in the Rat Liver   9
Discussion   9
References   15

Introduction

Chemical carcinogens in humans have been identified by epidemiological data. Such carcinogens are classified into Group 1 of the carcinogen classification of the International Agency for Research on Cancer (IARC). However, epidemiological data are not always available. Therefore, the most important issue for carcinogen risk assessment is to experimentally identify carcinogenicity of chemicals and to assess risks for such carcinogens to humans. Generally, detection of carcinogenicity of chemicals is performed using 2-year carcinogenicity tests in rodents, especially rats and mice. To obtain statistically acceptable data, the carcinogenicity tests of the chemicals are performed at high doses compared to

Thresholds of Genotoxic Carcinogens.
DOI: http://dx.doi.org/10.1016/B978-0-12-801663-3.00001-7

human exposure levels, including the maximum tolerated dose. To assess risk in humans, carcinogenic response curves from these tests are used. To quantify the carcinogenicity at very low doses, which are close to carcinogen exposure levels in humans, the extrapolation is usually done based on the carcinogenicity study obtained at high doses.

Generally carcinogens are classified into genotoxic and nongenotoxic types. For quantitatively assessing risks to humans of genotoxic carcinogens a linear nonthreshold approach is used. This "nonthreshold concept" of genotoxic carcinogenicity reflects the idea that a single genetic event caused by a genotoxic carcinogen positively influences cancer development. However, protective biological mechanisms exist in vivo, which suggest carcinogenic thresholds may exist even for genotoxic carcinogens.

Famous low-dose carcinogenicity studies have examined thresholds of genotoxic carcinogens in rodents. For instance, about 20,000 female BALB/cStCrlfC3Hctr mice were continuously fed 2-acetylaminofluorene (2-AAF) *ad libitum* in the diet at various doses from 30 to 150 ppm for a maximum of 33 months (ED_{01} study; "megamouse study") [1]. In this study, the incidences of neoplasms in the urinary bladder and the liver that are target organs for 2-AAF carcinogenicity were examined. While the lowest dose of 30 ppm and over induced liver neoplasms, the 30, 35, and 45 ppm doses had no effect on neoplasms of the urinary bladder. As a result, it was concluded that the data for urinary bladder neoplasms did not contradict the "nonthreshold theory" for 2-AAF carcinogenesis, while those for the liver carcinogenesis strongly supported it. However, it must be noted that the lowest dose of 2-AAF employed in this study was still high to examine "low-dose" carcinogenicity of 2-AAF. Moreover, Peto et al. [2] previously investigated the carcinogenicity of *N*-nitrosodiethylamine (DEN) using 2040 male and 2040 female Colworth rats. DEN at various doses from 0.033 to 16.896 ppm was administered to rats in their drinking water, and induction of liver tumors was found to be dependent on the doses of DEN. At lower doses a linear dose–tumor incidence relationship was observed. It was concluded that DEN carcinogenicity in the rat liver had no threshold. In this experiment, the lowest dose that was used in the study was still high for examination of a threshold of DEN carcinogenicity, when compared to human exposure levels.

Most genotoxic carcinogens must be metabolized to active ultimate carcinogens. The ultimate carcinogens bind covalently to DNA, forming adducts. Such DNA adducts are efficiently repaired. However, there is the possibility of misrepair or replication of damaged DNA, resulting in mutation and its fixation in the cell genome. Such irreversible mutations contribute to initiation of the carcinogenic process. Most mutated cells will die due to metabolic dysfunctions or be eliminated by apoptosis. However, some of them will survive as initiated cells. In the classical two-stage chemical carcinogenesis model, this sequence of events is thought to occur during the initiation stage. Cell proliferations from initiated cells form preneoplastic lesions and may develop into tumors, benign and malignant. There is evidence that, before developing into tumors, many preneoplastic lesions disappear spontaneously or do not change, presumably due to elimination by the immune system. The development from initiated cells into tumors is the promotion stage of two-stage chemical carcinogenesis. This mode of action of genotoxic carcinogens is generally accepted.

For hazard identification, the standard method is long-term carcinogenicity testing in two rodent species, such as rats and mice, with at least three dose levels, with a duration of 18 months for mice and 24 months for rats [3]. However, such tests are extremely time-consuming, laborious, and expensive. Therefore, alternative methods to long-term carcinogenicity testing have been developed and accepted as in vivo medium-term bioassays for carcinogenicity of chemicals. Preneoplastic lesions are accepted as endpoint markers for the assessment of carcinogenicity [4]. Results from such in vivo medium-term bioassays are obtained within weeks.

In the following, we present our own data on quantitative assessment of key events that are important in qualitative analysis of genotoxic carcinogens. We examined DNA adduct formation, oxidative stress and gene mutations, events cells typical for the move through the initiation stage of hepatocarcinogenesis in rats. Hepatocarcinogenicity was examined by quantitative analysis of glutathione *S*-transferase placental form (GST-P)-positive foci, which represent preneoplastic lesions in rat hepatocarcinogenesis and is the endpoint carcinogenic marker in the rat medium-term carcinogenicity bioassay [4].

Qualitative and Quantitative Analyses on Low-Dose Carcinogenicity of 2-Amino-3,8-dimethylimidazo[4,5-f]quinoxaline in the Rat Liver

2-Amino-3,8-dimethylimidazo[4,5-*f*]quinoxaline (MeIQx) is a heterocyclic amine contained in fried meat and fish. MeIQx, at doses of 100–400 ppm in the diet, is carcinogenic in the rat liver [5] and is classified into Group 2B by IARC [6]. To investigate the carcinogenic effect of exposure to low doses of MeIQx, 1145 twenty-one-day-old male F344 rats were divided into seven groups and administered MeIQx in the diet at doses of 0, 0.001, 0.01, 0.1, 1, 10 ppm (low-dose groups) and 100 ppm (high-dose group) for 4–32 weeks [7].

MeIQx is metabolized in the liver cells to an ultimate carcinogen capable of covalently binding DNA. MeIQx–DNA adducts are dose-dependently formed in the rat liver [8]. The formation of MeIQx–DNA adducts at week 4 was below the limit of detection in the 0 and 0.001 ppm groups. The adducts increased upon administration of 0.01 ppm and higher doses of MeIQx (Fig. 1.1A).

DNA is subject to constant oxidative damage from endogenous oxidants. 8-Hydroxy-2′-deoxyguanosine (8-OHdG) is an accepted marker for oxidative DNA damage [9], and its levels rise as a cell becomes more metabolically active. MeIQx administration increased the levels of 8-OHdG of rat liver in a dose-dependent manner. The 8-OHdG levels at week 4

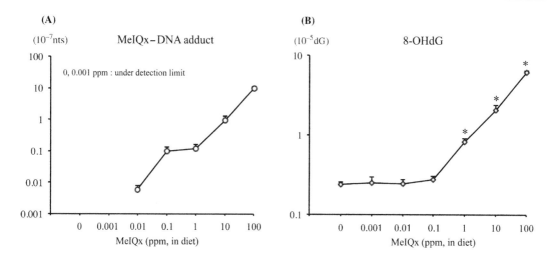

Figure 1.1

MeIQx–DNA adduct formation (A) and 8-OHdG levels (B) in the liver of F344 rats treated with MeIQx at various doses for 4 weeks. *$P < 0.01$ versus 0 ppm group.

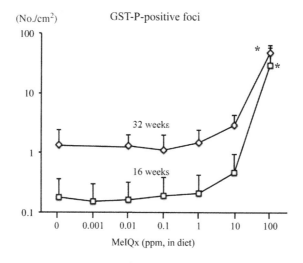

Figure 1.2

GST-P-positive foci in the livers of F344 rats treated with MeIQx at various doses for 16 and 32 weeks. *$P < 0.01$ versus respective 0 ppm group.

were unaffected by treatment with 0.001, 0.01, or 0.1 ppm MeIQx, but became statistically significantly elevated after treatment with MeIQx at doses of 1, 10, and 100 ppm (Fig. 1.1B).

The induction of liver GST-P-positive foci after treatment with various doses of MeIQx for 16 and 32 weeks is shown in Fig. 1.2. The numbers of GST-P-positive foci were not significantly elevated in the 0.001- to 10-ppm MeIQx groups, but a statistically significant increase was detected in the 100 ppm group. Similar results were observed when the treatment with MeIQx continued for 32 weeks.

Based on the results of MeIQx-related events in the present study, the no-observed-effect level (NOEL) was estimated to be 0.1 ppm for 8-OHdG and 10 ppm for GST-P-positive foci. Due to limitations in detection of DNA adducts, we were unable to determine a NOEL for MeIQx–DNA adduct formation. However, such adduct levels should be very low. The 8-OHdG formation level was higher than that of DNA adducts. The NOEL for 8-OHdG was lower than that for GST-P-positive foci.

We also examined mutation of the *lacI* gene and induction of GST-P-positive foci in livers of Big Blue rats [10]. Forty male Big Blue rats were divided into seven groups and administered MeIQx in the diet at doses of 0, 0.001, 0.01, 0.1, 1, 10, and 100 ppm for 16 weeks. A statistically significant elevation of the *lacI* gene mutation level was detected in the 10 and 100 ppm groups (Fig. 1.3A). The NOEL was 1 ppm. On the other hand, formation of GST-P-positive foci was statistically significantly induced by administration of 100 ppm but not 10 ppm or less MeIQx (Fig. 1.3B). Thus a significant increase of *lacI* gene mutation was lower than that of GST-P-positive foci.

Since NOEL of *lacI* gene mutation was obtained from MeIQx mutagenicity in rats, the initiation activity of MeIQx was examined in a two-stage hepatocarcinogenesis of rats using a typical promoter, phenobarbital, in the promotion stage [11]. A total of 850 twenty-one-day-old male F344 rats were administered MeIQx at doses of 0, 0.001, 0.01, 0.1, 1, 10, and 100 ppm for 4 weeks and followed by administration of 500 ppm phenobarbital in

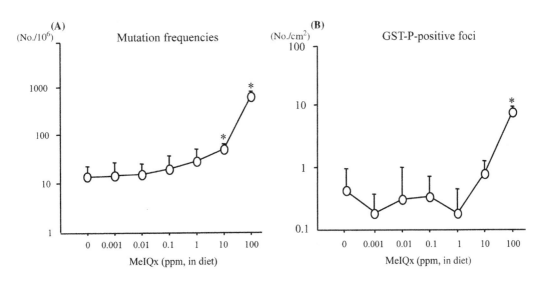

Figure 1.3

lacI gene mutation frequencies (A) and GST-P-positive foci (B) in the liver of Big Blue rats treated with MeIQx at various doses for 16 weeks. *$P < 0.001$ versus 0 ppm group.

the diet for 12 weeks. The numbers of GST-P-positive foci were not increased in MeIQx groups at doses of 0.001–1 ppm, but significant increases were observed at 10 and 100 ppm. The result indicates that the level of the initiation activity is the same to that of *lacI* gene mutation.

Research on factors such as disease status, genetic status, and lifestyle, which influence the ability to tolerate exposure to environmental stressors through activation of adaptive response is needed [12]. Little is known about differences in the low dose–response relationship of genotoxic carcinogens between undamaged and damaged liver. Therefore, we examined the low-dose carcinogenicity of MeIQx in damaged rat liver [13]. Two hundred and eighty male F344 rats were divided into 14 groups. Liver damage was induced by administration of 0.03% thioacetamide (TAA), a well-known hepatotoxin, in their drinking water for 12 weeks. After cessation of TAA treatment, the rats received 0, 0.001, 0.01, 0.1, 1, 10, and 100 ppm MeIQx in the diet for 16 weeks. A linear dose-dependent increase of MeIQx–DNA adduct in damaged liver was evident from 0.1 to 100 ppm: adduct formation in the 0, 0.001, and 0.01 ppm MeIQx groups was below the limit of detection (Fig. 1.4A). The levels of MeIQx–DNA adducts were virtually identical in undamaged and damaged livers. These results are consistent with previous data [7]. In both TAA-treated and -untreated groups, the lower doses (0.001–10 ppm) of MeIQx had no effect on the number of GST-P-positive foci, but a significant increase was observed in the 100-ppm MeIQx-administered groups (Fig. 1.4B). Using the maximum likelihood method to model these data, the numbers of GST-P-positive foci, in the presence or absence of TAA treatment, fitted a hockey stick regression model.

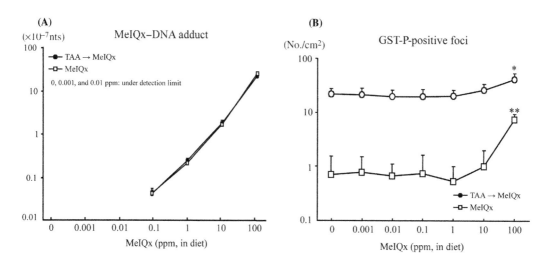

Figure 1.4

MeIQx–DNA adduct formation (A) and GST-P-positive foci (B) in the liver of F334 rats treated with MeIQx with or without thioacetamide. *$P < 0.01$ versus TAA initiation alone group; **$P < 0.01$ versus 0 ppm group.

These results are again consistent with the previous data [7] and support the existence of a no-effect level for MeIQx hepatocarcinogenicity in rats, even when there is a background of liver damage.

To know more about the influence of genetic factors, we examined the dose–response relationship of genotoxic carcinogens in different strains of rats. Male F344 and Brown Norway (BN) rats, 180 each, were administered MeIQx in the diet at doses of 0, 0.1, 1, 5, 10, and 100 ppm for 16 weeks [14]. The background levels of GST-P-positive foci in the control F344 rats were significantly lower than in the BN rats, and numbers of GST-P-positive foci in MeIQx-treated F344 rats were significantly lower in nearly all treatment groups compared with the corresponding BN strain groups. However, the effects of MeIQx on inductions of GST-P-positive foci in these two strains were the same. Lower doses of MeIQx, 0.1–10 ppm, had significant effects on the number of GST-P-positive foci compared to the corresponding controls, while a significant increase was detected at 100 ppm in both strains compared to the respective control groups.

Qualitative and Quantitative Analyses on Low-Dose Hepatocarcinogenicity of 2-Amino-3-methylimidazo[4,5-f]quinoline in the Rat Liver

The heterocyclic amine 2-amino-3-methylimidazo[4,5-*f*]quinoline (IQ) is a genotoxic carcinogen contained in seared meat and fish, exerting carcinogenicity in the rat liver and colon [15]. It is classified into Group 2A by IARC [16]. We investigated the hepatocarcinogenicity of IQ in rats at doses of 0.001–100 ppm [17]. A total of 1595 male F344 rats were divided into seven groups and administered with IQ at doses of 0, 0.001, 0.01, 0.1, 1, 10, and 100 ppm in the diet for 16 weeks.

IQ is a genotoxic compound, which is metabolized in target cells to an ultimate carcinogen capable of covalently binding DNA [18]. IQ–DNA adducts play an important role in this carcinogenicity. Formations of hepatic IQ–DNA adducts at week 4 were not detectable (due to limits of detection of the assay) in the control and 0.001 ppm groups, but were induced by administration of 0.01 ppm and higher doses of IQ (Fig. 1.5A). We found that IQ doses of 1 ppm and below did not increase GST-P-positive foci in the liver, while doses of 10 and 100 ppm significantly increased the foci (Fig. 1.5B). Thus, similarly to MeIQx, DNA adduct formation was observed after administration of low doses of IQ, while doses required to induce GST-P-positive foci were much higher.

We also examined the relative mRNA expression of a panel of genes involved in cell proliferation, cell cycle regulation, and DNA repair. A significant increase in the expression level of PCNA, which is a marker of cell proliferation was observed in the 100 ppm group, but not in the groups administered lower doses of IQ (Fig. 1.5C). Expression levels of p21[Cip1/WAF1], a negative cell cycle regulator, were significantly induced in the 0.01 ppm IQ

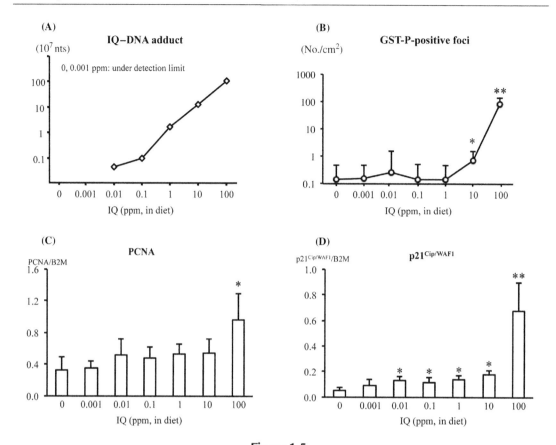

Figure 1.5

IQ–DNA adduct formation (A); GST-P-positive foci (B); and mRNA expression of PCNA (C) and p21$^{Cip1/WAF1}$ (D) in the livers of F344 rats treated with IQ at various doses for 16 weeks. *$P < 0.01$ versus 0 ppm group. **$P < 0.001$ versus 0 ppm group.

compared to the control group, and maximally induced in the 100 ppm group (Fig. 1.5D). The expression level of p21$^{Cip1/WAF1}$ in the 100 ppm IQ group was significantly higher than in the 10 ppm and lower-dose groups. There were no significant changes in p53 expression levels in the IQ-treated groups. These findings suggest that the hepatocytes have adequate capacity to cope with the type of damage that is repaired by the p21$^{Cip1/WAF1}$ pathway when exposed to low doses of IQ, but that the repair capacity of these hepatocytes, even in the presence of high p21$^{Cip1/WAF1}$ expression, can be overwhelmed when the cell is subjected to very high doses of IQ, resulting in cell proliferation at 100 ppm. It is reasonable to suggest that suppression of cell cycle progression by p21$^{Cip1/WAF1}$ followed by DNA repair is at least one of the mechanisms responsible for the observed no-effect of low doses of IQ in rats in this model.

Qualitative and Quantitative Analysis on Low-Dose Hepatocarcinogenicity of N-nitrosodiethylamine in the Rat Liver

N-nitroso compounds, such as DEN, are formed in the stomach through the reaction of secondary amines and nitrites in the diet. They are also found as contaminants of a variety of manufactured food products. Peto et al. [2] investigated the low-dose carcinogenicity of DEN. However, the doses used were still very high compared to human exposure levels.

We have therefore reexamined the carcinogenicity on rat liver at low doses of DEN [7]. Approximately 2000 twenty-one-day-old male F344 rats were administered DEN at doses ranging from 0.0001 to 10 ppm in their drinking water for 16 weeks. No increase in the number of GST-P-positive foci was found at DEN doses of 0.0001–0.01 ppm (Fig. 1.6). However, the number of GST-P-positive foci was statistically significantly elevated at 0.1 and 1 ppm DEN. In the 10 ppm group, the numbers of GST-P-positive foci were so numerous that quantitation was not possible.

Discussion

The mode of action in chemical carcinogenesis is an important aspect in the qualitative analysis of low-dose carcinogenicity of genotoxic carcinogens. Thereby, in the qualitative analysis, it is important to verify the exposure-related sequences of each key event in the initiation and promotion stages of the carcinogenesis.

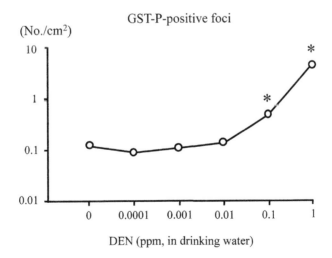

Figure 1.6
GST-P-positive foci in the livers of F344 rats treated with DEN at various doses for 16 weeks.
$*P < 0.01$ versus respective 0 ppm group.

It is clear that genetic alterations are key in genotoxic carcinogenesis. These include carcinogen–DNA adduct formation and mutation in the initiation process. DNA adduct formation is the first genetic key event caused by genotoxic carcinogens and has been accepted as being necessary for carcinogenesis. Therefore, quantitation of DNA adducts provides an indication of biologically effective doses of carcinogens [19]. Therefore, examination of the relationship between DNA adduct formation and mutation is a keystone for the mode of action of genotoxic carcinogenesis. Low-dose linearity is an important aspect for genotoxic carcinogens. However, there is no clear evidence that essential types of mutations are involved in MeIQx-induced hepatocarcinogenesis in rats. Therefore, the *lacI* gene mutation in the liver of Big Blue rats treated with MeIQx was examined [10]. Concerning the correlation between DNA adduct levels and mutation levels, our low-dose hepatocarcinogenicity study of rats treated with MeIQx indicated that levels of DNA adduct formation were much lower than alterations of *lacI* gene mutation frequency [7,10]. Krebs et al. [20] have provided evidence for different dose-responses of DNA adduct formation and gene mutation using transgenic Big Blue rats. Recently, Moeller et al. [21,22] reported that formaldehyde and acetaldehyde-derived exogenous adduct levels are insignificant compared to endogenous adduct levels at low external exposure concentrations. They argued that detoxification mechanisms lead to nonlinearity and even a threshold for DNA adduct formation. The cellular response to DNA adduct formation of genetic carcinogens at low doses may result in nonlinearity for generation of the mutation [23]. Taken together, it is clear that DNA adduct formation levels are lower than mutation levels. Williams et al. [24] emphasized that DNA adduct formation levels at low doses of genotoxic carcinogens are far below the quantities of spontaneous DNA modifications and may be considered unlikely to be of biological significance.

8-OHdG is the most abundant adduct associated with oxidative stress, which produces DNA damage and results in specific types of mutation. 8-OHdG is induced in nuclear DNA of target organs by both genotoxic and nongenotoxic carcinogens. Treatment with MeIQx to rats increases dose-dependently 8-OHdG levels in the liver, although it is unclear whether increases of 8-OHdG levels in the liver contribute to genotoxicity and carcinogenicity of MeIQx [25]. Interestingly, in our study of MeIQx carcinogenicity at low doses, 8-OHdG levels in the rat liver were observed at much lower levels compared to the levels of GST-P-positive foci. They were somewhat lower than mutation levels, but not much lower than the specific DNA adduct levels.

Considering relations between DNA adduct formation and carcinogenicity in this study, there were large differences in DNA adduct formation and development of GST-P-positive foci, preneoplastic lesions developed in promotion stage and the endpoint marker of hepatocarcinogenicity in rat liver after dosing MeIQx [7]. DNA adduct formations were quantitatively observed at very low levels while the induction of GST-P-positive foci was seen at the highest dose of the study only. Low-dose responses of DNA adduct formation and GST-P-positive foci induction by MeIQx in damaged livers of rats showed similarities [13]. There is similarity with the result on relation between and adduct formation and GST-P-positive foci development in the liver of rats treated with IQ [17]. The ED_{01} study of 2-AAF carcinogenicity showed that doses lower than 60 ppm did not induce urinary bladder neoplasms [1]. However, 2-AAF–DNA adduct formation increased lineally from the lowest dose (15 ppm) [26]. On the other hand, liver neoplasms increased from 30 ppm on, and the DNA adduct also increased lineally from less than 30 ppm. Thus, there is a clear quantitative difference between DNA adduct formation and tumor development of 2-AAF [1]. In the case of DEN, curves of DNA adduct formation and tumor incidence in rat liver were similar [26,27]. Williams et al. [28] examined DNA adduct formation and induction of GST-P-positive foci in rats treated with 2-AAF or DEN followed by phenobarbital (initiation and promotion protocol). They concluded that formation of DNA adducts was nonlinear, with a NOEL at lower doses; GST-P-positive foci showed a NOEL at higher doses and dose–response was supralinear. 4-Aminobiphenyl (4-ABP) induces urinary bladder and liver tumors in mice. When mice were given 4-ABP at various doses in drinking water chronically, incidences of urinary bladder tumors were higher than those of liver tumors. Levels of DNA adduct formation in the urinary bladder were higher than those in the liver, and both DNA adducts appeared at lower levels compared to tumor induction doses [29,30]. Poirier et al. [31] also indicated a linear correlation between adduct levels and the incidence of liver tumors in female mice treated with 4-ABP. However, in the urinary bladder of male mice, the relationship was markedly nonlinear. The data indicated that adduct formation alone is insufficient for carcinogenicity and indicative only of the extent of exposure. We previously examined correlations between DNA adduct formation and aberrant crypt foci (ACF), which are surrogate markers of colon carcinogenesis, in the colon of rats treated with 2-amino-1-methyl-6-phenylimidazo [5,6-*b*]pyridine (PhIP), and found that PhIP doses required to induce ACF were much (approximately 50,000 times) higher than those needed for PhIP–DNA adduct formation [32]. Taking together, DNA adduct formations of genotoxic carcinogens in target organs occur quantitatively at much lower doses, compared to carcinogenic doses.

Comparison of the doses capable of inducing gene mutation with the doses capable of inducing cancer (carcinogenesis) will facilitate a better understanding of the threshold for genotoxic carcinogens. In MeIQx rat hepatocarcinogenesis, a specific mutation induced by MeIQx is the best-documented event in the initiation stage. However, there are no data of the following gene mutation event. Therefore, we quantitatively examined the levels of *lacI* gene mutation and of GST-P-positive foci as markers using transgenic Big Blue rats. For MeIQx, doses for inducing the gene mutations were extremely lower compared to those for GST-P-positive liver foci [10]. It is worth noting that in a two-stage hepatocarcinogenesis study, MeIQx exerted initiation activity from the same level on that also induced the gene mutations [11]. Furthermore, H-ras mutation frequencies were elevated significantly at 10 and 100 ppm MeIQx, but not at 1 ppm or less in a 2-week experiment [33]. A similar relationship between the gene mutation and carcinogenesis was also observed in livers of rats treated with IQ (unpublished data, Fukushima Shoji). In renal carcinogenesis of rats induced by potassium bromate, an indirect-acting genotoxic carcinogen, *lacI* gene mutation levels of transgenic Big Blue rats were seen at a lower level, compared to the renal carcinogenic dose [34]. Therefore, we conclude that for genotoxic carcinogens the levels of carcinogen-induced mutations are much lower than carcinogenic dose levels.

Our 2-year carcinogenicity test of MeIQx in rats showed no hepatocarcinogenicity at doses of 0, 0.001, 1, and 10 ppm (low-dose groups) but there was hepatocarcinogenicity at 100 ppm (high-dose group) [35]. GST-P-positive foci were parallel to tumor incidences at various doses. No significant induction of neoplastic lesions was found in MeIQx-administered groups except for 100 ppm, confirming the result of 16- or 32-week studies for inductions of GST-P-positive foci. The relationship among MeIQx adduct, 8-OHdG, *lacI* mutation, and GST-P-positive foci in case of MeIQx is summarized in Fig. 1.7. Levels of MeIQx–DNA adducts increase starting from a very low dose, and then 8-OHdG, *lacI* gene mutation, and GST-P-positive foci develop. Therefore, in the case of exposure to genotoxic carcinogens at low doses, different no-effect levels exist for different parameters relevant to carcinogenesis. We emphasize that dose levels for induction of DNA adduct formation are not equal to dose levels for induction of mutations, and the dose levels for induction of mutations are not equal to those of induction of preneoplastic or neoplastic lesions. The Working Group on Quantitative Approaches to Genetic Toxicity Risk Assessment (QWG) of the International Workshop on Genotoxicity Testing (IWGT) emphasized to use a point of departure (PoD) methodology for determining acceptable exposure levels of genotoxic substances in humans [36], and the benchmark dose (BMD)

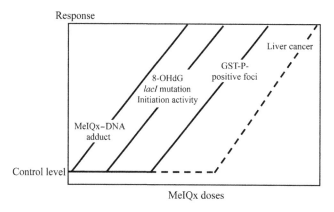

Figure 1.7
Risk of liver cancer: reaction curves for carcinogenesis markers are dependent on the dose of MeIQx.

approach has been recommended to derive a PoD for human health risk assessment. The BMDL, a lower statistical confidence bound on the BMD, was recommended as a suitable PoD. The IWGT Working Group calculated the BMDLs for the key events of genotoxicity and carcinogenicity of MeIQx in rats using our and Kushida's data [37], and indicated the following quantitative order of significant induction events: DNA adducts≪mutations<GST-P-positive foci≪cancer (Fig. 1.8) [38]. The IWGT Working Group also mentioned that earlier key events increased at earlier times and at lower doses than those closer to the apical endpoint of cancer induction [38].

It is of interest that biological adaptive responses, resulting in physiological protection of cells, have been recognized for radiation carcinogenesis at low doses [39,40]. This concept is also useful for understanding low-dose effects in chemical carcinogenesis, since adaptation may be expected to occur in response to low doses of all types of DNA-damaging agents [41]. Various factors, such as induction of enzymatic detoxification and DNA repair, cell cycle control, apoptosis, necrosis, and stimulation of immune system, could result in no carcinogenicity at low-dose exposures to genotoxic carcinogens. We have suggested that induction of $p21^{Cip1/WAF1}$ is indicative of NOELs of low doses of IQ in rats, as non-carcinogenic doses of IQ resulted in a moderate but significant induction of $p21^{Cip1/WAF1}$ [17]. Moreover, the increased cell proliferation accompanied with significantly higher inductions of $p21^{Cip1/WAF1}$ at carcinogenic doses of IQ likely reflects extensive genetic damage, which exceeds the repair capacity of the liver and consequently leads to preneoplastic lesions. A review by Hengstler et al. [42] concluded that many potential carcinogens seem to have a linear dose–response relationship with no observable thresholds; however, for several carcinogens, sufficient data provide an adequate base for the judgment that they operate by mechanisms that encounter a practical threshold. Some carcinogens, such as vinyl acetate and formaldehyde, show non-linear dose–response relationships indicating clear practical or possibly even real thresholds. Recently, Greim and Albertini [23] emphasized the importance of mechanisms which counterbalance interaction with DNA and DNA damage: (1) Toxicokinetic factors may operate to prevent a genotoxic chemical from ever reaching target cells. (2) Mammalian cells have developed mechanisms to ensure protection of the genome. (3) Due to a remarkable efficiency of the DNA repair mechanism, a small amount of DNA damage should be repaired equally efficiently and would not lead to an increase in mutations. Therefore, it was concluded that low exposure to genotoxic carcinogens is unlikely to lead to impairment of cellular homeostasis.

In conclusion, qualitative markers of carcinogenic mechanisms in vivo and quantitative analysis of genotoxicity and carcinogenicity dose–response point to a nonthreshold theory also for genotoxic carcinogens. Our low-dose carcinogenicity studies support that threshold, at least practical threshold exists for the carcinogenicity of genotoxic carcinogens. This is of direct impact to cancer risk assessment in humans.

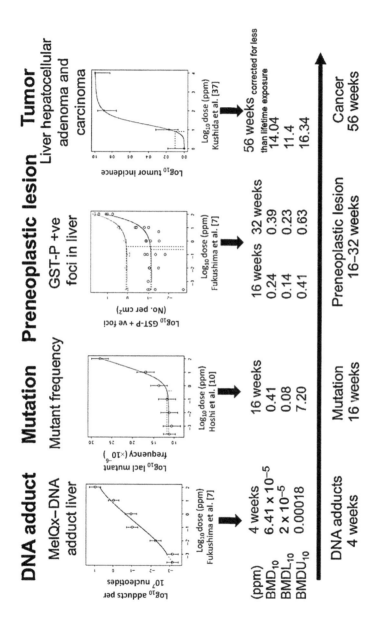

Figure 1.8

Dose-response plots and derived BMD values for DNA adducts, mutations, GST-P-positive foci, and liver hepatocellular adenoma and carcinoma in livers of F344 rats treated with MelQx at various doses. *Source: Data from MacGregor JT, Frotschl R, White PA, Crump KS, Eastmond DA, Fukushima S, et al. IWGT report on quantitative approaches to genotoxicity risk assessment II. Use of point-of-departure (PoD) metrics in defining acceptable exposure limits and assessing human risk. Mutat Res Genet Toxicol Environ Mutagen 2015;783:66–78.*

References

[1] Farmer JH, Kodell RL, Greenman DL, Shaw GW. Dose and time response models for the incidence of bladder and liver neoplasms in mice fed 2-acetylaminofluorene continuously. J Environ Pathol Toxicol 1980;3:55–68.

[2] Peto R, Gray R, Brantom P, Grasso P. Effects on 4080 rats of chronic ingestion of *N*-nitrosodiethylamine or *N*-nitrosodimethylamine: a detailed dose-response study. Cancer Res 1991;51:6415–51.

[3] OECD guideline for testing of chemicals: Carcinogenicity Studies, 451. Paris: OECD; 2009, available on the OECD public website for Test Guideline at <http://www.oecd-ilibrary.org/environment/oecd-guidelines-for-the-testing-of-chemicals-section-4-health-effects_20745788;jsessionid=b11peot04q1k h.x-oecd-live-02>.

[4] Ito N, Tamano S, Shirai T. A medium-term rat liver bioassay for rapid in vivo detection of carcinogenic potential of chemicals. Cancer Sci 2003;94:3–8.

[5] Kato T, Ohgaki H, Hasegawa H, Sato S, Takayama S, Sugimura T. Carcinogenicity in rats of a mutagenic compound, 2-amino-3,8-dimethylimidazo[4,5-*f*]quinoxaline. Carcinogenesis 1988;9:71–3.

[6] IARC Working Group on the Evaluation of Carcinogenic Risk to Humans MeIQx (2-amino-3,8-dimethylimidazo[4,5-*f*]quinoxaline IARC monographs on the evaluation of carcinogenic risks to humans: some naturally occurring substances: food items and constituents, heterocyclic aromatic amines and mycotoxins, vol. 56. Lyon: IARC; 1993, pp. 211–28

[7] Fukushima S, Wanibuchi H, Morimura K, Wei M, Nakae D, Konishi Y, et al. Lack of a dose-response relationship for carcinogenicity in the rat liver with low doses of 2-amino-3,8-dimethylimidazo[4,5-*f*] quinoxaline or *N*-nitrosodiethylamine. Jpn J Cancer Res 2002;93:1076–82.

[8] Yamashita K, Adachi M, Kato S, Nakagama H, Ochiai M, Wakabayashi K, et al. DNA adducts formed by 2-amino-3,8-dimethylimidazo[4,5-*f*]quinoxaline in rat liver: dose-response on chronic administration. Jpn J Cancer Res 1990;81:470–6.

[9] Kasai H, Nishimura S, Kurokawa Y, Hayashi Y. Oral administration of the renal carcinogen, potassium bromate, specifically produces 8-hydroxydeoxyguanosine in rat target organ DNA. Carcinogenesis 1987;8:1959–61.

[10] Hoshi M, Morimura K, Wanibuchi H, Wei M, Okochi E, Ushijima T, et al. No-observed effect levels for carcinogenicity and for in vivo mutagenicity of a genotoxic carcinogen. Toxicol Sci 2004;81:273–9.

[11] Fukushima S, Wanibuchi H, Morimura K, Wei M, Nakae D, Konishi Y, et al. Lack of initiation activity in rat liver of low doses of 2-amino-3,8-dimethylimidazo[4,5-*f*]quinoxaline. Cancer Lett 2003;191:35–40.

[12] Conolly RB, Gaylor DW, Lutz WK. Population variability in biological adaptive responses to DNA damage and the shapes of carcinogen dose-response curves. Toxicol Appl Pharmacol 2005;207:570–5.

[13] Kang JS, Wanibuchi H, Morimura K, Totsuka Y, Yoshimura I, Fukushima S. Existence of a no effect level for MeIQx hepatocarcinogenicity on a background of thioacetamide-induced liver damage in rats. Cancer Sci 2006;97:453–8.

[14] Wei M, Hori TA, Ichihara T, Wanibuchi H, Morimura K, Kang JS, et al. Existence of no-observed effect levels for 2-amino-3,8-dimethylimidazo[4,5-*f*]quinoxaline on hepatic preneoplastic lesion development in BN rats. Cancer Lett 2006;231:304–8.

[15] Ohgaki H, Hasegawa H, Kato T, Suenaga M, Ubukata M, Sato S, et al. Carcinogenicity in mice and rats of heterocyclic amines in cooked foods. Environ Health Perspect 1986;67:129–34.

[16] IARC Working Group on the Evaluation of Carcinogenic Risk to Humans IQ (2-amino-3-methylimidazo[4,5-f]quinoline) IARC monographs on the evaluation of carcinogenic risks to humans: some naturally occurring substances: food items and constituents, heterocyclic aromatic amines and mycotoxins, vol. 56. Lyon: IARC; 1993.165.95

[17] Wei M, Wanibuchi H, Nakae D, Tsuda H, Takahashi S, Hirose M, et al. Low-dose carcinogenicity of 2-amino-3-methylimidazo[4,5-*f*]quinoline in rats: evidence for the existence of no-effect levels and a mechanism involving p21(Cip/WAF1). Cancer Sci 2011;102:88–94.

[18] Schut HA, Snyderwine EG. DNA adducts of heterocyclic amine food mutagens: implications for mutagenesis and carcinogenesis. Carcinogenesis 1999;20:353–68.

[19] Yuspa SH, Poirier MC. Chemical carcinogenesis: from animal models to molecular models in one decade. Adv Cancer Res 1988;50:25–70.

[20] Krebs O, Schafer B, Wolff T, Oesterle D, Deml E, Sund M, et al. The DNA damaging drug cyproterone acetate causes gene mutations and induces glutathione-*S*-transferase P in the liver of female Big Blue transgenic F344 rats. Carcinogenesis 1998;19:241–5.

[21] Moeller BC, Recio L, Green A, Sun W, Wright FA, Bodnar WM, et al. Biomarkers of exposure and effect in human lymphoblastoid TK6 cells following [13C2]-acetaldehyde exposure. Toxicol Sci 2013;133:1–12.

[22] Moeller BC, Lu K, Doyle-Eisele M, McDonald J, Gigliotti A, Swenberg JA. Determination of N^2-hydroxymethyl-dG adducts in the nasal epithelium and bone marrow of nonhuman primates following $^{13}CD_2$-formaldehyde inhalation exposure. Chem Res Toxicol 2011;24:162–4.

[23] Greim H, Albertini R. Cellular response to the genotoxic insult: the question of threshold for genotoxic carcinogens. Toxicol Res 2015;4:36–45.

[24] Williams GM, Iatropoulos MJ, Jeffrey AM. Mechanistic basis for nonlinearities and thresholds in rat liver carcinogenesis by the DNA-reactive carcinogens 2-acetylaminofluorene and diethylnitrosamine. Toxicol Pathol 2000;28:388–95.

[25] Kato T, Hasegawa R, Nakae D, Hirose M, Yaono M, Cui L, et al. Dose-dependent induction of 8-hydroxyguanine and preneoplastic foci in rat liver by a food-derived carcinogen, 2-amino-3,8-dimethylimidazo[4,5-*f*]quinoxaline, at low dose levels. Jpn J Cancer Res 1996;87:127–33.

[26] Poirier MC, Beland FA. DNA adduct measurements and tumor incidence during chronic carcinogen exposure in animal models: implications for DNA adduct-based human cancer risk assessment. Chem Res Toxicol 1992;5:749–55.

[27] Boucheron JA, Richardson FC, Morgan PH, Swenberg JA. Molecular dosimetry of O_4-ethyldeoxythymidine in rats continuously exposed to diethylnitrosamine. Cancer Res 1987;47:1577–81.

[28] Williams GM, Iatropoulos MJ, Jeffrey AM. Thresholds for the effects of 2-acetylaminofluorene in rat liver. Toxicol Pathol 2004;32(Suppl. 2):85–91.

[29] Schieferstein GJ, Littlefield NA, Gaylor DW, Sheldon WG, Burger GT. Carcinogenesis of 4-aminobiphenyl in BALB/cStCrlfC3Hf/Nctr mice. Eur J Cancer Clin Oncol 1985;21:865–73.

[30] Beland FA, Fullerton NF, Smith BA, Poirier MC. DNA adduct formation and aromatic amine tumorigenesis. Prog Clin Biol Res 1992;374:79–92.

[31] Poirier MC, Fullerton NF, Smith BA, Beland FA. DNA adduct formation and tumorigenesis in mice during the chronic administration of 4-aminobiphenyl at multiple dose levels. Carcinogenesis 1995;16:2917–21.

[32] Fukushima S, Wanibuchi H, Morimura K, Iwai S, Nakae D, Kishida H, et al. Existence of a threshold for induction of aberrant crypt foci in the rat colon with low doses of 2-amino-1-methyl-6-phenolimidazo[4,5-*b*] pyridine. Toxicol Sci 2004;80:109–14.

[33] Yano Y, Yano T, Kinoshita A, Matoba A, Hasuma T, Wanibuchi H, et al. Sensitive quantitative assay for point mutations in the rat H-ras gene based on single nucleotide primer extension. Exp Ther Med 2010;1:657–61.

[34] Yamaguchi T, Wei M, Hagihara N, Omori M, Wanibuchi H, Fukushima S. Lack of mutagenic and toxic effects of low dose potassium bromate on kidneys in the Big Blue rat. Mutat Res 2008;652:1–11.

[35] Murai T, Mori S, Kang JS, Morimura K, Wanibuchi H, Totsuka Y, et al. Evidence of a threshold-effect for 2-amino-3,8-dimethylimidazo-[4,5-*f*]quinoxaline liver carcinogenicity in F344/DuCrj rats. Toxicol Pathol 2008;36:472–7.

[36] MacGregor JT, Frotschl R, White PA, Crump KS, Eastmond DA, Fukushima S, et al. IWGT report on quantitative approaches to genotoxicity risk assessment. I. Methods and metrics for defining exposure-response relationships and points of departure (PoDs). Mutat Res Genet Toxicol Environ Mutagen 2015;783:55–65.

[37] Kushida H, Wakabayashi K, Sato H, Katami M, Kurosaka R, Nagao M. Dose-response study of MeIQx carcinogenicity in F344 male rats. Cancer Lett 1994;83:31–5.

[38] MacGregor JT, Frotschl R, White PA, Crump KS, Eastmond DA, Fukushima S, et al. IWGT report on quantitative approaches to genotoxicity risk assessment II. Use of point-of-departure (PoD) metrics in defining acceptable exposure limits and assessing human risk. Mutat Res Genet Toxicol Environ Mutagen 2015;783:66–78.

[39] Wolff S. The adaptive response in radiobiology: evolving insights and implications. Environ Health Perspect 1998;106(Suppl. 1):277–83.

[40] Morgan WF. Communicating non-targeted effects of ionizing radiation to achieve adaptive homeostasis in tissues. Curr Mol Pharmacol 2011;4:135–40.

[41] Kleczkowska HE, Althaus FR. Response of human keratinocytes to extremely low concentrations of *N*-methyl-*N'*-nitro-*N*-nitrosoguanidine. Mutat Res 1996;367:151–9.

[42] Hengstler JG, Bogdanffy MS, Bolt HM, Oesch F. Challenging dogma: thresholds for genotoxic carcinogens? The case of vinyl acetate. Annu Rev Pharmacol Toxicol 2003;43:485–520.

CHAPTER 2

Thresholds for Hepatocarcinogenicity of DNA-Reactive Compounds

T. Kobets and G.M. Williams

Chemical Safety Program, Department of Pathology, New York Medical College, Valhalla, NY, United States

Chapter Outline

Introduction   19
Dose–Effect Studies of Initiation of Liver Carcinogenesis   22
Conclusions   28
Relevance to Humans   30
References   32

Introduction

The concept of thresholds or virtually safe doses for chemical carcinogens is an aspect of risk assessment which has long been under consideration [1–7]. Central to this issue is the chemical mode of action (MoA), from which carcinogens can be divided in two broad groups: epigenetic (nongenotoxic) compounds and DNA-reactive (genotoxic) compounds [6–14]. For epigenetic carcinogens, the MoA entails mechanisms that do not involve direct reaction of the chemical with target cell DNA, but rather derive from other cellular effects, including indirect genotoxicity, epigenetic changes to the genome (eg, alterations in global and gene-specific DNA methylation status, histone modification, miRNA expression), change in gene expression or paragenomic effects to other cellular components (eg, cytotoxicity), which are the basis for their carcinogenicity in target tissues (Fig. 2.1) [11,13,14]. Epigenetic carcinogens are widely accepted to have cancer thresholds [11,12,15–17] at exposures below which they do not elicit the cellular effects that underlie their carcinogenicity. For the other type of carcinogen, the DNA-reactive or genotoxic carcinogens, their MoA involves formation of a reactive electrophile, either through chemical transformation of the parent molecule or through its bioactivation by cellular systems. Electrophiles engage in direct reactions with cellular macromolecules, particularly DNA, in target tissues to form chemical-specific adducts or

Thresholds of Genotoxic Carcinogens.
DOI: http://dx.doi.org/10.1016/B978-0-12-801663-3.00002-9

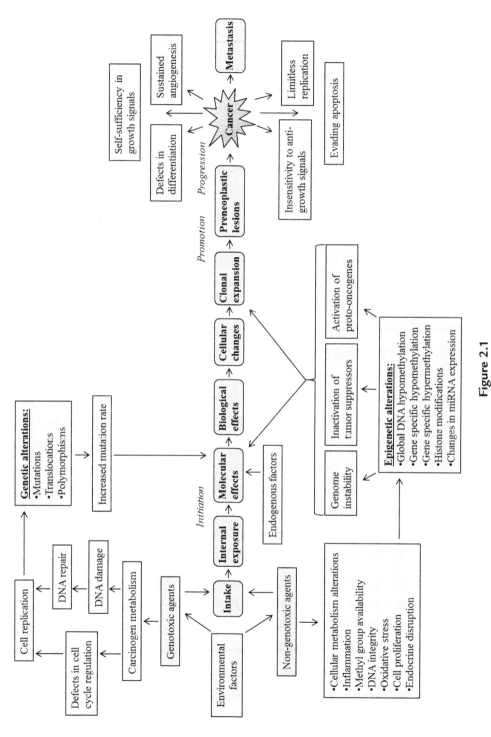

Figure 2.1

Carcinogenesis: triggers and mechanisms.

other DNA lesions, which in turn lead to procarcinogenic mutations in critical genes (Fig. 2.1) [14,18–21]. It has been postulated that a DNA-reactive MoA in mutagenesis and carcinogenesis might result from a single direct biochemical reaction, specifically, a single hit at a critical target in the DNA of a single target cell [22] and thus, no threshold would exist. Against this possibility is the fact that biological processes exist that protect against the genotoxicity of DNA-reactive carcinogens; these include limited uptake of the carcinogen, detoxication, reaction with macromolecules other than DNA, repair of DNA damage, and apoptosis [23–26]. Accordingly, thresholds have also been postulated for DNA-reactive carcinogens [4,12,24,25]. Currently, however, this type of carcinogen is not generally accepted as having thresholds for carcinogenicity, in part because of the nature of its MoA [11,22]. Indeed, most of the carcinogenicity studies of DNA-reactive agents that have used relatively low cumulative doses (CDs) have been interpreted as not showing a threshold [27–32], although some investigators have calculated "virtually safe doses" (level of exposure to a carcinogen that is not expected to induce an excess of cancer incidences beyond the level acceptable by society), "practical thresholds" (dose level below which any effect is considered to be biologically insignificant), or "no-observed-adverse-effect levels" (NOAEL) (the highest dose level that does not cause biologically significant adverse effects compared to the control population) [28,30]. Carcinogenicity studies, however, are limited in their ability to provide evidence of thresholds because they typically involve the quantification of infrequent neoplasms in chronic (2-year) rodent bioassays which do not incorporate the large number of animals required to establish the absence of a tumor increase at low doses. Even in a very large study by Bailey and colleagues [33] using 40,800 trout over an ultralow dose range of 0.45–225 ppm diet dibenzo[*a*]pyrene, which induced liver and stomach neoplasms, the authors concluded that "although the data were consistent with a threshold interpretation, even the use of over 30,000 animals did not provide *proof* that a threshold was reached, or would exist, in either target organ for this carcinogen." Thus, other approaches must be applied to determine whether thresholds exist for the tumorigenicity of DNA-reactive carcinogens. One approach involves measurements of bioindicators of effect such as DNA-adduct formation, cytotoxicity, enhanced cell proliferation, and induction of preneoplastic lesions [17].

In the present review, we focus on thresholds for DNA-reactive liver carcinogens. In this discussion we define a threshold for carcinogenicity as a CD below which there is a NOAEL for a necessary precursor event for cancer initiation (ie, preneoplastic lesions). Such NOAEL can be supported by NOAEL for other adverse effects, which should be differentiated from adaptive responses [34,35]. The experimental conditions can of course influence the results produced by identical CD. The observation of NOAEL allows for the possibility of practical thresholds [5]. In most dose–effect studies, the dose range to detect NOAEL is insufficient. For example, the ED_{01} study performed by NCTR [36], with 2-acetylaminofluorene, the dose range in mice was only 30–150 ppm in the diet. Nevertheless, these limitations can be overcome by using bioindicators of effect, such as DNA adducts, changes in cellular physiology(enzyme activities), cytotoxicity, induction of cell proliferation, and induction of preneoplastic lesions [17].

Dose–Effect Studies of Initiation of Liver Carcinogenesis

Hepatic preneoplastic lesions precede the development of neoplasms and have phenotypic and genomic alterations indicative of neoplastic potential. They have higher rates of development into neoplasms than do unaltered normal cells [37–39]. Accordingly, induction of preneoplastic lesions can be used as a bioindicator of initiation of carcinogenesis. Preneoplasia has proven useful for this purpose because it occurs at lower CD and with shorter durations of dosing than what is needed for tumor induction [39–41]. Immunohistochemical staining is a widely used technique for the detection of preneoplastic lesions which is more sensitive compared to simple H&E staining. The method uses antibodies that detect the presence and location of the specific marker proteins expressed in the altered cells.

In rodent liver carcinogenesis, hepatocellular altered foci (HAF) are recognized as preneoplastic lesions [38–41]. Dose–effect studies aimed at delineating NOAEL have been conducted with liver carcinogens using preneoplastic lesions, together with other bioindicators of effect, such as cytotoxicity and increased cell proliferation, as endpoints for measuring tumor initiation. The concept underlying this approach is that since a preneoplastic lesion is a prerequisite to a neoplasm, a NOAEL for induction of preneoplasia will necessarily be a threshold for neoplasia. This is supported by the demonstration in a series of studies [25,42–48] that administration of carcinogen for 8–16 weeks followed by tumor promotion with phenobarbital (PB) yielded neoplasms only with CD of carcinogen that produced preneoplastic effects. The sensitivity of an initiation/promotion protocol is demonstrated by the fact that it yields higher tumor incidences at lower CD than occur with chronic administration of carcinogen alone [46] (Table 2.1), reflecting the acceleration of tumor development by the promoter. Several dose–effect studies in rodent liver have been reported.

A dose–effect study of 3′-methyl-4-(dimethylamino)azobenzene (MDAB) was conducted by Hino and Kitagawa [50] using adenosine triphosphatase (ATPase) deficiency as a marker for HAF. MDAB was fed to groups of 5–9 male Donryu rats for 24 weeks at concentrations of 0, 1, 5, 10, 20, 60, 100, or 300 ppm. The incidences of HAF were dose-related with the highest dose producing a 23-fold increase over control. With doses of 1–20 ppm, the incidences of HAF were below the control background, which the authors suggested could be due to inhibition of background carcinogenesis by MDAB, an effect described as hormesis, which has been reviewed by Calabrese [51]. The data were interpreted to show a "practical threshold" between 20 and 60 ppm. In general, hormetic (low-dose) effects can either (depending on the target tissue) result from inhibitory signals that trigger stimulatory overcompensation hormesis, or stimulatory signals that trigger inhibitory overcompensation (hormoligosis) [52,53].

Table 2.1 Carcinogenicity in an initiation/promotion (I/P) protocol using phenobarbital[a] as promoter compared to that resulting from chronic administration.

Protocol and Dosage	Cumulative Dose (mg/kg)	Incidence of Liver Neoplasms (%)
Diethylnitrosamine (DEN)		
I/P protocol		
Williams et al.(1996) [42]		
0 mg/kg	0	0
0 mg/kg per P[a]	0	0
5 mg/kg[b]	50	0
5 mg/kg[b] per P[a]	50	3 (one adenoma only)
10 mg/kg[b]	100	9 (adenomas)
10 mg/kg[b] per P[a]	100	32 (adenomas and carcinomas)
20 mg/kg[b]	200	80 (adenomas and carcinomas)
20 mg/kg[b] per P[a]	200	100 (only carcinomas)
Continuous administration protocol		
Peto et al. (1991) [31,32]		
6.3 ppm[c]	287	45
16.9 ppm[c]	771	78
2-Acetylaminofluorene (AAF)		
I/P protocol		
Williams et al.(1998) [43]		
0 mg/kg per P[a]	0	0
1.1 mg/kg[b] per P[a]	94	3 (one adenoma only)
3.4 mg/kg[b] per P[a]	288	100 (adenomas and carcinomas)
Continuous administration protocol		
Williams et al.(1991) [49]		
50 ppm in diet[d]	1772	100

[a]Phenobarbital at 500 ppm.
[b]Intragastric instillation, for DEN once/week for 10 weeks, and for AAF 7 days/week for 12 weeks.
[c]In drinking water for 2.5 years.
[d]In diet for 76 weeks.

A dose–effect study of aflatoxin B_1 (AFB$_1$) was conducted by Root et al. [54] using γ-glutamyltransferase (GGTase) as a marker for HAF. AFB$_1$ was administered to groups of 10 male F344 rats by gavage for 10 days at daily doses of 50, 100, 150, 200, 250, or 350 µg/kg bw, after which rats were maintained for 12 weeks for development of HAF. AFB$_1$–guanine adduct levels were directly proportional to dose after the first dose, but after the 10th dose were much lower in the top three dose groups than after a single dose. The dose–effect relationship for HAF was sublinear, and at the highest dose, achieved over a 1000-fold increase in HAF. A threshold was claimed at the dose of about 150 µg/kg bw per day. From Fig. 5 of the paper, however, some values at 100 µg/kg bw per day are greater than those at 50 µg/kg bw per day, and thus a threshold may not have been identified, but rather a NOAEL. There is no mention of control rats and thus the incidence of background HAF in this study is unknown.

A dose–effect study of *N*-nitrosomorpholine (NNM) was conducted by Enzmann et al. [55] using glucose-6-phosphate dehydrogenase (G6PDH), glycogen phosphorylase (GP), and glycogen content measured by periodic acid-Schiff stain (PAS) as markers for HAF. NNM was administered to groups of 9–23 male Sprague–Dawley rats in the drinking water at concentrations of 0, 0.006, 0.06, 0.60, 6.0, or 60.0 mg/L for 6 or 12 weeks. The dose–effect curves were nonlinear with a slight positive slope at the low doses and a markedly increased slope at higher doses. Quantitation of hepatocellular replication by proliferating cell nuclear antigen (PCNA) at up to 6.0 mg/L revealed a dose-dependent increase at 12 weeks, but not 6 weeks. The apparent nonlinear shape of the dose–response curves of the HAF was interpreted to suggest that some mechanisms contribute to carcinogenesis over the whole dose range, whereas other mechanisms enhance carcinogenicity only at higher doses. Of the three HAF markers used, the $G6PDH^+$ and PAS^+ HAF were increased at ≥ 6 mg/L (at both 6- and 12-week intervals). In contrast, GP^+ HAF were not increased. Thus, $G6PDH^+$ and PAS^+ HAF incidence curves were suggested to indicate nonlinearity, but this, at least in part, was a consequence of log/log plotting of the data (Fig. 1 in the paper),with the background value not having been first subtracted. Based on a linear decrease in the HAF incidence from 4.4 cm^{-2} of liver tissue at 6 mg/L to 0.44 (0.22 if the background is first subtracted), at 0.6 mg/L, lower doses would not be expected to produce a measurable increase above the observed background value of 2.19 HAF/cm^2.

A dose–effect study of 2-amino-3,8-dimethylimidazo[4,5-*f*]quinoxaline (MeIQ$_x$) was conducted by Fukushima [56] using placental-type glutathione *S*-transferase (GST-P) as the marker for HAF. MeIQ$_x$ was administered to groups of 50–150 male F344 rats for 16 weeks at doses of 0, 0.001, 0.01, 0.1, 1.0, 10.0, or 100 ppm in the diet. The numbers of GST-P$^+$ HAF per cm^2 of the rat livers of the four groups administered up to 1 ppm of the carcinogen did not differ from the control value and hence were NOAEL. In contrast, a measurable increase was observed with 10 ppm and a substantial elevation with 100 ppm (both significant at $P < 0.001$). The apparent nonlinearity in the induction of HAF was, as noted above, at least in part, a consequence of a log/log plot of the data (Fig. 1 in the paper) in which there was a background value which was not first subtracted. Transplacental and breast-milk-mediated exposures resulting from feeding diets containing up to 10 ppm MeIQ$_x$ did not increase GST-P$^+$ HAF, whereas caloric restriction for 15 weeks reduced GST-P$^+$ HAF by 20%.

Fukushima et al. [57] conducted a longer duration dose–effect study of MeIQ$_x$ using GST-P as a marker for HAF. MeIQ$_x$ was administered in the diet to groups of 30–50 male F344 rats for 32 weeks at concentrations of 0, 0.001, 0.01, 0.1, 1.0, 10, or 100 ppm. The lowest dose was estimated to provide an intake equivalent to the daily intake of this carcinogen in humans [58]. The numbers of GST-P$^+$ HAF per cm^2 of the rat livers of the four groups receiving up to 1 ppm of the carcinogen did not differ from the control value and hence were NOAEL. In contrast, an increase was observed with 10 ppm and a substantial elevation ($P < 0.01$) with 100 ppm MeIQ$_x$. Thus, at doses below 10 ppm, MeIQ$_x$ did not induce a measurable increase in GST-P$^+$ HAF, but did form DNA adducts at 0.1 ppm and above. Moreover, as discussed above, the log/log plots (Fig. 1 in the paper) give deceptive-looking responses when control values are not subtracted. The effect at 10 ppm for total MeIQ$_x$-induced HAF (Table II in the paper), however, is significantly lower than would be projected from the 100 ppm values with a linear model. In a follow-up 2-year study with MeIQ$_x$ in male F344 rats using 0.001, 1, or 100 ppm in the diet, Murai et al. [59] reported increased frequency of hepatocellular carcinomas, adenomas, and GST-P$^+$ HAF, and increased levels of adducts at 100 ppm. With 0.001 and 1 ppm no significant inductions of hepatocellular preneoplastic or neoplastic lesions were evident, consistent with no significant increase in DNA adducts at 1 ppm. The authors state that 1 ppm may have been a NOAEL for MeIQ$_x$ carcinogenicity, although 10 ppm, which was not tested, would have been predicted by a linear model to have shown less than one tumor, that is, also a NOAEL.

Fukushima et al. [57] also conducted a dose–effect study of *N*-nitrosodiethylamine, also known as diethylnitrosamine (DEN), in which the carcinogen was administered in the drinking water to groups of 151–326 male F344 rats for 16 weeks at concentrations of 0, 0.0001, 0.001, 0.01, 0.1, 1, or 10 ppm. Numbers of GST-P$^+$ HAF in the liver in groups receiving DEN at 0.0001 ppm to 0.01 ppm were not different from those of the control, while the groups administered 0.1 or 1 ppm DEN showed significant increases in HAF. Extracting the data from Fig. 4 in the paper reveals that the effects at 0.1 and 1 ppm were approximately 0.48 and 5.8 GST-P$^+$ foci/cm^2, respectively. The projected value, based on a linear response, at 0.01 ppm would have been 0.05 while the observed value was 0.12, which is similar to the background value. Thus, the expected value was too small to add significantly to the background and thus provided a NOAEL, as the authors stated.

Two studies with vinyl chloride (VC) were conducted by Laib et al. [60] in which groups of 7–21 newborn Wistarand Sprague–Dawley rats were exposed to VC at 0, 2.5, 5, 10, 20, 40, 70, 80, 150, 500, or 2000 ppm by inhalation. In one, the exposure was for 10 weeks (8 h/day, 5 days/week),followed by 1 week of recovery and termination, and in the second, the exposure was for 3 weeks (8 h/day, 5 days/week), followed by 10 weeks of recovery before termination. Evaluation of hepatocellular ATPase-deficient HAF yielded a linear relationship between the dose of VC and the percent of induced HAF. No threshold for the induction of HAF by VC was observed [60].

Williams and coworkers provided further evidence of NOAEL for DNA-reactive carcinogens in male F344 rat liver in a series of studies, using the hepatocarcinogens DEN [25,42,44,45,61] and 2-acetylaminofluorene (AAF) [25,43,45,46,48]. In these investigations, the effects of DEN and AAF were quantified by measurement of DNA adducts, hepatocellular cytotoxicity, cell proliferation (quantified as the PCNA-positive replicating fraction), and formation of GST-P$^+$ HAF, in the initiation phase of carcinogenesis, with the use of PB promotion to elicit manifestation of initiation of liver carcinogenesis by the formation of

Table 2.2 Liver DNA adducts, hepatocellular percent replicating fraction (RF), and GST-P-positive HAF/cm^2 of liver tissue of rats exposed to diethylnitrosamine (DEN).

Cumulative Doses (CD) at 10 Weeks (mg/kg)		DNA Adducts (10^{8}nts)	RF	HAF/cm^2	Percent of Phenobarbital (PB) Promotable (for 24 weeks) Neoplasms	References
Control	0	3	4.6	0.1	0	[25,42,44]
CD1	25.5	14	4.7	3.7	0	[25,44]
CD2	51.1	203	5.8	7.3	3	[25,42,44]
CD3	102.2	287	5.8	12.8	32	[25,42,44]
CD4	204.4	434	7.0	36.5	100	[25,31,44]
CD5	306.6	5040	11.6	69.4	100	[25,42]

GST-P, glutathione S-transferase placental-type; HAF, hepatocellular altered foci. DEN was administered by intragastric instillation in 0.5% carboxymethylcellulose, once/week for 10 weeks, followed by 24 weeks of 500 ppm phenobarbital (PB) in the diet for 24 weeks.

neoplasms after 24 weeks. In these studies, both carcinogens were administered by gavage to achieve precise dosing on a body weight basis.

With DEN [25,42,44,61], the CD of 25.5 mg/kg bw (the lowest dose tested), delivered over 10 weeks, was a NOAEL for cell proliferation, but HAF were increased, although no promotable hepatocellular neoplasia was produced (Table 2.2). At this biological effect level, about 14 DNA adducts in 10^8 normal nucleotides (nts) were formed, and at 51.1 mg/kg bw, which yielded promotable neoplasia, 200 adducts/10^8 nts were formed. The adducts quantified by HPLC analysis with fluorescence detection were 7-ethylguanine and O^6-ethylguanine, the latter being an accepted miscoding lesion. A NOAEL for DNA adduct formation was not found.

With AAF [25,43,45,46], the CD of 28 mg/kg bw, delivered over 12 weeks, was a NOAEL, for both hepatocellular proliferation and GST-P$^+$ HAF (Table 2.3), as were three lower CDs. At 28 mg/kg, no promotable (with 24 weeks of PB) hepatocellular neoplasia was produced (Table 2.3), indicating absence of initiation. At this CD, however, about six DNA adducts in 10^8 nts were formed as measured by ^{32}P-postlabeling. Thus, a NOAEL for DNA adduct formation was not found in these studies. In a recent study to explore NOAEL for adducts [48], two further dose–effect experiments were conducted at lower repeat doses than those previously used. In addition, the specific types of DNA adducts formed were identified. AAF was administered orally to male F344 rats at repeat dosages, which in one experiment ranged from 0.01 to 2.24 mg/kg bw per day, 7 days/week for 12 weeks followed by recovery for 4 weeks, and in a second, at lower dosages of 0.0026 or 0.026 mg/kg bw per day 3 days per week for 16 weeks. Initially the nonacetylated guanine adduct, N-(deoxyguanosine-8-yl)-aminofluorene, predominated in the liver. With continued dosing, the pattern of adducts changed such that by 4 weeks more acetylated adducts, N-(deoxyguanosine-N^2-yl)-AAF and N-(deoxyguanosine-8-yl)-AAF, were present. In the first experiment, total adducts reached a maximum by 12 weeks with

Table 2.3 Liver DNA adducts, hepatocellular percent replicating fraction (RF), and GST-P-Positive HAF/cm² of liver tissue of rats exposed to 2-acetylaminofluorene (AAF).

Cumulative Doses (CD) at 12 Weeks (mg/kg)	DNA Adducts (10^8 nts)	RF	HAF/cm²	CD at16 Weeks (mg/kg)	DNA Adducts (10^8 nts)	RF	HAF/cm²	Percent of Phenobarbital (PB) Promotable (for 24 Weeks) Neoplasms	References
Control	0.2–3.1	0.9	0.2	0	0.2–1.2	1.4	1.1	0	[25,43,45]
CD1	0.094[a]	0.6	1.5	0.8	0.125	0.6	1.6	1.5	ND	[45]
CD2	0.94[a]	6.0	1.8	1.2	1.25	1.6	1.8	1.3	ND	[45]
CD3	9.41[b]	21.4	ND	ND	9.41[b]	11.4	ND	ND	0	[25,43]
CD4	28.0[c]	5.6	1.7	0.6	ND	ND	ND	ND	0	[43,45]
CD5	94.1[b,c]	29.6	1.9	1.1	94.1[b]	14.4	ND	ND	3	[43]
CD6	288.2[b,c]	31.7	8.2	19.4	288.2[b]	12.6	ND	ND	100	[43]

GST-P, glutathione S-transferase placental-type; HAF, hepatocellular altered foci; ND, not done.
AAF was administered by intragastric instillation in 0.5% carboxymethylcellulose either 3 days per week for up to 12 weeks.
[a]Followed by 4 weeks of recovery.
[b]Or 7 days per week for up to 12 weeks.
[c]Followed by 24 weeks of 500 ppm phenobarbital (PB) in the diet for 24 weeks.

levels of 6.0 adducts/10^8 nucleotides at the lowest CD. In the second, the total DNA adducts at the lowest CD was below the limit of detection at 12 weeks, and at 0.6 in 10^8 nucleotides at 16 weeks, a level within the background range of 1.0–3.1/10^8 nucleotides. Thus, the CD of 0.125 mg/kg bw over 16 weeks was concluded to be a NOAEL for adducts.

In these studies, as detailed above, DNA adducts were formed at CD that were below those that elicited measureable increases in either hepatocellular proliferation or HAF (Tables 2.2 and 2.3), as has been noted in other studies [54,56,57]. The adduct levels at NOAEL for other effects were at or below 1 in 10^9 nts [46].

Conclusions

Most of the experiments reviewed herein which monitored induction of preneoplasia in the rat liver demonstrated NOAEL for critical effects of the DNA-reactive carcinogens studied. Importantly NOAEL were found for induction of HAF, which are a prerequisite to the eventual development of liver neoplasms [40,62]. Quantification of HAF provides more robust data than does measurement of tumors, because, with hepatocarcinogen dosing, the numbers of HAF per liver greatly exceed the numbers of tumors [63]. We conclude that NOAEL for HAF can be considered NOAEL for liver tumor development. Moreover, NOAEL for induced cell proliferation, a response to hepatocellular injury and an enhancing factor in hepatocarcinogenesis [35,64,65], were demonstrated.

These NOAEL for HAF and increased proliferation were found at CD that still produced DNA adducts, some of which are potentially miscoding, that is, dG-N^2-AAF and O^6-ethylguanine, while others are at sites not involved in base pairing. This indicates that formation of adducts is a more sensitive bioindicator of effect and that there is a level of DNA adduct formation which appears not to be of biological significance. We have proposed this level to be at about 1 in 10^9 nts, which represents only about three adducts per cell, or about one adduct per 7000 genes [46]. Since only 1–2% of the genome is functionally active [66], most adducts would be in regions of DNA not coding for gene products, and not all adducts, even in transcriptually active sites, are miscoding. Moreover, this level of DNA modification is small compared to the level of endogenous DNA lesions per cell, estimated to be in the order of 10^4–10^6 per cell [67–69], much of which is oxidative damage resulting from cellular metabolism.

Cancer is considered to be a multihit and multistep process, involving changes in the structure or function of oncogenes and tumor suppression genes, leading to initiation of tumor development, which can be enhanced by promotion. Such changes require, in general, substantial and sustained exposures, although there are examples where a single large dose can be tumorigenic, especially with carcinogens that are not effectively detoxicated [70–72]. The possibility of multiple effective hits in critical genes at extremely low levels of DNA adduct formation is highly unlikely, although in the whole body 3.72×10^{13} cells (Table 2.4) are at risk for rare events. In spite of this, most cells are not actively replicating, and hence are not susceptible to mutagenesis.

Table 2.4 Estimated minimum dose of a chemical carcinogen needed to produce a liver neoplasm in humans.

Line, L	Value	Calculation	Value identification	Comments
1	3.72×10^{13}		Number of cells in human body [93]	
2	3.61×10^{11}		Liver total cell number [93]	
3	3.2×10^9		Number of bases in the human genome	
4	6×10^{23}		mol^{-1}, Avogadro's number	
5	$<3.61 \times 10^9$	$L2 \times 0.01$	Number of stem (replicating) cells in the liver	Less than 1% of liver population is in the cell cycle
6	0.6	$L2 \times 10^{12}/L4$	pmole carcinogen to distribute 1 molecule per liver cell, based on Avogadro's number	
7	0.18	$L6 \times 300/1000$	ng for 1 molecule per cell for a carcinogen with MW 300 g/mol	Assuming average MW for carcinogen is 300 g/mol
8	0.9	$L7 \times 100/20$	ng if 20% is bioactivated to a DNA-reactive metabolite	For some carcinogens all of the metabolism may be through a reactive intermediate while for others <1% may be bioactivated
9	1.8	$L8 \times 100/50$	ng if 50% of bioactivated carcinogen binds to DNA	Only a very small % will actually bind to DNA, usually <10%, assume 50%
10	5		Approximation of minimal number of genes needing to be mutated to induce a human neoplasm	Assuming half of ten identified hallmarks of cancer [94] is induced by chemicals and half is acquired
11	1–3		Number of sites at which a mutation can activate an oncogene	*ras*, for example, has three possible sites [95]
12	many		Sites at which a mutation can inactivate a tumor suppressor gene	Not all mutations will inactivate: some codon changes will not change amino acid sequence, and some amino acid changes will not affect
13	28.9	$L9 \times L3 \times L10 \times 10^{-9}$	g of carcinogen required over a lifetime to hit five critical bases per cell in liver	Assuming only one site per gene capable of activating critical bases per cell in liver an oncogene or inactivation of a tumor suppressor gene
14	1.13	$L5/L3$	More stem (labile) cells in the liver than bases in the genome	Multiple cells will have equivalent damage
15	25.6	$L13/L14$	g to hit the required five bases in one stem (labile) cell in the liver over a lifetime (70 years) exposure	Underestimated based on DNA repair; overestimated based on clonal expansion
16	1	$L15 \times 10^3/(70 \times 365)$	mg/day	~30 µg/day limit set for AFB$_1$ [96], a potent human liver carcinogen and provides a safety margin of ~33

Modified from Williams GM, Iatropoulos MJ, Jeffrey AM. Thresholds for DNA-reactive (genotoxic) organic carcinogens. J Toxicol Pathol 2005;18:69–77.

L indicate reference to the line number, plain text indicates numerical value.

Another approach to establish a threshold for genotoxic compounds, as well as epigenetic agents, is the analysis of the gene expression profile alterations induced by exposure to carcinogens. Analysis of genomic changes can potentially reveal NOAEL for gene expression alterations at doses significantly lower than those already established to be NOAEL for other effects. In particular, the absence of induction of genes related to DNA damage response would reinforce the threshold identified for DNA adducts.

Thus, the totality of the biological evidence supports the possibility of NOAEL and practical thresholds for DNA-reactive carcinogens, similar to those of epigenetic carcinogens, but generally at lower CD, because of their MoA. The possibility of a hormetic effect at low doses of hepatocarcinogen, resulting in decreased initiation, as reported in the study of Hino and Kitagawa [50], further supports the possibility of thresholds.

Relevance to Humans

Several considerations are involved in assessing the implications from the available experimental database to human relevance. In order to extrapolate meaningfully from rats to humans, differences in adult liver anatomy and physiology must be considered. For example, the rat liver accounts for 4.8% of body weight, whereas the human liver is only 2.8% of body weight [35]. Moreover, the absence of a gallbladder in the rat influences the intrahepatobiliary adaptive homeostasis, by enlargement of the periportal biliary plexus [35]. In addition, there are known to be important differences in xenobiotic biotransformation between rat and human livers. For example, tamoxifen, which is a potent rat hepatocarcinogen [73], has not been associated with liver cancer in humans [74], apparently owing to insufficient hepatic enzymatic sulfotransfcrasc activation in humans [75].

The epidemiology of chemical-induced cancer in humans demonstrates the need for sustained exposure, except in specific situations such as in utero exposure to the hormonal agent diethylstilbestrol (DES) [76]. All chemicals judged by the International Agency for Research on Cancer to be human carcinogens based on sufficient epidemiological evidence are characterized by repeat exposure to toxicologically significant levels which we calculated to be >1 mg/day (Table 2.4) [77], apart from the aforementioned DES. Thus, for the many DNA-reactive carcinogens for which there is human intake data, there are apparently conditions that pose no significant (or measurable) cancer risk, although this "virtually safe dose" can vary over several orders of magnitude, depending on how it is calculated [78].

For the estimation of intakes that do not convey a significant cancer risk, a procedure for calculating a "toxicologically insignificant daily intake" (TIDI) [12,17] is given in Table 2.5. For a DNA-reactive carcinogen, the molecular effect for which a NOAEL would be used to calculate the TIDI is DNA binding of less than 1 in 10^9 nts [12], which was concluded, as discussed above, to be biologically insignificant. Importantly, this assessment, applies only to exposures to a single carcinogen. It is well established experimentally that combinations of

Table 2.5 Toxicologically insignificant daily intake (TIDI) for carcinogens[a].

- No-observed-adverse-effect level (NOAEL) for molecular/cellular effect that is the basis for carcinogenicity
- Safety margin (SM)
  Multiple of uncertainty factors (UF)[b]
      10 for species to species extrapolation
      10 for individual variation
- TIDI is NOAEL divided by SM

[a]Based on Williams GM. Application of mode-of-action considerations in human cancer risk assessment. Toxicol Lett 2008;180:75–80.
[b]UF for short-term to long-term intake not needed if molecular/cellular effect has reached steady state.

DNA-reactive carcinogens given at effective levels can produce additive or synergistic effects [79,80]. Additionally, Schmähl [79] has described the phenomenon of "syncarcinogenesis" resulting from carcinogens given in sequence. For example, sequential administration of AAF and DEN, in either order, produced a syncarcinogenic effect in rat liver carcinogenicity [81,82]. These types of interactions indicate that overall cancer risk assessment in humans is more complex than simple modeling of dose–effect data from experimental animals administered single compounds. Whether such interactions would occur at TIDIs is unknown, but has been reported for teratogenicity [83].

Compounds that are noncarcinogenic also can enhance the experimental effects of carcinogens, a phenomenon known as cocarcinogenicity. As an example, benzo[e]pyrene (B[e]P), pyrene, and fluoranthene increase the carcinogenicity of benzo[a]pyrene (B[a]P) on mouse skin although they are not carcinogenic themselves [84]. The B[a]P/B[e]P result was confirmed by DiGiovanni et al. [85], who also noted that, in contrast, B[e]P inhibited the tumor-initiating activities of 7,12-dimethylbenz[a]anthracene and other polycyclic aromatic hydrocarbons [86]. In the few studies undertaken, these results correlate well with the levels of DNA adducts formed [86,87]. In addition, experimental promotion of neoplasia by a compound administered after a carcinogen is well recognized [80,84], and this can enhance the carcinogenicity of an initiating agent (Table 2.1).

Exposures of humans to trace levels of organic DNA-reactive (genotoxic) carcinogens occur through a variety of sources. Several types of DNA-reactive carcinogens are foodborne [88], including, for example, mycotoxins [58,89] and the heterocyclic amines formed during cooking of food [58]. Drinking water can contain minute amounts of reactive chlorination byproducts [90]. Environmental exposures also occur through other natural and industrial sources [91]. Most such exposures are less than a lifetime [76,92]. We have calculated that lifetime intake of up to 1 mg/day of a DNA-reactive carcinogen is unlikely to pose a human cancer risk (Table 2.4), bearing in mind that these calculations involve several assumptions [46]. For a specific carcinogen, the calculation of a TIDI based on adducts would likely yield a much lower value for a safe intake. The research reviewed here supports the conclusion that very low levels of intake of individual DNA-reactive carcinogens are unlikely to pose significant (>1 in 10^6) cancer risk, even assuming lifetime exposure, and thus may be practical thresholds. However, concurrent intakes of several carcinogens may occur, for example with cigarette smoking [84], and this must be factored into overall risk assessment.

References

[1]   Mantel N. The concept of threshold in carcinogenesis. Clin Pharmacol Ther 1963;4:104–9.
[2]   Brown CC. Mathematical aspects of dose-response studies in carcinogenesis—the concept of thresholds. Oncology 1976;33:62–5.
[3]   Carlborg FW. The threshold and the virtually safe dose. Food ChemToxicol 1982;20:219–21.
[4]   Lutz WK, Kopp-Schneider A. Threshold dose response for tumor induction by genotoxic carcinogens modeled via cell-cycle delay. Toxicol Sci 1999;49:110–5.
[5]   Slob W. Thresholds in toxicology and risk assessment. Int J Toxicol 1999;18:259–68.
[6]   Weisburger JH, Williams GM. Types and amounts of carcinogens as potential human cancer hazards. Cell Biol Toxicol 1989;5:377–91.
[7]   Williams GM. Mechanistic considerations in cancer risk assessment. Inhal Toxicol 1999;11:549–54.
[8]   Williams GM. Mechanisms of chemical carcinogenesis and application to human cancer risk assessment. Toxicology 2001;166:3–10.
[9]   Sonich-Mullin C, Fielder R, Wiltse J, Baetke K, Dempsey J, Fenner-Crisp P, et al. IPCS conceptual framework for evaluating a mode of action for chemical carcinogenesis. Regul Toxicol Pharmacol 2001;34:146–52.
[10] Meek ME, Bucher JR, Cohen SM, DeMarco V, Hill RN, Lehman-McKeeman LD, et al. A framework for human relevance analysis of information on carcinogenic modes of action. Crit Rev Toxicol 2003;33:591–654.
[11] Barlow S, Renwick AG, Kleiner J, Bridges JW, Busk L, Dybing E, et al. Introduction. In: Risk assessment of substances that are both genotoxic and carcinogenic, EFSA/WHO international conference with support of ILSI Europe, Brussels, Belgium, 2005, p. 1–286.
[12] Williams GM. Application of mode-of-action considerations in human cancer risk assessment. Toxicol Lett 2008;180:75–80.
[13] Weisburger JH, Williams GM. Classification of carcinogens as genotoxic and epigenetic as basis for improved toxicologic bioassay methods. In: Sugimura T, Kondo S, Takebe H, editors. Environmental mutagens and carcinogens. Tokyo: University of Tokyo Press. Alan R. Liss, Inc., New York; 1982. p. 283–94.
[14] Williams GM. DNA reactive and epigenetic carcinogens. Exp Toxicol Pathol 1992;44:457–64.
[15] Williams GM, Karbe E, Fenner-Crisp P, Iatropoulos MJ, Weisburger JH. Risk assessment of carcinogens in food with special consideration of non-genotoxic carcinogens: scientific arguments for use of risk assessment and for changing the Delaney Clause specifically. Exp Toxicol Pathol 1996;48:209–15.
[16] Dybing E, Doe J, Groten J, Kleiner J, O'Brien J, Renwick AG, et al. Hazard characterisation of chemicals in food and diet: dose response, mechanism and extrapolation issues. Food Chem Toxicol 2002;40:237–82.
[17] Williams GM, Iatropoulos MJ, Jeffrey AM. Dose-effect relationships for DNA-reactive liver carcinogens. In: Greim H, Albertini RJ, editors. The cellular response to the genotoxic insult: the question of threshold for genotoxic carcinogens. Royal Society of Chemistry Issues in Toxicology Series; 2012. p. 33–51.
[18] Nestmann ER, Bryant DW, Carr CJ, Fennell TT, Gallagher JE, Gorelick NJ, et al. Toxicological significance of DNA adducts: summary of discussion with an expert panel. Regul Toxicol Pharmacol 1996;24:9–18.
[19] Preston RJ, Williams GM. DNA-reactive carcinogens: mode of action and human cancer hazard. Crit Rev Toxicol 2005;35:673–83.
[20] Jarabek AM, Pottenger LH, Andrews LS, Casciano D, Embry MR, Kim JH, et al. Creating context for the use of DNA adduct data in cancer risk assessment: I. Data Organization. Crit Rev Toxicol 2009;39: 659–78.

[21] Pottenger LH, Carmichael N, Banton M, Boogaard P, Kim J, Kirkland D, et al. ECETOC workshop on the biological significance of DNA adducts: follow-up from an expert panel meeting. Mutat Res 2009;678:152–7.

[22] Kirsch-Volders M, Aardema M, Elhajouji A. Concepts of threshold in mutagenesis and carcinogenesis. Mutat Res 2000;464:3–11.

[23] Swenberg JA, La DK, Scheller NA, Wu KY. Dose-response relationships for carcinogens. Toxicol Lett 1995;82–83:751–6.

[24] Oesch F, Herrero ME, Hengstler JG, Lohmann M, Arand M. Metabolic detoxification: implications for thresholds. Toxicol Pathol 2000;28:382–7.

[25] Williams GM, Iatropoulos MJ, Jeffrey AM. Mechanistic basis for nonlinearities and thresholds in rat liver carcinogenesis by the DNA-reactive carcinogens 2-acetylaminofluorene and diethylnitrosamine. Toxicol Pathol 2000;28:388–95.

[26] Hengstler JG, Bogdanffy MS, Bolt HM, Oesch F. Challenging dogma: thresholds for genotoxic carcinogens? The case of vinyl acetate. Annu Rev Pharmacol Toxicol 2003;43:485–520.

[27] Farmer JH, Kodell RL, Greenman DL, Shaw GW. Dose and time responses models for the incidence of bladder and liver neoplasms in mice fed 2-acetylamino-fluorene continuously. J Environ Pathol Toxicol 1980;3:55–68.

[28] Maekawa A, Ogiu T, Matsuoka C, Onodera H, Furuta K, Kurokawa Y, et al. Carcinogenicity of low doses of N-ethyl-N-nitrosourea in F344 rats: a dose-response study. Gann 1984;75:117–25.

[29] Lijinsky W, Kovatch RM, Riggs CW, Walters PT. Dose-response study with N-nitrosomorpholine in drinking water of F-344 rats. Cancer Res 1988;48:2089–95.

[30] Maekawa A, Onodera H, Matsushima Y, Nagaoka T, Todate A, Shibutani M, et al. Dose-response carcinogenicity in rats on low-dose levels of N-ethyl-N-nitrosourethane. Jpn J Cancer Res 1989;80:632–6.

[31] Peto R, Gray R, Brantom P, Grasso P. Effects on 4080 rats of chronic ingestion of N-nitrosodiethylamine or N-nitrosodimethylamine: a detailed dose-response study. Cancer Res 1991;51:6415–51.

[32] Peto R, Gray R, Brantom P, Grasso P. Dose and time relationships for tumor induction in the liver and esophagus of 4080 inbred rats by chronic ingestion of N-nitrosodiethylamine or N-nitrosodimethylamine. Cancer Res 1991;51:6452–69.

[33] Bailey GS, Reddy AP, Pereira CB, Harttig V, Baird W, Spitzbergen JM, et al. Nonlinear cancer response of ultralow dose: a 40,800-animal ED$_{001}$ tumor and biomarker study. Chem Res Toxicol 2009;22:1264–76.

[34] Lewis RW, Billington R, Debryune E, Gamer A, Lang B, Carpanini F. Recognition of adverse and nonadverse effects in toxicity studies. Toxicol Pathol 2002;30:66–74.

[35] Williams GM, Iatropoulos MJ. Alteration of liver cell function and proliferation: differentiation between adaptation and toxicity. Toxicol Pathol 2002;30:41–53.

[36] Littlefield NA, Farmer JH, Gaylor DW, Sheldon WG. Effects of dose and time in a long-term, low-dose carcinogenic study. J Environ Pathol Toxicol 1979;3:17–34.

[37] Williams GM. Functional markers and growth behavior of preneoplastic hepatocytes. Cancer Res 1976;36:2540–3.

[38] Bannasch P. Preneoplastic lesions as end points in carcinogenicity testing. I. Hepatic preneoplasia. Carcinogenesis 1986;7:689–95.

[39] Williams GM. Chemically induced rodent preneoplastic lesions as indicators of carcinogenic activity. In: McGregor DB, Rice JM, Venitt S, editors. The use of short- and medium-term tests for carcinogens and data on genetic effects in carcinogenic hazard evaluation. Lyon, France: IARC Scientific Publications No. 146; 1999. p. 185–202.

[40] Williams GM. The significance of chemically-induced hepatocellular altered foci in rat liver and application to carcinogen detection. Toxicol Pathol 1989;17:663–74.

[41] Tsuda H, Fukushima S, Wanibuchi H, Morimura K, Nakae D, Imaida K, et al. Value of GST-P positive preneoplastic hepatic foci in dose-response studies of hepatocarcinogenesis: evidence for practical thresholds with both genotoxic and nongenotoxic carcinogens. A review of recent work. Toxicol Pathol 2003;31:80–6.

[42] Williams GM, Iatropoulos MJ, Wang CX, Ali N, Rivenson A, Peterson LA, et al. Diethylnitrosamine exposure-responses for DNA damage, centrilobular cytotoxicity, cell proliferation and carcinogenesis in rat liver exhibit some non-linearities. Carcinogenesis 1996;17:2253–8.

[43] Williams GM, Iatropoulos MJ, Wang CX, Jeffrey AM, Thompson S, Pittman B, et al. Non-linearities in 2-acetylaminofluorene exposure-responses for genotoxic and epigenetic effects leading to initiation of carcinogenesis in rat liver. Toxicol Sci 1998;45:152–61.

[44] Williams GM, Iatropoulos MJ, Jeffrey AM, Luo FQ, Wang CX, Thompson S, et al. Diethylnitrosamine exposure-responses for DNA ethylation, hepatocellular proliferation and initiation of carcinogenesis in rat liver display non-lincarities and thresholds. Arch Toxicol 1999;73:394–402.

[45] Williams GM, Iatropoulos MJ, Jeffrey AM. Thresholds for the effects of 2-acetylaminofluorene in rat liver. Toxicol Pathol 2004;32(Suppl. 2):85–91.

[46] Williams GM, Iatropoulos MJ, Jeffrey AM. Thresholds for DNA-reactive (genotoxic) organic carcinogens. J Toxicol Pathol 2005;18:69–77.

[47] Williams GM, Iatropoulos MJ, Jeffrey A, Duan J-D. Methyleugenol hepatocellular cancer initiating effects in rat liver. Food Chem Toxicol 2013;53:187–96.

[48] Williams GM, Duan J-D, Iatropoulos MJ, Kobets T. A no observed adverse effect level for DNA adduct formation in rat liver with repeat prolonged dosing of the hepatocarcinogen 2-acetylaminofluorene. Toxicol Res 2015;4:233–40.

[49] Williams GM, Tanaka T, Maruyama H, Maeura Y, Weisburger JH, Zang E. Modulation by butylated hydroxytoluene of liver and bladder carcinogenesis induced by chronic low level exposure to 2-acetylaminofluorene. Cancer Res 1991;51:6224–30.

[50] Hino O, Kitagawa T. Existence of a practical threshold dose for the hepatocarcinogen 3'-methyl-4-(dimethylamino) azobenzene in rat liver. Gann 1981;72:637–8.

[51] Calabrese EJ. Hormesis is central to toxicology, pharmacology and risk assessment. Hum Exp Toxicol 2010;29:249–61.

[52] Rozman KK, Doull J. Scientific foundations of hormesis. Part 2. Maturation, strengths, limitations, and possible applications in toxicology, pharmacology, and epidemiology. Crit Rev Toxicol 2003;33:451–62.

[53] Rozman KK. Hormesis and risk assessment. Hum Exp Toxicol 2005;24:255–7.

[54] Root M, Lange T, Campbell TC. Dissimilarity in aflatoxin dose-response relationships between DNA adduct formation and development of preneoplastic foci in rat liver. Chem Biol Interact 1997;106:213–27.

[55] Enzmann H, Zerban H, Kopp-Schneider A, Loser E, Bannach P. Effects of low doses of N-nitrosomorpholine on the development of early stages of hepatocarcinogenesis. Carcinogenesis 1995;16:1513–8.

[56] Fukushima S. Low-dose carcinogenicity of a heterocyclic amine, 2-amino-3,8-dimethylimidazo[4,5-f] quinoxaline: relevance to risk assessment. Cancer Lett 1999;143:157–9.

[57] Fukushima S, Wanibuchi H, Morimura K, Wei M, Nakae D, Konishi Y, et al. Lack of a dose-response relationship for carcinogenicity in the rat liver with low doses of 2-amino-3,8-dimethylimidazo[4,5-f] quinoxaline or N-nitrosodiethylamine. Jpn J Cancer Res 2002;93:1076–82.

[58] International Agency for Research on Cancer (IARC). Some naturally occurring substances: food items and constituents, heterocyclic aromatic amines and mycotoxins. In: IARC, vol. 56. Lyon, France; 1993. p. 1–599.

[59] Murai T, Mori S, Kang JS, Morimura K, Wanibuchi H, Totsuka Y, et al. Evidence of a threshold-effect for 2-amino-3,8-dimethylimidazo[4,5-f]quinoxaline liver carcinogenicity in F344/DuCrj rats. Toxicol Pathol 2008;36:472–7.

[60] Laib RJ, Pellio T, Wünschel VM, Zimmermann N, Bolt HM. The rat liver foci bioassay: II. Investigations on the dose-dependent induction of ATPase-deficient foci by vinyl chloride at very low doses. Carcinogenesis 1985;6:69–72.

[61] Williams GM, Gebhardt R, Sirma H, Stenbäck F. Non-linearity of neoplastic conversion induced in rat liver by low exposures to diethylnitrosamine. Carcinogenesis 1993;14:2149–56.

[62] Williams GM. Chemicals with carcinogenic activity in rodent liver Comprehensive toxicology, vol. 9. Oxford: Academic Press; 2010. p. 221–50.

[63] Williams GM, Watanabe K. Quantitative kinetics of development of *N*-2-fluroenylacetanide-induced altered (hyperplastic) hepatocellular foci resistant to iron accumulation and of their reversion or persistence following removal of carcinogen. J Natl Cancer Inst 1978;61:113–21.

[64] Loury DJ, Goldsworthy TL, Butterworth BE. The value of measuring cell replication as a predictive index of tissue-specific tumorigenic potential. In: Butterworth BE, Slaga TJ, editors. Nongenotoxic mechanisms in carcinogenesis. NY: The Banbury Report, Cold Spring Harbor Laboratory; 1987. p. 119–36.

[65] Cohen SM, Ellwein LB. Genetic errors, cell proliferation, and carcinogenesis. Cancer Res 1991;51:6493–505.

[66] Biémont C. A brief history of the status of transposable elements: from junk DNA to major players in evolution. Genetics 2010;186:1085–93.

[67] Lindahl T. Instability and decay of the primary structure of DNA. Nature 1993;362:709–15.

[68] Marnett LJ, Burcham PC. Endogenous DNA adducts: potential and paradox. Chem Res Toxicol 1993;6:771–85.

[69] Povey AC. DNA adducts: endogenous and induced. Toxicol Pathol 2000;28:405–14.

[70] Druckrey H, Steinhoff D, Preussmann R, Ivankovic S. Induction of cancer by a single dose of methylnitrosourea and various dialkylnitrosamines in rats. Z Krebsforsch 1964;66:1–10.

[71] Pitot HC, Barsness L, Goldworthy T, Kitagawa T. Biochemical characterization of stages of hepatocarcinogenesis after a single dose of diethylnitrosamine. Nature 1978;271:456–8.

[72] Tanaka T, Mori H, Hirota N, Furuya K, Williams GM. Effect of DNA synthesis on induction of preneoplastic and neoplastic lesions in rat liver by a single dose of methoxyazoxymethanol acetate. Chem Biol Interact 1986;58:13–27.

[73] Williams GM, Iatropoulos MJ, Djordjevic MV, Kaltenberg OP. The triphenylethylene drug, tamoxifen is a strong liver carcinogen in the rat. Carcinogenesis 1993;14:315–7.

[74] International Agency for Research on Cancer (IARC). Evaluation of carcinogenic risks to humans: some pharmaceutical drugs, Tamoxifen. In: IARC, vol. 66. Lyon, France; 1996. p. 367–88.

[75] Glatt H, Davis W, Meinl W, Hermersdörfer H, Venitt S, Phillips DH. Rat, but not human, sulfotransferase activates a tamoxifen metabolite to produce DNA adducts and gene mutations in bacteria and mammalian cells in culture. Carcinogenesis 1998;19:1709–13.

[76] Williams GM, Reiss B, Weisburger JH. A comparison of the animal and human carcinogenicity of several environmental, occupational and therapeutic chemicals. In: Flamm G, Lorentzen R, editors. Mechanisms and toxicology of chemical carcinogens and mutagens, vol. IX. Princeton, NJ: Princeton Scientific Publishers; 1985. p. 207–48.

[77] Deleted in review.

[78] Williams DE, Orner G, Willard KD, Tilton S, Hendricks JD, Pereira C, et al. Rainbow trout (*Oncorhynchus mykiss*) and ultra-low dose cancer studies. Comp Biochem Physiol Toxicol Pharmacol 2009;149:175–81.

[79] Schmähl D. Combination effects in chemical carcinogenesis. Arch Toxicol Suppl 1980;4.29–40.

[80] Williams GM. Interactive carcinogenesis in the liver. In: Bannasch P, Keppler D, Weber G, editors. Falk symposium: liver cell carcinoma, vol. 51. Boston, MA: Academic Press; 1989. p. 197–216.

[81] Williams GM, Katayama S, Ohmori T. Enhancement of hepatocarcinogenesis by sequential administration of chemicals: summation versus promotion effects. Carcinogenesis 1981;2:1111–7.

[82] Williams GM, Furuya K. Distinction between liver neoplasm promoting and syncarcinogenic effects demonstrated by exposure to phenobarbital or diethylnitrosamine either before or after *N*-2-fluorenylacetamide. Carcinogenesis 1984;5:171–4.

[83] Mayura K, Parker P, Berndt WO, Philips TD. Effect of simultaneous prenatal exposure to ochratoxin A and citrinin in the rat. J Toxicol Environ Health 1984;13:553–61.

[84] Van Duren BL, Goldschmidt BM. Carcinogenic and tumor-promoting agents in tobacco carcinogenesis. J Natl Cancer Inst 1976;56:1237–42.

[85] DiGiovanni J, Rymer J, Slaga TJ, Boutwell RK. Anticarcinogenis and cocarcinogenic effects of benzo[*e*]pyrene and dibenz[*a,c*]anthracene on skin tumor initiation by polycyclic hydrocarbons. Carcinogenesis 1982;3:371–5.

[86] Smolarek TA, Baird WM, Fisher EP, DiGiovanni J. Benzo(*e*)pyrene-induced alterations in the binding of benzo(*a*)pyrene and 7,12-dimethylbenz(*a*)anthracene to DNA in Sencar mouse epidermis. Cancer Res 1987;47:3701–6.

[87] Rice JE, Hosted TJ, Lavoie EJ. Fluoranthene and pyrene enhance benzo[*a*]pyrene-DNA adduct formation in vivo in mouse skin. Cancer Lett 1984;24:327–33.

[88] Williams GM. Food-borne carcinogens. Prog Clin Biol Res 1986;206:73–81.

[89] International Agency for Research on Cancer (IARC). Some traditional herbal medicines, some mycotoxins, naphthalene and styrene. In: IARC, vol. 82. Lyon, France; 2002. p. 169–275.

[90] Koivusalo M, Vartiainen T. Drinking water chlorination by-products and cancer. Rev Environ Health 1997;12:81–90.

[91] Meijers JMM, Swaen GMH, Bloemen LJN. The predictive value of animal data in human cancer risk assessment. Regul Toxicol Pharmacol 1997;25:94–102.

[92] Felter S, Conolly R, Bercu J, Bolger P, Boobis A, Bos P, et al. A proposed framework for assessing risk from less-than lifetime exposures to carcinogens. Crit Rev Toxicol 2011;41:507–44.

[93] Bianconi E, Piovesan A, Facchin F, Beraudi A, Casadei R, Frabetti F, et al. An estimation of the number of cells in the human body. Ann Hum Biol 2013;40:463–71.

[94] Hanahan D, Weinberg RA. Hallmarks of cancer: the next generation. Cell 2011;144:646–74.

[95] Prior IA, Lewis PD, Mattos C. A comprehensive survey of Ras mutations in cancer. Cancer Res 2012;72:2457–67.

[96] International Agency for Research on Cancer (IARC). Evaluation of carcinogenic risks to humans: some traditional herbal medicines, some mycotoxins, naphthalene and styrene, Vol 82. Lyone, France: IARC; 2002;171–300.

CHAPTER 3

Interaction of Low-Dose Radiation and Chemicals in Cancer Risk

Shizuko Kakinuma, Benjamin J. Blyth and Yoshiya Shimada

Radiobiology for Children's Health Program, Research Center for Radiation Protection, National Institute of Radiological Sciences, Chiba, Japan

Chapter Outline

Epidemiological Analysis of Cancer Risk   38
    Solid Cancer   38
    Leukemia   40
Interaction of Radiation and Other Carcinogens   41
Data From Animal Experiments   42
    Skin Tumors   42
    Thymic Lymphoma   43
Conclusion   46
Acknowledgments   46
References   46

Accurate prediction of radiation-induced cancer risk at the low radiation exposure levels relevant to the general public is key to addressing considerable public concern [1]. While epidemiology data show overall cancer risk increases linearly with radiation dose, the relationship is more difficult to define as doses approach natural background levels, and there remains considerable heterogeneity by organ site, with some tissues refractory to radiation-induced cancer or showing an apparent threshold.

Since natural and man-made carcinogens in tobacco, food, and inflammatory pathogens in the environment are major contributors to cancer development, the small additional risk posed by low-dose radiation in isolation is difficult to estimate precisely and should be considered in the context of combined exposures with these other environmental carcinogens. For instance, the risk of radiation-induced lung cancer is profoundly modified by smoking status, with the additional risk negligible for heavy smokers, while for light smokers it increases in a synergistic fashion.

Thresholds of Genotoxic Carcinogens.
DOI: http://dx.doi.org/10.1016/B978-0-12-801663-3.00003-0

Table 3.1 Defining absolute, excess, and relative risks.

	Group A	Group B
Baseline rate (per 10^4 person years)	20	100
Absolute risk (AR) (per 10^4 person years)	40	120
Excess absolute risk (EAR) (per 10^4 person years)	20	20
Relative risk (RR)	2	1.2
Excess relative risk (ERR)	1	0.2

EAR, AR − Baseline; RR, AR/Baseline; ERR = EAR/Baseline. Groups A and B, which could, for example, represent different genders or ages, have different baseline rates (in unexposed populations) for a particular tumor type. The absolute risks (the risk in the exposed populations) are also different for both groups, but subtracting the baseline shows the same excess absolute risk. However, there is a greater relative risk following exposure in Group A (where the baseline is lower) which can also be expressed as an excess relative risk, by dividing the induced risk by the baseline rate. Since the risk (absolute or relative) can change with exposure level, the EAR and ERR are often quoted per unit dose (eg, ERR/Gy).

Experimental studies using animal models have demonstrated that the carcinogenic effects of radiation when combined with other carcinogens show synergy, additivity, or antagonism, depending on the dose, order, and timing of exposures. Given the variety of potential carcinogenic mechanisms involved, the data available to explain the differing natures of the interactions are quite limited. We review here the combined effect of radiation and chemical carcinogens focusing on low doses of radiation, and introduce our recent study on the molecular mechanism of T-cell lymphomagenesis after combined exposure to X-rays and N-ethyl-N-nitrosourea (ENU).

Epidemiological Analysis of Cancer Risk

Solid Cancer

Of all the studies which have contributed to our understanding of the effects of low-dose radiation, the Life Span Study (LSS) of Japanese atomic bomb survivors from Hiroshima and Nagasaki remains the gold standard, providing data on the late health effects of single acute exposures. The risk of solid cancer deaths (see Table 3.1) is positively associated with radiation dose [2]. A linear model provided the best fit when the linear (L), linear-quadratic (LQ), and quadratic (Q) models for the rate of all solid cancer mortality were compared over the full radiation dose range, giving a sex-averaged excess relative risk (ERR) per Gy of 0.42 (95% confidence interval (CI): 0.32, 0.53) for all solid cancer at age 70, after exposure at age 30 (Fig. 3.1). The lowest dose range with a significant ERR for all solid cancer mortality was from 0 to 0.2 Gy, while a formal dose–threshold analysis indicated no threshold; that is, zero dose was the best estimate of the threshold. Similarly, solid cancer *incidence* data from the A-bomb survivor cohort was best fit by a simple linear model [3].

When cancer mortality risk was subdivided by organ site, higher excess risk per unit dose (both for ERR and excess absolute risk (EAR)) was obtained for breast, bladder, ovary, lung, colon,

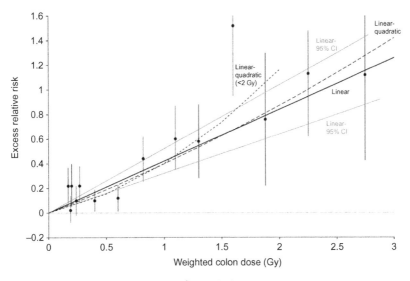

Figure 3.1

Excess relative risk (ERR) for all solid cancer mortality by radiation exposure categories. The black circles and bars represent ERR and 95% CI for each dose category. Overlaid are the best fit with 95% CI (thin grey lines) for a linear model (thick black line) and fits for alternative linear-quadratic (LQ) models over the full dose range (long dashed line) or restricted to doses <2 Gy (short dashed line). *This figure was made by modification of Fig. 3.4 of Ozasa et al. [2], with permission.*

and bone marrow, compared to no significant radiation-induced risk in rectum, gallbladder, uterus, prostate, and kidney at 1 Gy. Nonmelanoma skin cancer was the only cancer that had a dose response consistent with a threshold. The radiation risk of skin cancer among the atomic bomb survivors has been recently revised [4]. Each skin cancer was pathologically reviewed, and radiation risk of the primary skin cancer was analyzed by histological subtype. Classifications included basal cell carcinoma (BCC), squamous cell carcinoma (SCC), SCC in situ, Paget disease, and malignant melanoma. The shape of the dose response for BCC fits best to a threshold model with threshold dose of 0.63 Gy (95% CI: 0.32, 0.89). The ERR slope over the threshold dose was estimated to be 2.0 per Gy (95% CI: 0.69, 4.3) (Fig. 3.2). The ERR for SCC in situ appears to have a threshold dose (>1 Gy). However, there were no significant dose responses for malignant melanoma, SCC, Paget disease, or other skin cancers.

It is well known that the carcinogenic effect of radiation can be reduced by dose fractionation and/or exposure at a low-dose rate. When high cumulative lung doses were received across a very large number of chest fluoroscopies (each delivering about 10 mGy) in cohorts of Canadian and Massachusetts tuberculosis patients, there was no evidence of any positive association between the risk of lung cancer and radiation dose, with a relative risk (RR) ≤1 in dose groups below 2 Sv [5,6]. The difference between these results and the data from the LSS, where a clear significant lung cancer dose response was found, suggests that fractionation significantly reduced the cancer risk and introduced an effective threshold. In contrast, the same fluoroscopy cohort data do show an increase in breast cancer after the repeated low-dose

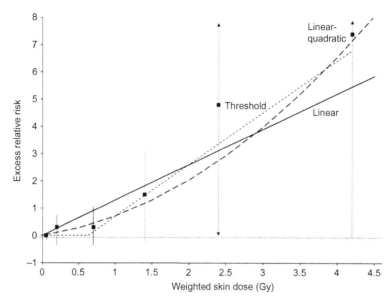

Figure 3.2
Basal cell carcinoma radiation dose–response data (black boxes) with curves shown for linear
(solid line), linear-quadratic (long dashed line), and threshold models (short dashed line):
the models include gender, period at diagnosis, and attained age as background parameters,
with age at the time of bombing as an effect modifier. *This figure was made by modification of
Fig. 3.1 of Sugiyama et al. [4], with permission.*

irradiations, albeit reduced compared to acute exposures. This serves to highlight the different
responses of organs not just to dose, but also to the effects of other modifying parameters.

Cohort studies in high background radiation areas (nonradon) in India and China have
concluded that low dose–rate radiation is unlikely to increase cancer mortality, even in
populations receiving up to 14.4 mGy/year with lifetime accumulated doses up to 600 mSv
[7]. However, in a metaanalysis of 14 studies on occupational and environmental exposures
to low-dose and low dose–rate radiation, 6 show significant increases in RR/Sv despite their
relatively low statistical power and associated increased chance of false-negative results [8].

Leukemia

The risk of leukemia after radiation exposure is higher compared to the risk of solid cancers,
with acute myeloid leukemia (AML), acute lymphocytic leukemia (ALL), and chronic
myeloid leukemia (CML) each exhibiting a strong association with radiation exposure.
In contrast, no association is observed between radiation exposure and the risk of chronic
lymphocytic leukemia (CLL), an indolent chronic disease seen in elderly patients. Many of
the excess leukemia cases occur within the first two decades after exposure, particularly for
those irradiated at young ages. There is clear evidence of nonlinearity in the dose response

for leukemia, most strikingly for AML; with the risk per unit dose lower in the lower dose range. Analysis of leukemia incidence data demonstrated a significant improvement in fit when a threshold is incorporated in a linear-quadratic RR model [9]. However, the analysis of mortality data by the same authors demonstrated that the threshold was not significantly different from zero [10], although the best estimate of threshold was 90 mGy.

Interaction of Radiation and Other Carcinogens

In A-bomb survivors, lung cancer risk increased linearly with dose over the 0–2 Gy range [3]. However, a case–control study of A-bomb survivors to account for smoking [11] found that the effect of smoking was complex, being modified by the age, extent, and duration of smoking with additional effects for those who had quit smoking. The interaction effect of radiation exposure and smoking appeared to be super-multiplicative for those smoking up to 10 cigarettes a day who showed a marked increase in radiation-related excess risk, which was lost in those smoking more than a pack a day (who had a much higher background risk without radiation) implying a practical threshold (Fig. 3.3). Although complex models which

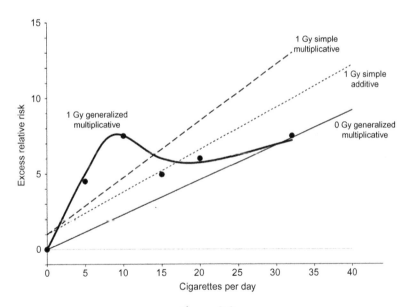

Figure 3.3

Variation of the excess relative risk (ERR) with smoking intensity. The data for excess relative lung cancer risk by smoking intensity are shown (black circles). The dotted line at ERR = 0 represents the baseline risk of nonexposed, nonsmokers, with the additional risk posed by smoking alone shown above (thin solid line, 0 Gy generalized multiplicative). The combined effect in smokers of exposure to 1 Gy is shown using an additive model (short dashed line, 1 Gy simple additive) or multiplicative model (long dashed line, 1 Gy simple multiplicative). However, when the effects of 1 Gy radiation were allowed to vary with smoking intensity, the model showed much better fit to the data (thick solid line, 1 Gy generalized multiplicative). *This figure was made by modification of Panel A of Fig. 3.4 of Furukawa et al. [11], with permission.*

allowed the radiation effect to vary with smoking status provided the best fit for all lung cancer and showed a similar response for the different subtypes, there was no clear improvement in fit against simpler linear models when the subtypes were analyzed individually [12].

Inhalation of the radioactive progeny of radon gas is the most important natural source of human exposure to ionizing radiation. An early ecological study of cancer rates and radon concentrations by geographical area showed a negative correlation between radon and lung cancer [13] but suffered from many limitations, including absence of area-specific tobacco use. Now, radon is recognized to be the second leading cause of lung cancer death after smoking. The ERR per WLM (working level month, an industry radon exposure measurement unit) from a combined analysis of 11 occupational cohort studies on miners indicates a linear dose response [14]. Several studies have been conducted to estimate the risks from residential radon for the general population, and although the individual studies failed to show a statistically significant effect, together they were consistent with a small excess lung cancer risk due to residential radon [15]. The BEIR VI Committee concluded that lung cancer risks from smoking and radon combined to produce a submultiplicative risk (greater than additive, but less than multiplicative) [16]. The difference in the interaction between smoking and radon inhalation, and smoking and the A-bomb radiation exposures could be due to differences in the quality of radiation (alpha-particles vs gamma-rays) or the mode of exposure (chronic vs acute).

The WISMUT cohort is the largest single study (about 59,000 male workers) on the health risks associated with radon and silica dust inhaled by uranium miners [17] and showed that lung cancer mortality increased linearly with cumulative radon exposure (RR = 0.19/100 WLM, 95% CI: 0.16–0.22) [18]. In contrast, the excess risk of lung cancer from silica exposure showed a linear function with a threshold of $10 \, mg/m^3$ per year. Adjustment for smoking led to only marginal changes, indicating that smoking was not a major confounder of the radon-associated lung cancer risk. However, when this case–control study was merged with two other European uranium miner studies, there was evidence for a submultiplicative interaction between radon and smoking [19] consistent with the earlier US studies [14].

Data From Animal Experiments

As in humans, the susceptibility to radiation carcinogenesis in laboratory rodents is tissue-/organ-dependent, which is in turn specific to each strain of laboratory mice and rats. Generally, the skin, thymus (immature T cells), ovaries, and kidneys are refractory to tumor induction by low-dose radiation below individual threshold doses [20].

Skin Tumors

Radiation-induced skin cancer has been studied using mice and rats, and shows clear thresholds below which no skin tumors are induced. Mice develop skin and bone tumors with 100% efficiency after repeated β-ray exposure to 1 Gy three times a week, yet with

0.5-Gy fractions no skin tumors develop over a lifetime even with a total dose of 150 Gy over 2 years [21]. However, β-irradiation, which was alone insufficient to induce skin tumors, was effective for skin tumor induction when combined with subsequent promotion using topical 4-nitroquinoline 1-oxide [22]. Likewise, UV exposure is also capable of converting X-ray-initiated cells into skin tumors [23], where with maximal UV promotion the threshold response became a simple linear one. These findings illustrate the ability of thresholds for radiation exposure to be bypassed when accompanied by other carcinogenic agents.

Thymic Lymphoma

Thymic lymphoma (TL) is another murine-specific tumor which shows a threshold dose, around 2–4 Gy for C57BL and BALB/c mice [24,25]. The RFM strain is more susceptible with even 0.2-Gy gamma-rays increasing the incidence of TL, but still displaying a threshold at 0.1 Gy [26]. Severe combined immune deficiency (SCID) mutant mice carry a defective DNA-dependent protein kinase catalytic subunit (*DNA-PKcs*) [27]. SCID mice are extremely susceptible to the induction of spontaneous and radiation-induced TL (TL incidence 75% with 1 Gy, compared to 2% in wild-type mice) and yet our study still found a threshold at 0.1 Gy [28]. These results highlight the important difference between the loss of a threshold response and a dramatic decrease in the threshold, which requires sufficient data and statistical power to differentiate.

We previously studied the combined effect of X-rays with ENU, a potent carcinogen for inducing TL. Mice were given weekly exposure to X-rays for 4 consecutive weeks (Kaplan's method). No TL was induced by 0.4 Gy/fraction (1.6 Gy in total) or by ENU treatment at 100 ppm in drinking water for 4 weeks, implying these exposures were below an apparent threshold [29] (Fig. 3.4). Combined exposure (Fig. 3.5) to X-rays and ENU where both were below these thresholds also did not induce TL. Yet, with combined exposure to X-rays

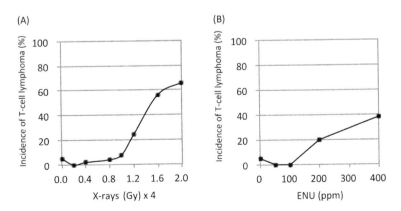

Figure 3.4
Dose–response curve of incidence of T-cell lymphoma (TL) induction by X-rays (A) or ENU (B).

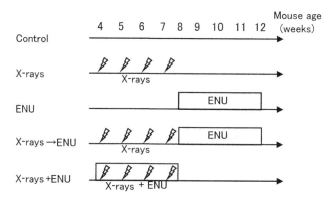

Figure 3.5
Experimental protocol for combined exposure to X-rays followed by ENU (X-rays→ENU) and simultaneous exposure of X-rays and ENU (X-rays + ENU). Mice were exposed to X-rays every week (lightning bolts) starting at age of 4 weeks. ENU treatment was started at age 4 or 8 weeks.

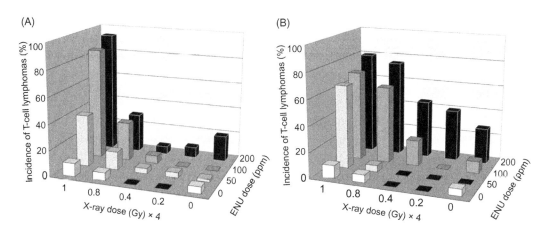

Figure 3.6
Incidence of T-cell lymphoma (TL) induction by combined exposure to X-rays followed by ENU (X-rays→ENU) (A) and simultaneous exposure of X-rays and ENU (X-rays + ENU) (B).

followed by ENU, X-ray doses above the threshold acted synergistically with ENU to promote lymphoma development, whereas radiation doses below the threshold antagonized ENU-induced lymphoma development when ENU treatment was above the threshold (Fig. 3.6A). None of the combined exposure regimens appeared to modify the threshold dose for X-rays, implying a hard limit which may represent a nonredundant step which cannot be bypassed by the action of ENU.

Later work showed that for simultaneous X-ray exposure and ENU treatment (X-rays + ENU), radiation doses above an apparent threshold showed a synergistic effect, but lower doses did not show any antagonistic effect (Fig. 3.6B) [30]. When delivered simultaneously, the exposures at the threshold (0.4 Gy X-rays and 100 ppm ENU) were now able to induce TL, but when either or both exposures were below the threshold no TL were induced.

Mechanism of combined exposure in thymic lymphomagenesis

We next investigated carcinogen-associated molecular changes in the induced tumors to delineate the carcinogenic pathways involved in combined exposure. We previously reported that the frequency of loss of heterozygosity (LOH) at the Ikaros locus and the mutation spectrum of *Ikaros* distinguishes X-ray-induced lymphomas from ENU-induced lymphomas [31,32]. X-ray-induced lymphomas harbored four types of *Ikaros* alterations (point mutation, insertion or deletion, null expression, and altered splicing); point mutations were predominantly G:C to A:T substitutions at CpG sites and A:T to G:C substitutions, which were accompanied by LOH. In contrast, ENU-induced lymphomas showed mainly *Ikaros* point mutations with A:T to G:C substitutions, and without LOH.

Analysis of lymphomas induced by combined exposure to 0.8 Gy/week (3.2 Gy in total) and ENU treatment showed the most frequent *Ikaros* mutations were point mutations, for both X-rays followed by ENU (42%) and X-rays concurrent with ENU (51%). The spectrum of point mutations for X-rays followed by ENU was base substitutions (A:T to G:C, G:C to A:T at non-CpG, G:C to T:A, and A:T to T:A) sometimes (18%) accompanied by LOH [29]. In contrast, concurrent X-ray and ENU treatment resulted in A:T to G:C and G:C to A:T at non-CpG sites, more frequently (40%) accompanied by LOH [30]. The results suggest that sequential exposure activated an ENU-induced mutagenic pathway, while simultaneous exposure activated both radiation- and ENU-induced mutagenic pathways, indicating the importance of treatment order in determining the mutation spectrum.

The mechanism of antagonism of ENU-induced lymphoma observed with prior subthreshold irradiation is difficult to determine given the low frequency of tumors; however, we have shown that prior exposure to subthreshold X-rays decreased the rate of *gpt*-mutation in the thymocytes recovered from *gpt* delta mice treated with ENU [33]. Analogously, combined chronic radiation exposure (1.5 mGy/h) with 4-(methylnitrosoamino)-1-(3-pyridyl)-1-butanone (NNK) has been demonstrated to reduce large deletions in lung cells as detected by the Spi^- assay compared to radiation alone [34]. These results together with others suggest that combined exposure of radiation and chemicals can protect cells from mutation induction, known as cross-adaptation [35]. Upregulation of DNA/cellular repair genes by radiation pretreatment may protect from damage during ENU treatment. Three genes important in protective responses: O^6-methylguanine-DNA methyltransferase (*Mgmt*) [36], pituitary tumor-transforming 1 (*Pttg1*) [37], and apurine/apyrimidine endonuclease (*Apex1*) [38], showed sustained upregulation through to the end of ENU treatment (200 ppm) after 0.2 Gy irradiation, but were dampened after prior exposure to 1 Gy [28]. Differential modulation of gene expression by radiation dose may explain the paradoxical suppression and enhancement of ENU carcinogenesis by prior irradiation, and the inflection point for gene regulation may correlate with the dose that marks the threshold. Whether such "cross-adaptation" responses can be generalized to other carcinogen combinations remains to be elucidated.

In summary, these data highlight the importance of not only the carcinogen doses, but also the order and timing of their delivery for combined exposures. Further studies like this one, which help us to understand the interplay of multiple carcinogen exposures will be crucial to developing a comprehensive framework for the assessment of cancer risk in people exposed to environmental carcinogens.

Conclusion

1. The linear nonthreshold model is generally accepted for radiation protection purposes.
2. The dose–response relationships, however, differ among tissues with examples of linear, linear-quadratic, and linear with threshold relationships as well as unresponsive tissues.
3. The radiation effect is profoundly affected by confounding factors, such as radiation and smoking for lung cancer induction.
4. The combined effect may differ by radiation quality and exposure regimen (A-bomb vs radon).
5. Combined exposure of carcinogens at subthreshold doses may not interact to induce cancer.
6. The mode of the interaction (synergistic, additive, or antagonistic) is dependent on the dose and order of exposure.
7. The order of combined exposure can drive distinct pathways for carcinogenesis.

Acknowledgments

We thank Dr Nohmi of National Institute of Health Sciences for giving us a chance to write this review. We thank all laboratory members for their encouragement throughout this work. This study was supported in part by grant of Grants-in-Aid for Scientific Research (S.K. 18510053 and 15H01834, Y.S. 21610029), a grant of Long-range Research Initiative (LRI) by Japan Chemical Industry Association to Y.S. and S.K (2003CC03-2005CC03 and 2006CC03-2010CC03).

References

[1] Sugimoto T, Shinozaki T, Naruse T, Miyamoto Y. Who was concerned about radiation, food safety, and natural disasters after the great East Japan earthquake and Fukushima catastrophe? A nationwide cross-sectional survey in 2012. PLoS One 2014;9:e106377.
[2] Ozasa K, Shimizu Y, Suyama A, Kasagi F, Soda M, Grant EJ, et al. Studies of the mortality of atomic bomb survivors, Report 14, 1950-2003: an overview of cancer and noncancer diseases. Radiat Res 2012;177:229–43.

[3] Preston DL, Ron E, Tokuoka S, Funamoto S, Nishi N, Soda M, et al. Solid cancer incidence in atomic bomb survivors: 1958–1998. Radiat Res 2007;168:1–64.

[4] Sugiyama H, Misumi M, Kishikawa M, Iseki M, Yonehara S, Hayashi T, et al. Skin cancer incidence among atomic bomb survivors from 1958 to 1996. Radiat Res 2014;181:531–9.

[5] Howe GR. Lung cancer mortality between 1950 and 1987 after exposure to fractionated moderate-dose-rate ionizing radiation in the Canadian fluoroscopy cohort study and a comparison with lung cancer mortality in the Atomic Bomb survivors study. Radiat Res 1995;142:295–304.

[6] Davis FG, Boice Jr. JD, Hrubec Z, Monson RR. Cancer mortality in a radiation-exposed cohort of Massachusetts tuberculosis patients. Cancer Res 1989;49:6130–6.

[7] Nair RR, Rajan B, Akiba S, Jayalekshmi P, Nair MK, Gangadharan P, et al. Background radiation and cancer incidence in Kerala, India-Karanagappally cohort study. Health Phys 2009;96:55–66.

[8] Shore RE. Implications of radiation epidemiologic data for risk assessment and radiation protection. Health Phys 2011;100:306–8.

[9] Little MP, Muirhead CR. Curvilinearity in the dose-response curve for cancer in Japanese atomic bomb survivors. Environ Health Perspect 1997;105(Suppl. 6):1505–9.

[10] Little MP, Muirhead CR. Curvature in the cancer mortality dose response in Japanese atomic bomb survivors: absence of evidence of threshold. Int J Radiat Biol 1998;74:471–80.

[11] Furukawa K, Preston DL, Lonn S, Funamoto S, Yonehara S, Matsuo T, et al. Radiation and smoking effects on lung cancer incidence among atomic bomb survivors. Radiat Res 2010;174:72–82.

[12] Egawa H, Furukawa K, Preston D, Funamoto S, Yonehara S, Matsuo T, et al. Radiation and smoking effects on lung cancer incidence by histological types among atomic bomb survivors. Radiat Res 2012;178:191–201.

[13] Cohen BL. Test of the linear-no threshold theory of radiation carcinogenesis for inhaled radon decay products. Health Phys 1995;68:157–74.

[14] Lubin JH, Steindorf K. Cigarette use and the estimation of lung cancer attributable to radon in the United States. Radiat Res 1995;141:79–85.

[15] Darby S, Hill D, Auvinen A, Barros-Dios JM, Baysson H, Bochicchio F, et al. Radon in homes and risk of lung cancer: collaborative analysis of individual data from 13 European case-control studies. BMJ 2005;330:223.

[16] National Research Council, Committee on the Biological Effects of Ionizing Radiation Health effects of exposure to radon (BEIR VI). Washington, DC: National Academy Press; 1999.

[17] Kreuzer M, Schnelzer M, Tschcnsc A, Walsh L, Grosche B. Cohort profile: the German uranium miners cohort study (WISMUT cohort), 1946–2003. Int J Epidemiol 2010;39:980–7.

[18] Walsh L, Tschense A, Schnelzer M, Dufey F, Grosche B, Kreuzer M. The influence of radon exposures on lung cancer mortality in German uranium miners, 1946–2003. Radiat Res 2010;173:79–90.

[19] Walsh L, Grosche B, Schnelzer M, Tschense A, Sogl M, Kreuzer M. A review of the results from the German Wismut uranium miners cohort. Radiat Prot Dosimetry 2015;164:147–53.

[20] Tanooka H. Threshold dose-response in radiation carcinogenesis: an approach from chronic beta-irradiation experiments and a review of non-tumour doses. Int J Radiat Biol 2001;77:541–51.

[21] Tanooka H, Ootsuyama A. Radiation carcinogenesis in mouse skin and its threshold-like response. J Radiat Res 1991;32(Suppl. 2):195–201.

[22] Hoshino H, Tanooka H. Interval effect of beta-irradiation and subsequent 4-nitroquinoline 1-oxide painting on skin tumor induction in mice. Cancer Res 1975;35:3663–6.

[23] Fry RJ, Storer JB, Burns FJ. Radiation induction of cancer of the skin. Br J Radiol Suppl 1986;19:58–60.

[24] Maisin JR, Wambersie A, Gerber GB, Mattelin G, Lambiet-Collier M, De Coster B, et al. Life-shortening and disease incidence in C57Bl mice after single and fractionated gamma and high-energy neutron exposure. Radiat Res 1988;113:300–17.

[25] Maisin JR, Wambersie A, Gerber GB, Mattelin G, Lambiet-Collier M, Gueulette J. The effects of a fractionated gamma irradiation on life shortening and disease incidence in BALB/c mice. Radiat Res 1983;94:359–73.

[26] Ullrich RL, Storer JB. Influence of gamma irradiation on the development of neoplastic disease in mice. I. Reticular tissue tumors. Radiat Res 1979;80:303–16.

[27] Blunt T, Gell D, Fox M, Taccioli GE, Lehmann AR, Jackson SP, et al. Identification of a nonsense mutation in the carboxyl-terminal region of DNA-dependent protein kinase catalytic subunit in the scid mouse. Proc Natl Acad Sci USA 1996;93:10285–90.

[28] Ishii-Ohba H, Kobayashi S, Nishimura M, Shimada Y, Tsuji H, Sado T, et al. Existence of a threshold-like dose for gamma-ray induction of thymic lymphomas and no susceptibility to radiation-induced solid tumors in SCID mice. Mutat Res 2007;619:124–33.

[29] Kakinuma S, Nishimura M, Amasaki Y, Takada M, Yamauchi K, Sudo S, et al. Combined exposure to X-irradiation followed by N-ethyl-N-nitrosourea treatment alters the frequency and spectrum of Ikaros point mutations in murine T-cell lymphoma. Mutat Res 2012;737:43–50.

[30] Hirano S, Kakinuma S, Amasaki Y, Nishimura M, Imaoka T, Fujimoto S, et al. Ikaros is a critical target during simultaneous exposure to X-rays and N-ethyl-N-nitrosourea in mouse T-cell lymphomagenesis. Int J Cancer 2013;132:259–68.

[31] Shimada Y, Nishimura M, Kakinuma S, Okumoto M, Shiroishi T, Clifton KH, et al. Radiation-associated loss of heterozygosity at the Znfn1a1 (Ikaros) locus on chromosome 11 in murine thymic lymphomas. Radiat Res 2000;154:293–300.

[32] Kakinuma S, Nishimura M, Sasanuma S, Mita K, Suzuki G, Katsura Y, et al. Spectrum of Znfn1a1 (Ikaros) inactivation and its association with loss of heterozygosity in radiogenic T-cell lymphomas in susceptible B6C3F1 mice. Radiat Res 2002;157:331–40.

[33] Yamauchi K, Kakinuma S, Sudo S, Kito S, Ohta Y, Nohmi T, et al. Differential effects of low- and high-dose X-rays on N-ethyl-N-nitrosourea-induced mutagenesis in thymocytes of B6C3F1 gpt-delta mice. Mutat Res 2008;640:27–37.

[34] Ikeda M, Masumura K, Sakamoto Y, Wang B, Nenoi M, Sakuma K, et al. Combined genotoxic effects of radiation and a tobacco-specific nitrosamine in the lung of gpt delta transgenic mice. Mutat Res 2007;626:15–25.

[35] Kakinuma S, Yamauchi K, Amasaki Y, Nishimura M, Shimada Y. Low-dose radiation attenuates chemical mutagenesis in vivo. J Radiat Res 2009;50:401–5.

[36] Kaina B, Christmann M, Naumann S, Roos WP. MGMT: key node in the battle against genotoxicity, carcinogenicity and apoptosis induced by alkylating agents. DNA Repair (Amst) 2007;6:1079–99.

[37] Romero F, Multon MC, Ramos-Morales F, Dominguez A, Bernal JA, Pintor-Toro JA, et al. Human securin, hPTTG, is associated with Ku heterodimer, the regulatory subunit of the DNA-dependent protein kinase. Nucleic Acids Res 2001;29:1300–7.

[38] Roos WP, Christmann M, Fraser ST, Kaina B. Mouse embryonic stem cells are hypersensitive to apoptosis triggered by the DNA damage O(6)-methylguanine due to high E2F1 regulated mismatch repair. Cell Death Differ 2007;14:1422–32.

Possible Mechanisms Underlying Genotoxic Thresholds: DNA Repair and Translesion DNA Synthesis

Takehiko Nohmi[1] and Teruhisa Tsuzuki[2]

[1]Biological Safety Research Center, National Institute of Health Sciences, Setagaya-ku, Tokyo, Japan
[2]Department of Medical Biophysics and Radiation Biology, Faculty of Medical Sciences, Kyushu University, Higashi-ku, Fukuoka, Japan

Chapter Outline
Introduction   49
Challenges in Identification of Genotoxicity of Chemicals   52
Possible Mechanisms Underlying Genotoxic Thresholds   54
Significance of DNA Repair Mechanisms in the Suppression of Mutagenesis and
    Tumorigenesis in Mammals   55
TLS as a Critical Factor for Mutagenesis   58
Future Perspectives   62
Acknowledgments   63
References   63

Introduction

Human DNA is continuously exposed to a variety of endogenous and exogenous chemicals. Some of these chemicals are DNA reactive, thereby inducing DNA damage such as base modifications, abasic sites, single- or double-strand breaks in DNA [1]. Although all cells possess defense systems against DNA damage, some damage escapes from the DNA repair mechanisms and induces mutations upon DNA replication. The frequency of mutations will be more enhanced when the genomic DNA is exposed to the adverse chemicals more extensively. If the mutations occur in critical genes for genomic integrity such as *TP53* or *RAS*, the cells may step forward for carcinogenesis and finally attack the host organisms [2].

To reduce the cancer risk associated with chemical exposure, international committees set up a variety of regulations on chemicals. The examples are guidelines recommended by the

Thresholds of Genotoxic Carcinogens.
DOI: http://dx.doi.org/10.1016/B978-0-12-801663-3.00004-2

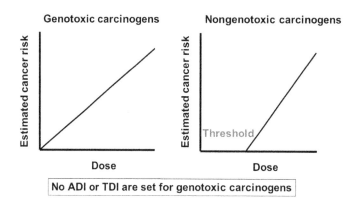

Figure 4.1
Modeled dose–responses of genotoxic carcinogens and nongenotoxic carcinogens.
Genotoxic carcinogens have no threshold for the cancer risk, while nongenotoxic
carcinogens have a threshold. *ADI*, acceptable daily intake; *TDI*, tolerable daily intake.

International Conference on Harmonisation of Technical Requirements for Registration of
Pharmaceuticals for Human Use (ICH) for pharmaceuticals (http://www.ich.org/products/
guidelines/safety/article/safety-guidelines.html) and those by the Organization for Economic
Co-operation and Development (OECD) for industrial chemicals (http://www.oecd-ilibrary.
org/environment/oecd-guidelines-for-the-testing-of-chemicals-section-4-health-effects_
20745788;jsessionid=2nh0sdqgrmcbe.x-oecd-live-01). Although details are different in each
guideline, a common default assumption is that genotoxic carcinogens have no safe level or
thresholds for the action (Fig. 4.1). It is assumed that genotoxic carcinogens impose cancer
risk on human population even at very low doses [3]. This is in contrast to regulatory policy
for nongenotoxic chemicals in that the chemicals have thresholds for the toxic effects and
thus can be used in society below the threshold level.

The term "genotoxic carcinogens" was coined in the late 1980s when a survey of the National
Toxicology Program revealed that about 40% of rodent carcinogens were negative in Ames
test (bacterial mutation assay) and had no structural alerts to interact with DNA [4] (Fig. 4.2).
These Ames-negative carcinogens were referred to as "nongenotoxic carcinogens," while
Ames-positive carcinogens with the structural alerts were named "genotoxic carcinogens."
Nongenotoxic carcinogens are usually carcinogenic in single species of rodents and induce
tumors in single organs while genotoxic carcinogens are in general carcinogenic in both rats and
mice and induce tumors in multiple organs. Nongenotoxic carcinogens induce tumors in rodents
through a variety of mechanisms other than genotoxicity, such as hormonal effects, cytotoxicity,
and cell proliferation. In contract, genotoxic carcinogens induce tumors through DNA damage
and mutations. This classification, that is, genotoxic and nongenotoxic carcinogens, has strong
implications in regulation of chemicals because no acceptable daily intake (ADI) or tolerable

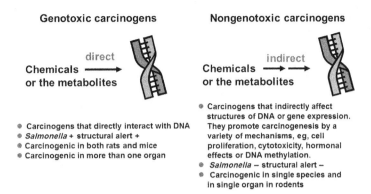

Figure 4.2

Characteristics of genotoxic carcinogens and nongenotoxic carcinogens. Genotoxic carcinogens
are chemicals that interact with DNA and induce mutations, thereby inducing cancer in rodents.
If the chemicals need metabolic activation, the metabolites interact with DNA, causing mutations.
In contrast, nongenotoxic carcinogens and the metabolites do not interact with DNA. They induce
cancer via nongenotoxic mechanisms such as hormonal effects, cell proliferation, and cell toxicity.

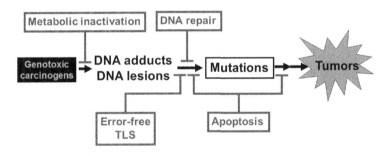

Figure 4.3

Self-defense mechanisms may suppress carcinogenic effects of genotoxic carcinogens.
The mechanisms may reduce the carcinogenicity of chemicals below spontaneous
levels, thereby establishing practical thresholds. *TLS*, translesion DNA synthesis.

daily intake (TDI) can be set for genotoxic carcinogens, while nongenotoxic carcinogens can be
used in the society if the dose is lower than the threshold or no-observed-adverse-effect levels
(NOAEL) (Fig. 4.1). ADI is a safety limit of daily intake for chemicals that are intentionally
added to food such as food additives, pesticides, and medicines for animal use, and TDI is the
same but for chemicals that are not deliberately added, such as contaminants in food (http://
www.inchem.org/documents/harmproj/harmproj/harmproj1.pdf). However, this paradigm that
genotoxic carcinogens have no thresholds has been challenged by experimental and theoretical
approaches in a last few decades [5,6]. In fact, this paradigm is counterintuitive because
all organisms including humans possess a number of self-defense mechanisms (Fig. 4.3).

The defense mechanisms include antioxidants, detoxication metabolism, DNA repair, error-free translesion DNA synthesis (TLS), apoptosis, and so on. These mechanisms may suppress the genotoxic effects of chemicals at low doses to the spontaneous levels and constitute a practical threshold. The term "practical threshold" is defined in this chapter as the doses below which no statistical increase in mutation frequencies is detected.

In this chapter, we at first discuss challenges of identification of genotoxicity of chemicals. Ames test and DNA reactivity are two gold standards for genotoxicity [4]. However, Ames-positive compounds are not necessarily positive in vivo. For example, they may be detoxified in whole-body systems. We emphasize the importance of in vivo gene mutation assay for identification of genotoxicity of chemicals. Then we discuss possible roles of DNA repair and TLS in practical thresholds and finally discuss the future perspective for genotoxic thresholds.

Challenges in Identification of Genotoxicity of Chemicals

At present, more than 100 genotoxicity assays are available, and representative assays are listed in Table 4.1. The assays employ a variety of organisms such as phage, bacteria, yeast, cultured mammalian cells, fruit fly, mice, and rats. Therefore, it is not uncommon that one chemical provides conflicting results in different genotoxicity assays, that is, positive results in one assay and negative results in another assay. Among the various assays, the results of "mutagenicity assays" are more important than "indicator assays" to evaluate the genotoxic risk, because "mutagenicity assays" detect irreversible heritable genetic changes such as mutations, while "indicator assays" detect transient DNA damage such as DNA adducts or DNA strand breaks [7]. In addition, the results of in vivo assays are more important than those of in vitro assays for the final decision of whether the chemical is genotoxic or not. For pharmaceuticals, Ames test, chromosome aberration test, or gene mutation tests with cultured mammalian cells and micronucleus test with mice or rats are a standard set for genotoxicity assays [8]. However, each test has its own shortcomings. For example, some chemicals that are positive in vivo mutagenicity tests, such as urethane (ethyl carbamate), acrylamide, and procarbazine, are negative or weakly positive in Ames tests because of inefficient metabolic activation of the chemicals in vitro. However, these chemicals are classified as class 2A carcinogens (probably carcinogenic to humans) by the International Agency for Research on Cancer (http://monographs.iarc.fr/ENG/Classification/). To mimic in vivo metabolism, Ames tests and other in vitro genotoxicity assays use liver $9000 \times g$ supernatant (S9) prepared from rats pretreated with either phenobarbital plus 5,6-benzoflavone or polychlorinated biphenyls. S9 contains several isoforms of cytochrome P-450 (CYP enzymes) and other drug-metabolizing enzymes. However, some chemicals such as those described above are not effectively activated. On the contrary, some nitro compounds, such as metronidazole, are strongly positive in Ames test but mostly negative or weakly positive in vivo tests including the micronucleus assay [9]. This is partly because nitro aromatics are effectively activated

Table 4.1 Representative genotoxicity assays.

	In Vitro Test	**In Vivo Test**
Mutagenicity Assay		
Gene mutation	Bacterial reverse mutation test (Ames test) Mammalian gene mutation test, eg, mouse lymphoma *TK* gene mutation assay	Transgenic rodent gene mutation test Mouse spot test Reverse mutation test with *Drosophila melanogaster*
Chromosome aberration	In vitro chromosome aberration test In vitro micronucleus test	Chromosome aberration test Micronucleus test (mouse, rat)
Indicator Assay		
DNA adduct DNA damage and killing DNA damage and gene expression	^{32}P-post labeling method Rec assay with *Bacillus subtilis* SOS test with *Escherichia coli*	^{32}P-post labeling method
DNA strand break DNA strand break	Alkaline elution Comet assay (single-cell gel electrophoresis)	Alkaline elution Comet assay (single-cell gel electrophoresis)
Chromosome aberration DNA damage and repair	Sister chromatid exchange (SCE) Unscheduled DNA synthesis (UDS)	Sister chromatid exchange (SCE) Unscheduled DNA synthesis (UDS)
Germ Cell Genotoxicity Assay		
Gene mutation Chromosome aberration		Transgenic rodent gene mutation test Mouse-specific locus test Sex-linked recessive lethal test with *Drosophila* ESTR mutation Dominant lethal test Heritable translocation test
Others	Cell transformation assay	

by bacterial nitro reductases. However, there are some reports that metronidazole induces chromosome aberrations in human patients [10,11]. Therefore, it is still controversial whether metronidazole is genotoxic and carcinogenic to humans or not [12,13]. Chromosome aberration tests and gene mutation tests with mammalian cells often give "false-positive" results at high doses where cell survival was substantially decreased [14,15]. Therefore, the revised ICH and OECD test guidelines recommend reduction of the top doses for the tests [16]. Besides, in the revised ICH guideline S2 (R1), in vitro mammalian assays can be skipped and the second in vivo assay such as in vivo comet assay or transgenic gene mutation assays may be conducted along with an in vivo micronucleus test. The false-positive results with cultured mammalian cells can be corrected or reevaluated by an in vivo micronucleus test. However, micronucleus tests employ bone marrow or peripheral blood for identification of aberrant cells. Thus, several liver carcinogens such as 2,4-diaminotoluene and diethylnitrosamine are negative or equivocal in the test probably because the active metabolites generated in the liver do not reach the bone marrow [17,18]. To compensate for this shortcoming, the micronucleus test with liver of mice and rats is being developed [19]. Another pitfall of the micronucleus test is that transient hypothermia causes micronucleus induction in the bone marrow of mice and rats without damage to DNA. Chlorpromazine is such a chemical that is negative in an in vitro chromosome aberration test but is "positive" in the micronucleus test in mice and rats because of the hypothermic effects [20,21]. Thus, caution should be taken to interpret the results of the micronucleus test.

In rodent carcinogenicity tests, species differences are sometimes observed to influence the results. For example, aflatoxin B_1 is a liver carcinogen in rats and humans but its carcinogenic effects are weak or negligible in mice [22]. Therefore, it is desirable to examine the mutagenicity of chemicals in the target organs of rodents used for 2-year cancer bioassay. In this respect, gene mutation assays with transgenic rodents are quite useful [23]. They can detect point mutations and some types of deletions in any organ of rodents such as liver, colon, lung, and testis [24]. In addition, sequence analyses provide insights into the mechanisms underlying the mutations detected. In mice, several transgenic models have been established [25]. Cao et al. used *gpt* delta mice for in vivo mutagenicity of ethyl methanesulfonate at low doses and suggested that the practical thresholds were lower in *gpt* delta mice than in Muta Mouse because of the lower background mutation frequency [26]. In rats, *gpt* delta rats have been developed in genetic backgrounds of Sprague–Dawley (SD) and Fisher 344 (F-344) [27,28]. Because F-344 rats are used more often than SD rats for 2-year cancer bioassay, F-344 *gpt* delta rats have been used to establish the standard protocol of transgenic rodent gene mutation assays for OECD test guideline TG488 [29–31]. Recently, Umemura et al. revealed that ochratoxin A, a mycotoxin that induces renal tumors in rats, and is a possible causing factor for urinary tract tumors in humans, induces deletion mutations in the renal outer medulla, specifically in the S3 segment, in male F-344 *gpt* delta rats [32,33]. However, ochratoxin A is negative in Ames test and has no structural alerts to interact with DNA [34]. The mechanism of action of ochratoxin A in the target organ for carcinogenesis remains to be solved. The findings raise questions of whether ochratoxin A is a genotoxic carcinogen or not. This relates to a question in regulation whether TDI can be set for this mycotoxin or not. Mechanistic understanding of tumor induction is critically important for regulation of chemicals.

Possible Mechanisms Underlying Genotoxic Thresholds

In recent years, the paradigm that a linear relationship exists between exposed doses of DNA-reactive genotoxins and mutations even at low doses has been challenged. It is expected that various cellular defense mechanisms may constitute the practical thresholds even for DNA-reactive genotoxic chemicals. Nevertheless, there is still limited experimental data that suggest the threshold doses for genotoxic carcinogens. Here, we discuss the possible involvement of DNA repair and TLS in genotoxic thresholds.

Significance of DNA Repair Mechanisms in the Suppression of Mutagenesis and Tumorigenesis in Mammals

DNA repair mechanisms generally involve the removal of damaged or incorrect bases in chromosomal DNA. Reactive oxygen species (ROS) are produced through normal cellular metabolism, and the formation of such radicals is further enhanced by radiation and by various chemicals. ROS attack DNA and its precursor nucleotides, and consequently bases with various modifications are introduced into the DNA of normally growing cells. One such modified base, 8-oxo-7,8-dihydroguanine (8-oxoG) is highly mutagenic because of its ambiguous pairing property. Three enzymes, MTH1, OGG1, and MUTYH, play important roles in avoiding 8-oxoG-related mutagenesis in mammalian cells (Fig. 4.4) [35–38].

We have been studying these three proteins; MTH1, MUTYH, and OGG1 together with MSH2 as factors involved in the avoiding mechanisms for 8-oxoG-related mutagenesis. Here we focus on MUTYH, in relation to the control of spontaneous and oxidative stress-induced mutagenesis and tumorigenesis. We established the *Mutyh*-deficient mouse lines by gene targeting. Pathological examination revealed a statistically significant difference in the incidence of spontaneous tumors between wild-type and *Mutyh*-deficient mice after 1½ years of observation. *Mutyh*-deficient mice showed a marked predisposition to intestinal adenoma/adenocarcinoma. Using the *rpsL* (forward mutation detection) system [39], we analyzed the frequency and the spectra of spontaneous mutations in *Mutyh*-deficient mice. Crossing with the transgenic mice carrying approximately 100 copies of the reporter gene, *rpsL* of *Escherichia coli*, we first examined the mutation frequency. The overall spontaneous mutation frequency observed in small intestine samples from *Mutyh*-deficient mice at the age of 24 weeks, showed no dramatic increase compared to the value of wild-type mice; approximately 1×10^{-5}. However, there are distinct differences in the mutational spectra between the two genotypes; an increase in frequency of G:C to T:A transversion was evident in *Mutyh*-deficient mice (Yamauchi K, et al., in preparation). Thus we have established an experimental system for oxidative DNA-damage-induced mutagenesis and tumorigenesis in the gastrointestinal tracts of mice [40]. Oral administration of an oxidizing reagent, potassium bromate (KBrO$_3$), effectively induced G:C to T:A transversions and epithelial tumors in the small intestines of *Mutyh*-deficient mice, implying the significance of MUTYH in the suppression of mutagenesis and tumorigenesis induced by oxidative stress. We performed mutation analysis of the tumor-associated genes amplified from the intestinal tumors developed in four mutant mice that had been treated with KBrO$_3$. Many tumors had G:C to T:A transversions in either *Apc* or *Ctnnb1*. No mutations were found in either

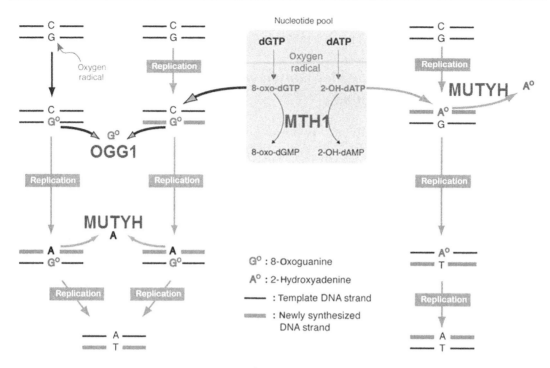

Figure 4.4

Oxidative damage-related mutagenesis and its avoiding mechanisms in mammals.
Among the various types of oxidative damage in DNA, the oxidized forms of guanine and adenine,
8-oxo-7,8-dihydroguanine (8-oxoguanine) and 1,2-dihydro-2-oxoadenine (2-hydroxyadenine), can
form relatively stable base pairs with either adenine or guanine in DNA, respectively. During DNA
replication, they are thought to induce spontaneous mutagenesis, such as A:T to C:G and G:C
to T:A transversions. The direct oxidation of DNA by reactive oxygen species has been reported
to generate a substantial amount of 8-oxoguanine but little 2-hydroxyadenine. In contrast,
2-hydroxyadenine is generated exclusively by the oxidation of dATP in the nucleotide pool. Studies
on mutator mutants have revealed that *Escherichia coli* has several error-avoiding mechanisms that
minimize the deleterious effects of 8-oxoguanine and in which MutT, MutM, and MutY proteins
play important roles. MutT protein hydrolyzes 8-oxo-dGTP to 8-oxo-dGMP and pyrophosphate,
thus avoiding the occurrence of A:T to C:G transversion mutations during DNA replication. MutM
and MutY proteins are DNA glycosylases, the former excises 8-oxoG paired with cytosine, whereas
the latter removes adenine paired with 8-oxoguanine. Mammalian cells are also equipped with
elaborate error-preventing mechanisms similar to those found in prokaryotes; MTH1 as a MutT
homolog, OGG1 as a functional homolog for MutM, and MUTYH (MYH) as a MutY homolog.
Recent studies showed that MTH1 effectively hydrolyzes 2-OH-dATP as well as 8-oxo-dGTP, while
MUTYH has the ability to excise 2-hydroxyadenine inserted opposite guanine in the template strand
as well as the ability to remove adenine incorporated opposite 8-oxoguanine in the template.
As a result of the cooperative action among MTH1/OGG1/MUTYH and other repair pathways,
mammalian cells effectively protect the occurrence of spontaneous mutations such as A:T to
C:G and G:C to T:A transversions, which are caused by 8-oxoguanine and 2-hydroxyadenine.

K-ras (exon 2) or *Trp53* (exon 5–8) [41]. Our findings confirm the association between MUTYH deficiency and the recessive form of hereditary multiple colorectal adenoma/carcinoma in humans, known as MUTYH-associated familial adenomatous polyposis [42], with the characteristic feature; G:C to T:A transversions in the GAA sequence context. Also, our results suggest that the abnormality in Wnt signal transduction pathway is causatively associated with oxidative stress-induced tumorigenesis in the small intestines of *Mutyh*-deficient mice. In addition, the multiple formation of tumor in the small intestines of *Mutyh*-deficient mice provides a suitable model system to investigate the processes of intestinal tumorigenesis.

To assess the dose-dependent relation between the level of oxidative stress and tumor incidence, we performed oxidative stress–induced intestinal tumorigenesis experiments using *Mutyh*-deficient mice as well as the wild-type controls. Mice were divided into five groups and received different doses of $KBrO_3$; 0%, 0.05%, 0.1%, 0.15%, 0.2%, in drinking water for 16 weeks. No tumors were developed in untreated *Mutyh*-deficient mice or those treated at the dose of 0.05%, whereas a number of tumors were observed in the small intestine of all of the mice treated at 0.1% or higher (Ohno M, et al., in preparation). The results suggest that the intestinal tumorigenesis correlates to the level of oxidative stress in *Mutyh*-deficient mice. Accordingly, we found a practical threshold in the dose–response relationship for the oxidative stress–induced intestinal tumorigenesis in *Mutyh*-deficient mice. Analyses of oxidative stress–induced mutation at different doses of $KBrO_3$ at the *rpsL* gene in transgenic mice, wild-type mice and *Mutyh*-deficient mice, are currently in progress. Preliminary mutation analyses revealed that a 4-week administration of $KBrO_3$ dramatically increased the incidence of G:C to T:A transversion mutations, especially in the small intestines of *Mutyh*-deficient mice in relation to the dose applied; 0.05%, 0.1%, and 0.15%. This result might reflect that the higher dose of $KBrO_3$ treatment effectively induces more oxidative DNA damage, mainly resulting in G:C to T:A transversions, in the small intestines. These results suggest that cells are able to correctly repair oxidative DNA lesions resulting from exposure to a certain level of low doses of endogenous and exogenous chemicals with oxidizing property, and thus are less likely to be transformed to the neoplastic phenotype.

It is of interest that among the repair factors so far examined, only MUTYH [40,41] and MSH2 [36,43] were shown to play a significant role in the suppression of $KBrO_3$-induced intestinal tumorigenesis in mice. Increasing evidence suggests that mismatch repair is involved in both the repair and cell death caused by oxidative DNA damages. Recently, we reported the involvement of MUTYH in cell death caused by oxidative DNA damage [44]. Thus, a defect in either MUTYH or MSH2 in mice would simultaneously compromise both DNA repair and cell death caused by oxidative DNA damage (Fig. 4.5). This notion may explain why among many DNA repair factors, only MUTYH and mismatch repair factors are, so far, identified to be associated with hereditary colorectal cancers in humans.

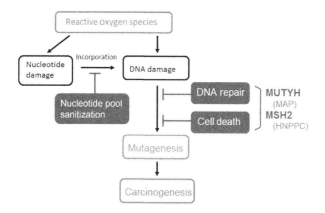

Figure 4.5
The roles of MUTYH and mismatch repair (MSH2) in the avoiding
mechanisms for ROS-induced mutagenesis and carcinogenesis.
The defects in MUTYH or in MSH2 simultaneously compromise both DNA repair
and cell death induced by oxidative DNA damage. Thus, the defect in MUTYH or in
MSH2 makes mice highly susceptible to oxidative stress–induced tumorigenesis.

TLS as a Critical Factor for Mutagenesis

TLS is a short DNA synthesis across DNA lesions [45]. DNA damage such as DNA adducts, DNA inter- and intrastrand cross-links, block progress of DNA replication and may generate a single-strand region downstream of the lesion and induce strand breaks in DNA. To circumvent the genotoxic consequences of the lesions, cells possess multiple specialized DNA polymerases (Pol) that can continue DNA synthesis across the lesion [46]. These Pols are specialized in that they may have partly overlapping but basically distinct specificity to DNA lesions that they can bypass [47]. The specialized Pols are much less processive than replicative Pol, such as Pol δ or ε. Processivity is an ability of DNA polymerases to catalyze consecutive polymerization without falling off from DNA substrates. Therefore, the specialized Pols can synthesize only short stretches of DNA. The specialized Pols are in general error-prone, that is, low fidelity of DNA synthesis, in contrast to the high fidelity of replicative Pols [48]. If correct dNTPs are inserted opposite the damaged base during TLS, it will be an error-free DNA synthesis and no mutation will occur (Fig. 4.6). However, when incorrect dNTPs are inserted opposite the lesion, the TLS will be an error-prone DNA synthesis and generate mutations. Therefore, TLS is a critical biochemical step for reduction and induction of mutations induced by DNA damage. It may be worth noting that unlike DNA repair, which removes DNA lesions, TLS does not remove DNA damage but continues DNA replication beyond the lesion, thereby enhancing cellular survival. It is often said that TLS is a double-edged sword because it may enhance survival of cells with concomitant induction of mutations.

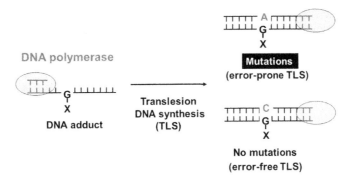

Figure 4.6
Translesion DNA synthesis (TLS). TLS is a biochemical process where DNA polymerases (in most cases, specialized DNA polymerases) continue DNA synthesis across lesions in DNA. TLS can be classified to either error-free or error-prone TLS across the lesions. The error-free TLS suppresses induction of mutations, while the error-prone TLS induces mutations. DNA polymerases are presented as oval shapes.

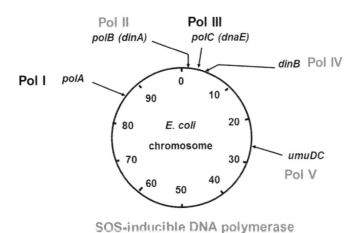

Figure 4.7
Genetic map position of DNA polymerases in *Escherichia coli*. DNA polymerase II (Pol II), DNA polymerase IV (Pol IV), and DNA polymerase V (Pol V) are specialized DNA polymerases. These polymerases are SOS-inducible, that is, the expression is enhanced when the bacterial chromosome DNA is damaged.

In *E. coli* and *Salmonella typhimurium*, which are used in bacterial mutation assays, there are two replicative Pols, Pol I and Pol III, and three specialized Pols, Pol II, IV, and V, in the genome (Fig. 4.7) [47]. These specialized Pols are SOS-inducible, that is, the expression is induced when the bacterial chromosome DNA is damaged. To examine the specificity of bacterial specialized Pols, Pol II, Pol IV, and Pol V-homolog, that is, Pol RI encoded by the *mucAB* genes in plasmid pKM101 [49], were expressed from plasmids

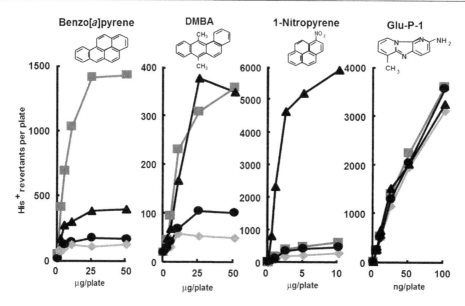

Figure 4.8

Typical dose-responses of *Salmonella typhimurium* TA1538 expressing specialized DNA polymerases [50]. The specialized DNA polymerases are DNA polymerase II (diamonds), DNA polymerase IV (DinB) (squares) and DNA polymerase R1 (triangles). The polymerases were overexpressed from plasmid pYG787, pYG768, or pKM101 introduced in the host strain. The dose–response curves of *S. typhimurium* TA1538 without plasmid are represented with circles.

in *S. typhimurium* TA1538, a standard tester strain of Ames test, and the effects of the expression on the mutability of the host strain were examined for 30 chemicals (Fig. 4.8) [50]. Interestingly, Pol IV and Pol RI displayed a partly overlapping but distinct substrate specificity. The mutagenicity of benzo[*a*]pyrene and another seven chemicals was very much enhanced when Pol IV was expressed. The mutagenicity was only slightly enhanced by the expression of Pol RI. In contrast, the mutagenicity of 1-nitropyrene and 11 other chemicals was strongly enhanced by Pol RI but not by Pol IV. Dimethylbenz[*a*]anthracene and other five chemicals seem to be intermediates because both Pol IV and Pol RI almost equally enhanced the mutagenicity. Pol II was inactive as far as the chemicals were tested. Unexpectedly, the mutagenicity of Glu-P-1 and the other five chemicals was not enhanced at all by the expression of any of the specialized Pols. The results suggest that the replicative Pols are responsible for the induction of mutations, which may be due to the target DNA sequence in *S. typhimurium* TA1538, that is, CGCGCGCG, for − 2 frameshift mutations. In such a repetitive sequence, even replicative Pols may skip some lesions such as those induced by active metabolites of Glu-P-1 and continue DNA replication. Collectively, the results highlight the importance of TLS mediated by the specialized and replicative Pols for induction of mutations.

Table 4.2 DNA polymerases in humans.

Name	Gene	DNA Polymerase Family	Function(s)
Pol γ	POLG	A	Mitochondria DNA replication and repair
Pol θ	POLQ	A	Somatic hypermutation at G:C sites
Pol ν	POLN	A	Translesion DNA synthesis
Pol α	POLA	B	Priming DNA synthesis
Pol δ	POLD1	B	DNA replication and repair
Pol ε	POLE1	B	DNA replication and repair
Pol ζ	REV3L	B	Translesion DNA synthesis
Pol β	POLB	X	Base excision repair
Pol λ	POLL	X	Base excision repair, nonhomologous recombination
Pol μ	POLM	X	Base excision repair, nonhomologous recombination
TdT	DNTT	X	Nonhomologous recombination
Pol σ	POLS	X	Sister chromatid cohesion
Pol η	POLH	Y	Translesion DNA synthesis
Pol ι	POLI	Y	Translesion DNA synthesis
Pol κ	POLK	Y	Translesion DNA synthesis
Rev1	REV1	Y	Translesion DNA synthesis
Primase and polymerase (DNA-directed)	PRIMPOL	AEP[a]	Translesion DNA synthesis

[a]AEP, archaeo-eukaryotic primases.

In humans, there are more than 10 Pols and about half of them are suggested to be involved in TLS (Table 4.2) [51,52]. The fact that cells possess a number of specialized Pols implies that the human genome is exposed to a variety of DNA-damaging agents. The genome size of humans is more than 1000 times larger than that of bacteria and thus it is almost impossible to remove all DNA damage before DNA replication. Thus, TLS may be more important in humans than in bacteria to protect the genome from a variety of DNA-damaging agents. Among various human specialized Pols, Pol ζ, a B-family Pol, and four Y-family Pols, that is, Pol η, Pol ι, Pol κ, and REV1, appear to be key enzymes in TLS. The homozygous knockout of mouse Rev3L encoding Pol ζ leads to embryonic lethality, suggesting the essential role of Pol ζ in protection of genome DNA from endogenous DNA damage during embryogenesis [53]. Human Pol η is responsible for the human genetic disorder, *Xeroderma pigmentosum variant* (XPV), and is proficient in error-free TLS across thymine dimer induced by ultraviolet light and cisplatin-induced intrastrand cross-links [54,55]. The role of Pol ι in TLS is still elusive, but suppression of expression of Pol ι makes the cells sensitive to oxidizing agents such as hydrogen peroxide and menadione [56]. Pol κ is an ortholog of bacterial Pol IV and may play a variety role in TLS. Pol κ appears to bypass N^2-guanyl DNA adducts induced by benzo[*a*]pyrene diolepoxide and other lesions such as intra- and interstrand cross-links in DNA. However, most of the characterization has been done in biochemistry and it remains largely uncertain what roles it plays in vivo. Recently, *gpt* delta mice expressing an inactive Pol κ have been established and exposed to mitomycin C, an anticancer drug that induces inter- and intrastrand cross-links in DNA [57]. The mice were more sensitive to the mutagenicity and clastogenicity of mitomycin C in bone marrow than *gpt* delta mice expressing the wild-type Pol κ, suggesting the in vivo protective role of Pol κ from the DNA cross-linker. The mice seem appropriate to elucidate the role of Pol κ in protection of genomic DNA from genotoxic effects of chemicals at low doses. The last member of Y-family Pols is REV1, which plays an important role as a scaffold of multiple Pols because it interacts with Pol ζ, Pol η, Pol ι, and Pol κ [58].

In summary, TLS mainly mediated by specialized Pols plays a pivotal role in the reduction and induction of mutations. It is evident that each specialized Pol has a partly overlapping but distinct substrate (or DNA lesion) specificity for TLS. However, experimental data related to the role of TLS in the kinetics of mutation induction at low-dose regions are missing and further work is necessary to elucidate the role in the practical threshold in genotoxicity.

Future Perspectives

In this chapter, we first discussed the challenges in identification of genotoxicity of chemicals. WHO/IPCS defined the term "mutation" as permanent changes in the structure and/or amount of the genetic material of an organism that can lead to heritable changes in its function [7]. The term "mutation" includes structural and numerical chromosome alterations as well as gene mutations. In contrast, "genotoxicity" refers to the capability of substances to damage DNA and/or cellular components regulating the fidelity of the genome, such as the spindle apparatus and topoisomerases, and includes all adverse effects on genetic information. Therefore, "genotoxicity" is a broader term than "mutagenicity." Because several of the non-DNA-reactive "genotoxicants," such as topoisomerase II inhibitors, exhibit threshold-like dose-responses, it is generally accepted that topoisomerase inhibitors have NOAEL, and also that ADI or TDI can be set for the chemicals [59]. However, some of the topoisomerase inhibitors, such as berenil, inhibit the activity of topoisomerase through binding to AT-selective minor groove in DNA [60]. The altered DNA conformation changes the topological structure of DNA, thereby inhibiting the binding of topoisomerase II. Thus, it is a DNA-reactive topoisomerase inhibitor. It is questionable, therefore, whether ADI can be set for the chemical. As such, mechanisms of action should be carefully examined when ADI or TDI is set for chemicals.

Recently, the concept of "threshold of toxicological concern" (TTC) has been proposed for regulation of genotoxic carcinogens [61]. In the ICH M7 guideline (http://www.ich.org/products/guidelines/multidisciplinary/article/multidisciplinary-guidelines.html), a value of 1.5 μg/day per person is proposed as the acceptable limit of mutagenic impurities in drug substances and drug products, which corresponds to a theoretical 10^{-5} excess lifetime risk of cancer. The value can be increased when the drug is used less than a life time. For example, 120 µg/day per person of mutagenic impurities is considered to be protective for daily intake when the drug is used for less than 1 month. Although the multiple mutagenic impurities from one drug are considered in the guideline, people, in particular senior citizens, may intake multiple drugs daily. Therefore, it may be possible that the person is exposed to mutagenic impurities over the TTC levels. Multiple exposures may be more serious in food rather than pharmaceuticals because people take a variety of foods in everyday life. It is demonstrated that multiple mutagenic heterocyclic amines that are not detectably mutagenic at each low dose become mutagenic when they are combined [62]. The result highlights the limit of risk evaluation of single mutagenic chemicals. Approaches for evaluation of genotoxic and carcinogenic risk of multiple exposure of chemicals are expected to be developed to achieve more comprehensive protection of the human genome from a variety of environmental genotoxic and carcinogenic agents.

Acknowledgments

The authors thank the members of our laboratories for discussion and for their technical assistance. This study was financially supported in part by grants-in-aid for scientific research (26281029 for TN and 25241012 for TT) from the Japan Society for the Promotion of Science and the Food Safety Commission.

References

[1] Friedberg EC, Walker GC, Siede W, Wood RD, Schultz RA, Ellenberger T. DNA repair and mutagenesis. 2nd ed. Washington, DC: ASM Press; 2006. p. 1–1118.

[2] Hanahan D, Weinberg RA. Hallmarks of cancer: the next generation. Cell 2011;144:646–74.

[3] Kirsch-Volders M, Aardema M, Elhajouji A. Concepts of threshold in mutagenesis and carcinogenesis. Mutat Res 2000;464:3–11.

[4] Ashby J, Tennant RW. Chemical structure, *Salmonella* mutagenicity and extent of carcinogenicity as indicators of genotoxic carcinogenesis among 222 chemicals tested in rodents by the U.S. NCI/NTP. Mutat Res 1988;204:17–115.

[5] Fukushima S, Wanibuchi H, Morimura K, Iwai S, Nakae D, Kishida H, et al. Existence of a threshold for induction of aberrant crypt foci in the rat colon with low doses of 2-amino-1-methyl-6-phenolimidazo[4,5-*b*] pyridine. Toxicol Sci 2004;80:109–14.

[6] Nohmi T, Toyoda-Hokaiwado N, Yamada M, Masumura K, Honma M, Fukushima S. International symposium on genotoxic and carcinogenic thresholds. Genes Environ 2008;30:101–7.

[7] Eastmond DA, Hartwig A, Anderson D, Anwar WA, Cimino MC, Dobrev I, et al. Mutagenicity testing for chemical risk assessment: update of the WHO/IPCS Harmonized Scheme. Mutagenesis 2009;24:341–9.

[8] Food and Drug Administration, HHS International Conference on Harmonisation; guidance on S2(R1) Genotoxicity Testing and Data Interpretation for Pharmaceuticals intended for Human Use; availability. Notice. Fed Regist 2012;77:33748–9.

[9] International Agency for Research on Cancer. Metronidazole IARC monographs on the evaluation of carcinogenic risk of chemicals to human use, suppl. 7, IARC, Lyon, 1987;250–2.

[10] Elizondo G, Gonsebatt ME, Salazar AM, Lares I, Santiago P, Herrera J, et al. Genotoxic effects of metronidazole. Mutat Res 1996;370:75–80.

[11] Menendez D, Rojas E, Herrera LA, Lopez MC, Sordo M, Elizondo G, et al. DNA breakage due to metronidazole treatment. Mutat Res 2001;478:153–8.

[12] Fahrig R, Engelke M. Reinvestigation of in vivo genotoxicity studies in man. I. No induction of DNA strand breaks in peripheral lymphocytes after metronidazole therapy. Mutat Res 1997;395:215–21.

[13] Bendesky A, Menendez D, Ostrosky-Wegman P. Is metronidazole carcinogenic? Mutat Res 2002;511:133–44.

[14] Kirkland D, Aardema M, Henderson L, Muller L. Evaluation of the ability of a battery of three in vitro genotoxicity tests to discriminate rodent carcinogens and non-carcinogens I. Sensitivity, specificity and relative predictivity. Mutat Res 2005;584:1–256.

[15] Morita T, Honma M, Morikawa K. Effect of reducing the top concentration used in the in vitro chromosomal aberration test in CHL cells on the evaluation of industrial chemical genotoxicity. Mutat Res 2012;741:32–56.

[16] Galloway S, Lorge E, Aardema MJ, Eastmond D, Fellows M, Heflich R, et al. Workshop summary: top concentration for in vitro mammalian cell genotoxicity assays; and report from working group on toxicity measures and top concentration for in vitro cytogenetics assays (chromosome aberrations and micronucleus). Mutat Res 2011;723:77–83.

[17] Morita T, Asano N, Awogi T, Sasaki YF, Sato S, Shimada H, et al. Evaluation of the rodent micronucleus assay in the screening of IARC carcinogens (groups 1, 2A and 2B) the summary report of the 6th collaborative study by CSGMT/JEMS MMS. Collaborative Study of the Micronucleus Group Test. Mammalian Mutagenicity Study Group. Mutat Res 1997;389:3–122.

[18] George E, Westmoreland C. Evaluation of the in vivo genotoxicity of the structural analogues 2,6-diaminotoluene and 2,4-diaminotoluene using the rat micronucleus test and rat liver UDS assay. Carcinogenesis 1991;12:2233–7.

[19] Narumi K, Ashizawa K, Takashima R, Takasawa H, Katayama S, Tsuzuki Y, et al. Development of a repeated-dose liver micronucleus assay using adult rats: an investigation of diethylnitrosamine and 2,4-diaminotoluene. Mutat Res 2012;747:234–9.

[20] Asanami S, Shimono K, Kaneda S. Transient hypothermia induces micronuclei in mice. Mutat Res 1998;413:7–14.

[21] Asanami S, Shimono K. Effects of chemically- and environmentally-induced hypothermia on micronucleus induction in rats. Mutat Res 2000;471:81–6.

[22] Dycaico MJ, Stuart GR, Tobal GM, de Boer JG, Glickman BW, Provost GS. Species-specific differences in hepatic mutant frequency and mutational spectrum among lambda/lacI transgenic rats and mice following exposure to aflatoxin B1. Carcinogenesis 1996;17:2347–56.

[23] Nohmi T, Yamada M, Masumura K. In vivo approaches to identify mutations and in vitro research to reveal underlying mechanisms of genotoxic thresholds. Genes Environ 2012;34:146–52.

[24] Nohmi T, Suzuki T, Masumura K. Recent advances in the protocols of transgenic mouse mutation assays. Mutat Res 2000;455:191–215.

[25] Thybaud V, Dean S, Nohmi T, de BJ, Douglas GR, Glickman BW, et al. In vivo transgenic mutation assays. Mutat Res 2003;540:141–51.

[26] Cao X, Mittelstaedt RA, Pearce MG, Allen BC, Soeteman-Hernandez LG, Johnson GE, et al. Quantitative dose-response analysis of ethyl methanesulfonate genotoxicity in adult *gpt* delta transgenic mice. Environ Mol Mutagen 2014;55:385–99.

[27] Hayashi H, Kondo H, Masumura K, Shindo Y, Nohmi T. Novel transgenic rat for in vivo genotoxicity assays using 6-thioguanine and Spi⁻ selection. Environ Mol Mutagen 2003;41:253–9.

[28] Toyoda-Hokaiwado N, Inoue T, Masumura K, Hayashi H, Kawamura Y, Kurata Y, et al. Integration of in vivo genotoxicity and short-term carcinogenicity assays using F344 *gpt* delta transgenic rats: in vivo mutagenicity of 2,4-diaminotoluene and 2,6-diaminotoluene structural isomers. Toxicol Sci 2010;114:71–8.

[29] Kamigaito T, Noguchi T, Narumi K, Takashima R, Hamada S, Sanada H, et al. Evaluation of the in vivo mutagenicity of nickel subsulfide in the lung of F344 *gpt* delta transgenic rats exposed by intratracheal

instillation: a collaborative study for the gpt delta transgenic rat mutation assay. Genes Environ 2012;34:34–44.

[30]   Sui H, Ohta R, Shiragiku T, Akahori A, Suzuki K, Nakajima M, et al. Evaluation of in vivo mutagenicity by 2,4-diaminotoluene and 2,6-diaminotoluene in liver of F344 *gpt* delta transgenic rat dosed for 28 days: a collaborative study of the *gpt* delta transgenic rat mutation assay. Genes Environ 2012;34:25–33.

[31]   Kawamura Y, Hayashi H, Tajima O, Yamada S, Takayanagi T, Hori H, et al. Evaluation of the genotoxicity of aristolochic acid in the kidney and liver of F344 *gpt* delta transgenic rat using a 28-day repeated-dose protocol: a collaborative study of the *gpt* delta transgenic rat mutation assay. Genes Environ 2012;34:18–24.

[32]   Hibi D, Suzuki Y, Ishii Y, Jin M, Watanabe M, Sugita-Konishi Y, et al. Site-specific in vivo mutagenicity in the kidney of *gpt* delta rats given a carcinogenic dose of ochratoxin A. Toxicol Sci 2011;122:406–14.

[33]   Kuroda K, Hibi D, Ishii Y, Takasu S, Kijima A, Matsushita K, et al. Ochratoxin A induces DNA double-strand breaks and large deletion mutations in the carcinogenic target site of *gpt* delta rats. Mutagenesis 2014;29:27–36.

[34]   Bendele AM, Neal SB, Oberly TJ, Thompson CZ, Bewsey BJ, Hill LE, et al. Evaluation of ochratoxin A for mutagenicity in a battery of bacterial and mammalian cell assays. Food Chem Toxicol 1985;23:911–8.

[35]   Sekiguchi M, Tsuzuki T. Oxidative nucleotide damage: consequences and prevention. Oncogene 2002;21:8895–904.

[36]   Tsuzuki T, Nakatsu Y, Nakabeppu Y. Significance of error-avoiding mechanisms for oxidative DNA damage in carcinogenesis. Cancer Sci 2007;98:465–70.

[37]   Tsuzuki T, Egashira A, Igarashi H, Iwakuma T, Nakatsuru Y, Tominaga Y, et al. Spontaneous tumorigenesis in mice defective in the *MTH1* gene encoding 8-oxo-dGTPase. Proc Natl Acad Sci USA 2001;98:11456–61.

[38]   Sakumi K, Tominaga Y, Furuichi M, Xu P, Tsuzuki T, Sekiguchi M, et al. *Ogg1* knockout-associated lung tumorigenesis and its suppression by Mth1 gene disruption. Cancer Res 2003;63:902–5.

[39]   Gondo Y, Shioyama Y, Nakao K, Katsuki M. A novel positive detection system of in vivo mutations in *rpsL* (strA) transgenic mice. Mutat Res 1996;360:1–14.

[40]   Sakamoto K, Tominaga Y, Yamauchi K, Nakatsu Y, Sakumi K, Yoshiyama K, et al. MUTYH-null mice are susceptible to spontaneous and oxidative stress induced intestinal tumorigenesis. Cancer Res 2007;67:6599–604.

[41]   Isoda T, Nakatsu Y, Yamauchi K, Piao J, Yao T, Honda H, et al. Abnormality in Wnt signaling is causatively associated with oxidative stress-induced intestinal tumorigenesis in MUTYH-null mice. Int J Biol Sci 2014;10:940–7.

[42]   Al-Tassan N, Chmiel NH, Maynard J, Fleming N, Livingston AL, Williams GT, et al. Inherited variants of MYH associated with somatic G:C-- > T:A mutations in colorectal tumors. Nat Genet 2002;30:227–32.

[43]   Piao J, Nakatsu Y, Ohno M, Taguchi K, Tsuzuki T. Mismatch repair deficient mice show susceptibility to oxidative stress-induced intestinal carcinogenesis. Int J Biol Sci 2013;10:73–9.

[44]   Oka S, Ohno M, Tsuchimoto D, Sakumi K, Furuichi M, Nakabeppu Y. Two distinct pathways of cell death triggered by oxidative damage to nuclear and mitochondrial DNAs. EMBO J 2008;27:421–32.

[45]   Nohmi T. Novel DNA polymerases and novel genotoxicity assays. Genes Environ 2007;29:75–88.

[46]   Friedberg EC, Wagner R, Radman M. Specialized DNA polymerases, cellular survival, and the genesis of mutations. Science 2002;296:1627–30.

[47]   Nohmi T. Environmental stress and lesion-bypass DNA polymerases. Annu Rev Microbiol 2006;60:231–53.

[48]   McCulloch SD, Kunkel TA. The fidelity of DNA synthesis by eukaryotic replicative and translesion synthesis polymerases. Cell Res 2008;18:148–61.

[49]   Goldsmith M, Sarov-Blat L, Livneh Z. Plasmid-encoded MucB protein is a DNA polymerase (pol RI) specialized for lesion bypass in the presence of MucA', RecA, and SSB. Proc Natl Acad Sci USA 2000;97:11227–31.

[50]   Matsui K, Yamada M, Imai M, Yamamoto K, Nohmi T. Specificity of replicative and SOS-inducible DNA polymerases in frameshift mutagenesis: mutability of *Salmonella typhimurium* strains overexpressing SOS-inducible DNA polymerases to 30 chemical mutagens. DNA Repair (Amst) 2006;5:465–78.

[51]   Burgers PM, Koonin EV, Bruford E, Blanco L, Burtis KC, Christman MF, et al. Eukaryotic DNA polymerases: proposal for a revised nomenclature. J Biol Chem 2001;276:43487–90.

[52] Lange SS, Takata K, Wood RD. DNA polymerases and cancer. Nat Rev Cancer 2011;11:96–110.
[53] Wittschieben J, Shivji MK, Lalani E, Jacobs MA, Marini F, Gearhart PJ, et al. Disruption of the developmentally regulated *Rev3l* gene causes embryonic lethality. Curr Biol 2000;10:1217–20.
[54] Masutani C, Kusumoto R, Yamada A, Dohmae N, Yokoi M, Yuasa M, et al. The *XPV* (Xeroderma pigmentosum variant) gene encodes human DNA polymerase eta. Nature 1999;399:700–4.
[55] Vaisman A, Masutani C, Hanaoka F, Chaney SG. Efficient translesion replication past oxaliplatin and cisplatin GpG adducts by human DNA polymerase eta. Biochemistry 2000;39:4575–80.
[56] Zlatanou A, Despras E, Braz-Petta T, Boubakour-Azzouz I, Pouvelle C, Stewart GS, et al. The hMsh2-hMsh6 complex acts in concert with monoubiquitinated PCNA and Pol eta in response to oxidative DNA damage in human cells. Mol Cell 2011;43:649–62.
[57] Takeiri A, Wada NA, Motoyama S, Matsuzaki K, Tateishi H, Matsumoto K, et al. In vivo evidence that DNA polymerase kappa is responsible for error-free bypass across DNA cross-links induced by mitomycin C. DNA Repair (Amst) 2014;24:113–21.
[58] Ohashi E, Murakumo Y, Kanjo N, Akagi J, Masutani C, Hanaoka F, et al. Interaction of hREV1 with three human Y-family DNA polymerases. Genes Cells 2004;9:523–31.
[59] Lynch A, Harvey J, Aylott M, Nicholas E, Burman M, Siddiqui A, et al. Investigations into the concept of a threshold for topoisomerase inhibitor-induced clastgenicity. Mutagenesis 2003;18:345–53.
[60] Abu-Daya A, Brown PM, Fox KR. DNA sequence preferences of several AT-selective minor groove binding ligands. Nucleic Acids Res 1995;23:3385–92.
[61] Pratt I, Barlow S, Kleiner J, Larsen JC. The influence of thresholds on the risk assessment of carcinogens in food. Mutat Res 2009;678:113–7.
[62] Ohta T. Mutagenic activity of a mixture of heterocyclic amines at doses below the biological threshold level of each. Genes Environ 2006;28:181–4.

DNA Repair and Its Influence on Points of Departure for Alkylating Agent Genotoxicity

Adam D. Thomas and George E. Johnson

DNA Damage Research Group, Institute of Life Science, College of Medicine, Swansea University, Swansea, United Kingdom

Chapter Outline

Introduction   67
The Paradigm Shift in Response to Low Doses of Alkylating Agents   69
Alkylating Agent Mechanism of Action   70
DNA Repair of Alkyl Adducts: Potential Influences on PoDs   71
Mechanistic Evidence Supporting a PoD for EMS   74
Mechanistic Evidence Supporting a PoD for ENU   75
Mechanistic Evidence Supporting a PoD for MMS   76
Mechanistic Evidence Supporting a PoD for MNU   76
Concluding Remarks   77
References   77

Introduction

For alkylating agents, the precautionary linear hypothesis has been applied by default, given their high mutagenic potential. However, this linear assumption does not fit experimentally derived data at low doses. A wealth of data exist, particularly for alkylating agents, to support nonlinear mutation responses. Such data have been used to derive metrics, that is, points of departure (PoDs) including breakpoint doses (BPDs), previously called threshold doses [1,2], benchmark doses (BMD) [3], and no-observed (genotoxic) effect levels (NO(G)ELs). These PoDs are actual data points or estimated points based on experimental observations and are defined by different statistical and analytical methods (Table 5.1). A PoD is an important parameter for assessing risk, where it is used to derive margins of exposure and safety limits for the human population.

Thresholds of Genotoxic Carcinogens.
DOI: http://dx.doi.org/10.1016/B978-0-12-801663-3.00005-4

Table 5.1 PoD metrics and their definitions.

PoD Metric	Full Name	Method of Calculation	Definition
NO(G)EL	No-observed genotoxic effect level	Dunnett's, Dunn's	Highest dose with no statistically significant response
BPD	Breakpoint dose	Hockey stick (bilinear) modeling	The dose at which the slope changes from zero (horizontal) to positive, with its standard error forming the confidence bounds (90% CI)
BMD_{10}	Benchmark dose 10	PROAST	An estimated dose that elicits a 10% increase in adverse endpoint over background levels

Source: Information obtained from Johnson GE, Soeteman-Hernandez LG, Gollapudi BB, Bodger OG, Dearfield KL, Heflich RH, et al. Derivation of pot of departure (PoD) estimates in genetic toxicology studies and their potential applications in risk assessment. Environ Mol Mutagen 2014;55:609–23.

A nonlinear dose-response shows that low doses of genotoxic carcinogens cause fewer adverse effects (which so far include chromosome breaks, mutations, and tumor incidence) than linear responses would predict. This suggests that low doses can be tolerated without causing an increase in effect, to the cell or organism, compared to the background rate. With such important ramifications in human health risk assessments, these nonlinear dose-responses need to be substantiated with strong mechanistic understanding that will examine the biological relevance of low doses. Are they truly safe or an artifact of an inability to detect increases in adverse endpoints?

To be able to answer this question, one must consider the mechanism of genotoxic action; understand the nature of DNA damage and how it can be converted into gene or chromosomal changes, as well as potential DNA repair, detoxification, or other protective mechanisms [4–6] that may prevent such genotoxic events at low doses, thus explaining the observed nonlinearity. This needs to be understood for each chemical, on a case-by-case basis, to contribute to a weight of evidence (WOE) in support of low-dose nonlinear responses for regulatory purposes.

There are broadly two subtypes of alkylating agents, monofunctional (simple) alkylating agents and bifunctional alkylating agents such as the nitrogen mustards. However, most attention has been given to monofunctional agents at low doses (the focus here) due to their relevance in regulatory toxicology, particularly following the incident where a monofunctional alkylator (ethyl methanesulfonate (EMS)) contaminated a batch of a well-used HIV drug [7,8]. We will focus on four alkylating agents that have been heavily investigated for their genotoxicity at low doses; these are EMS, *N*-ethyl-*N*-nitrosourea (ENU), methyl methanesulfonate (MMS), and *N*-methyl-*N*-nitrosourea (MNU). These four agents are colloquially referred to as the G4 compounds as they represent four different mechanisms of action and mutagenic potential [1,5,9].

The mechanism of genotoxicity for these alkylating agents is through a S_N1 or S_N2 mechanism of nucleophilic substitution onto DNA, forming potentially mutagenic and carcinogenic DNA adducts. Many sites exist for alkylation within DNA, including the oxygen (O), phosphate (P), and nitrogen (N) atoms of bases and within the phosphotriester backbone of DNA. Therefore, a spectrum of alky adducts is produced following DNA reaction. The composition is determined by the chemistry of alkylating agent and is, therefore, agent-specific. The three most abundant adducts within an alkylating agent's adduct spectrum are N7-alkylguanine (N7alkG), O^6-alkylguanine (O^6alkG), and N3-alkyladenine (N3alkA), although many more exist. Each adduct possesses a different insult to genome integrity, whereas N3AlkA is a clastogen as a *direct* block to replication and transcription [10,11], N7MeG and O^6alkG are *converted* into clastogenic and mutagenic events, respectively [12], but are also cytotoxic particularly at higher levels [13]. The chemistry of DNA reaction and the resulting mutagenicity, clastogenicity, and toxicity of alkyl damage is very well defined, stemming from their use as chemotherapeutic agents against a number of cancers, where their toxic potential is exploited in fast replicating tumor cells [14]. As a result, there has been a thorough investigation into the repair of alkyl adducts in order to understand tumor resistance [15] and improve the efficacy of cancer treatment [16]. However, the role of DNA repair against alkylating agent–induced damage has only recently been investigated as a protective mechanism responsible for nonlinear dose-responses at the low-dose region.

In this chapter, we will discuss the WOE in support of PoDs for the G4 monofunctional alkylating agents (henceforth referred to as alkylating agents) and examine recent reports on the potential influence of DNA repair for such PoDs in alkylating agent genotoxicity.

The Paradigm Shift in Response to Low Doses of Alkylating Agents

The validity of the linear assumption at low doses was first questioned for alkylating agents in the 1980s. In an informative paper by Jenssen and Ramel [17], hypoxanthine phosphoribosyltransferase (HPRT) mutant frequencies with low doses of the G4 compounds (EMS, ENU, MMS, and MNU) were experimentally determined in V79 cells using the HPRT mutation assay. These actual values were compared to theoretical frequencies calculated from a linear extrapolation from higher doses. The authors found that the linear hypothesis *overestimated* mutant frequencies for low doses of MMS and MNU but not for EMS or ENU. Even at these early times, DNA repair was hypothesized to be involved [18] but it is only recently being substantiated by experimental proof, which will be discussed later. Additional, putative nonlinear dose-responses were published [19] for mutagenic and clastogenic events in V79 cells following treatment with MNU and N-methyl-N'-nitro-N-nitrosoguanidine (MNNG). However, it wasn't until 2007 that the argument for nonlinearity gained momentum, particularly for alkylating agents. Since then, a wealth of data has emerged reporting PoDs for all the G4 compounds in a variety of genetic toxicity systems (discussed in detail case-by-case).

With increasing evidence of PoDs, attention now turns to the mechanism which may be in operation to prevent low-dose mutagenesis and possibly cancer.

Alkylating Agent Mechanism of Action

A catalyst for the study of mechanisms came from Doak and colleagues [20] that directly compared the G4 alkylating agents in two in vitro test systems, a strategy that compared different genotoxic potentials [21], mechanisms of action, and DNA repair processes. Each of the G4 chemicals represents a different chemistry of DNA reaction and mechanism of action (Table 5.2) leading to different spectrums of DNA alkylation [21] and, consequently, different mutagenic potencies and spectra [23]. The methylating agents (MNU and MMS) are 20-fold more reactive than the ethylating agents (ENU and EMS) [5]. However, the ethyl adducts, induced by ENU and EMS, are repaired less efficiently than the methylating adducts of MNU and MMS [5,22,24]. At equitoxic doses (LD_{37}), MNU is the most mutagenic of the four, producing 400 6-thioguanine (6-TG)-resistant mutants per 10^5 cells, MMS being the least mutagenic (15 mutants/10^5 cells), whereas there were 300 and 140 mutants/10^5 cells for ENU and EMS, respectively [1,25].

Agents, such as the alkyl nitrosoureas, with a lower Swain–Scott (s) constant target sites with higher nucleophilic potential, such as oxygen, and therefore have a higher O^6alkG to $N7$alkG ratio. As a result they tend to be mutagenic, whereas agents (the alkyl alkanesulfonates) with higher s constants, have a lower O^6alkG:$N7$alkG ratio are clastogenic. Of course, other adducts cannot be ignored, as they are also hazardous to genome integrity. For example, O^4-alkylthymine (O^4AlkT) has miscoding potential and, therefore, may contribute to alkylating agent–induced base substitutions [26]. ENU, in particular, induces a more diverse adduct spectra with higher levels of less well-defined adducts [22]. However, O^6alkG and $N7$AlkG are the most abundant in the adduct spectra and their mechanism of action is perhaps the best defined.

Table 5.2 The chemistry of the G4 alkylating agents.

Alkylating Agent	Type	Alkyl Group	Swain–Scott Constant (s)	Nucleophilic Substitution	Adduct Spectra
MNU	Alkyl nitrosourea	Methyl	Low (0.42)	S_N1	$N7$MeG: 65–70 O^6MeG: 6–8 $N3$MeA: 8–9
ENU	Alkyl nitrosourea	Ethyl	Low (0.26)	S_N1	$N7$EthG: 11–12 O^6EthG: 8–10 $N3$EthA: 3–6
MMS	Alkanesulfonate	Methyl	High (>0.83)	S_N2	$N7$MeG: 81–83 O^6MeG: 0.3 $N3$MeA: 0.6
EMS	Alkanesulfonate	Ethyl	High (0.67)	S_N2	$N7$EthG: 58–65 O^6EthG: 2 $N3$EthA: 4–5

Source: Adduct values are proportions (%) taken from Jenkins GJS, Doak SH, Johnson GE, Quick E, Water EM, Parry JM. Do dose response thresholds exist for genotoxic alkylating agents? Mutagenesis 2005;20(6):389–98; Beranek T. Distribution of methyl and ethyl adducts following alkylation with monofunctional alkylating agents. Mutat Res 1990;231:11–30
Three most abundant and apparently critical adducts are shown.

Alkylation of the exocyclic oxygen of guanine (O^6G) disrupts the third hydrogen bond between guanine (G) and cytosine (C) so that there are only two hydrogen bonds between O^6alkG and C. The replicating polymerase mistakes this adducted purine for an adenine (A) and, during the first posttreatment S-phase, an O^6AlkG:thymine (T) mispair forms, which is subsequently replicated into an A:T transition mutation [27] during the second replication cycle. These mutations are tumor-initiating lesions, implicated in the oncogenic transformation of *Ras* protooncogenes by MNU [28,29]. Whether this is prevented at low doses remains to be seen. It should be noted that O^6MeG is recombinogenic through its erroneous processing by mismatch repair (MMR) into double-strand breaks (DSBs), a primary lesion in the formation of structural chromosomal aberrations [30].

On the other hand, *N*7alkG adducts are clastogenic but also weakly mutagenic. *N*7MeG is labile to spontaneous and enzymatic hydrolysis, which leaves an apurinic (AP) site. This lesion attracts the action of apurinic endonuclease (APE) as part of the multienzyme, base excision repair (BER) pathway, which is discussed in the section entitled *DNA Repair of Alkyl Adducts: Potential Influences on PoDs*. The action of APE removes the AP site and leaves a single-strand gap, one nucleotide in length, in the DNA backbone. This poses a problem to the replicating polymerase, either directly or following the recruitment of downstream BER proteins [31], which forms a steric block to the polymerase [32], leading to fork stall and possible collapse into DSBs. A mechanism is also proposed whereby the ensuing AP sites are mutagenic during replication, where the replicating polymerase is switched for a translesion synthesis (TLS) polymerase that will circumvent polymerase stall but will preferentially insert an A opposite an AP site thereby, *N*7AlkG:C may be converted to T:A transition mutations [33,34]. Despite this, the biological relevance of *N*7MeG is questionable since a high background naturally exists [35], a key consideration in low-dose toxicity. The discrimination of endogenous and exogenous adducts is critically important in determining low-dose mechanisms and, although endogenous alkyl adducts remain relatively constant, exogenous alkyl adducts increase with a linear dose-response, even at submutagenic doses [36,37]. This heavily focuses the attention to the repair of adducts before they are fixed into mutations.

DNA Repair of Alkyl Adducts: Potential Influences on PoDs

A prominent barrier to adduct-induced genetic change is DNA repair that counteracts adduct mutagenicity and carcinogenicity by removing the damage before replication. Methylguanine-DNA methyltransferase (MGMT) is an error-free mechanism and is a primary defensive player against O^6 alkylating agent–induced mutagenesis and toxicity. MGMT removes a number of alkyl adducts (namely methyl, ethyl, but also larger alkyl groups such as 2-hydroxyethyl upon exposure to ethylene oxide (a metabolite of cigarette smoke)) and *n*-butyl groups (from *n*-butyl methanesulfonate (BMS) exposure) from O^6G [38]. Additionally, Sassanfar and colleagues [39] provide evidence that methyl groups on oxygen of thymine (O^4T) are substrates for removal by mammalian MGMT. MGMT-mediated O^6alkG repair has been implicated in the protection against MNU, EMS [40], and ENU [41].

In a direct reversal repair mechanism, MGMT restores the original DNA sequence by transferring the alkyl adduct to an internal cysteine residue (cys145) within the active site [42,43]. After repair, the (now-methylated) protein is tagged with ubiquitin [44,45] and targeted for proteolytic degradation by the 26S proteasome [42], through the ubiquitin-proteasome system leading to MGMT degradation [46]. Therefore, MGMT is more commonly referred to as a suicide enzyme, since its methyltransferase action is only available for one reaction. The repair is therefore stoichiometric. Using MGMT knockdown/knockout and overexpressing models [47], the role of MGMT in cancer etiology has received much attention for its ability to prevent alkylating agent–induced oncogenic mutations in normal cells [48] but also as a source of chemotherapy resistance in cancer [49]. Murine models that overexpress tissue-specific MGMT have significantly enhanced protection against alkylating agent–induced tumorigenesis within that tissue, including MNU-induced lymphogenesis [50], skin papillomas [51–53] and, interestingly, spontaneous hepatomas [54]. Conversely, loss of MGMT increases cancer susceptibility [55,56] and may even be an initiating event in colon carcinogenesis [57].

Since the majority of evidence states that MGMT is not inducible in human cells following alkylation stress [58], it is reasonable to state that the repair that MGMT offers is limited and it seems likely that it depends upon the basal expression level, and in turn, the basal activity of MGMT. Importantly, this means that MGMT is easily saturated at higher demands for repair and may explain the PoD for mutation induction by O^6 alkylating agents. Therefore, the PoD for mutations caused by MGMT repairable adducts depends upon the basal level of MGMT protein and activity. Therefore, cells with higher MGMT expression levels, such as the liver, will have increased MGMT repair capacity, increased tolerance and therefore, a higher PoD ([59]). For other *traditional* repair enzymes, the PoD may be dependent upon the V_{max} kinetics, although this needs substantiation.

MMR is also important in O^6alkG repair and may prevent mutagenesis by correcting the O^6alkG:thymine mispair, in the first postreplicative treatment cell cycle, but may also contribute to chromosomal instability [60,61]. On the other hand, MMR proteins may directly signal the activation of apoptosis [62–64]. Therefore, MMR may be protective by repairing mismatches and preventing mutagenesis or signaling to cell death, whether this occurs at low doses remains to be seen.

The other adducts within an agent's spectrum are substrates for repair by other mechanisms. Of the other two most abundant adducts, the N-alkylpurines ($N7$alkG and $N3$alkA), BER plays an important protective role in preventing their erroneous conversion into DSBs [65] and mutations [66]. BER is a multienzyme pathway, the specifics are beyond the scope of this chapter but the reader is directed to a review by Robertson and coworkers [67]. $N7$alkG and $N3$alkA are subject to enzymatic hydrolysis by a monofunctional glycosylase

N-methylpurine-DNA glycosylase (MPG, alias AAG), leaving an AP site, a lesion for downstream BER processing. As mentioned previously, this lesion is mutagenic, through TLS bypass replication, and clastogenic. This has been substantiated in an MPG overexpressing system, which showed increased genomic instability due to increased MPG-mediated hydrolysis of *N*7alkG and formation of AP sites [68]. Conversely, MPG null cells are alkylating resistant [69]. This situation is different to MGMT since BER involves the concerted effort of many proteins, and so, the overexpression of one enzyme may imbalance the system and contribute to genome instability, particularly within repair processes with mutagenic intermediates. Therefore, inferring the protective role of BER at low doses by either increasing or decreasing individual enzyme levels may be difficult.

MGMT and BER are perhaps the most documented repair pathways for alkyl damage, particularly at low doses (discussed later). Although other repair pathways exist and may play a role in alkyl adduct repair [60], namely recombinational repair (error-free homologous recombination (HR) and error-prone nonhomologous end-joining of DSBs, reviewed in Refs. [70,71], respectively), nucleotide excision repair (NER) and also the wider DNA damage response (DDR) signaling that limits the propensity for aberration caused by erroneous processing alkyl adducts previously discussed. Here, ataxia telangiectasia mutated (ATM) and ATM and Rad 3-related (ATR) kinases sense strand breaks or fork stalling events and initiate the DDR, which transduces the damage signal to effector proteins, of which p53 plays a central role [72], to orchestrate cell cycle arrest and DNA repair by HR in S and G2 phase [73] but also to induce apoptotic cell death [74], the desired outcome of alkylating chemotherapy [75].

Both processes of recombination repair have been theoretically implicated in nonlinear dose-responses, particularly for chromosomal damage due to their involvement in DSB resolution [76] resulting from erroneous processing of alkyl adducts. This has been observed for MMS-induced chromosomal aberrations in cell lines differing in recombination repair status [77]. However, experimental evidence is lacking. Since DSBs are a critically toxic lesion, perhaps their involvement would be within the toxic range [78]. In that case, HR would permit cell survival and may therefore propagate other mutagenic damage. NER has been implicated in the repair of bulky adducts and interstrand cross-links [79] such as those induced by bifunctional alkylating agents [80] but not for smaller alkyl groups like those of ENU [41]. However, this needs to be reassessed since the cells are not isogenic clones and the methods used to clarify their repair status may currently have greater sensitivity.

In the context of low-dose protection, the role of excision repair pathways (BER, MMR, and also NER) may be confused, where repair intermediates may exacerbate fork stalling, recombination events and contribute to mutagenesis. Nevertheless, evidence exists for the role of DNA repair in dose-responses for alkylating agent–induced chromosome and gene alterations and will be discussed in turn for each G4 agent.

Mechanistic Evidence Supporting a PoD for EMS

Of the four G4 compounds, EMS became the central focus of in vivo studies into the low-dose region because it contaminated an HIV therapeutic agent, Viracept. Extensive analysis of chromosome damage (in vivo bone marrow micronucleus test) and gene mutation in bone marrow, liver, and gut (*lacZ* transgenic Mutamouse mutation assay) by EMS was performed [81,82]. The shape of the dose-response for EMS was distinctly nonlinear, in all systems and cell types, with remarkably similar PoD and threshold metrics. For example, the NOEL for mutant frequency in liver was 50.0 mg EMS/kg with a threshold dose of 51.3 mg EMS/kg. To substantiate this, a BPD of 21.9 mg/kg has been identified in the *Pig-a* mutation assay in blood cells following a 28-day repeat treatment schedule in rats [83]. Further PoDs and BPDs have been found in vivo, in the liver, kidney, spleen, bone marrow, and small intestine using the *gpt* and *Pig-a* gene mutation assays and micronucleus bone marrow test [59]. Incidentally, this study was extended through the sequence analysis of *gpt* spleen cell mutants following EMS treatment and the proportion of GC to AT transitions was plotted as a function of dose. Identifying the base substitutions that increase nonlinearly over dose would prove to be an effective method of identifying the critical mutations and the adducts responsible. This evidence of nonlinear mutation induction by EMS substantiates the in vitro studies using human lymphoblastoid cells, more specifically in the HPRT mutation assay and micronucleus assay [20, 84]. This evidence highlighted the nonlinear induction of chromosome breaks and mutations by EMS. Furthermore, the role of MPG-initiated BER in the nonlinear dose-response for micronuclei through the repair of *N*7-ethylguanine (*N*7EtG) was substantiated [85]. By RNA interference, the authors knocked down the level of MPG in AHH-1 cells. The PoD was reduced from 1.25 to 1 mg/mL EMS, but, crucially, the spontaneous level of micronuclei does not change. This supports the hypothesis of MPG as a tolerance mechanism in nonlinear dose-responses since its removal lowers the cellular tolerance limits to EMS. Such a modest difference may be explained by the confused role of MPG as a repair enzyme that stimulates formation of a genotoxic intermediate. One rationale could be the knockdown of MPG would lower the abundance of enzymatically induced AP sites and would therefore lower the clastogenic potential of *N*7MeG. Of course, since MPG also acts on *N*3alkA, the repair of this adduct cannot be ignored in the nonlinear dose-response to EMS-induced clastogenicity. Pertinently, the knockdown did not affect the tolerance to O^6EtG mutagenesis and expectedly demonstrates that MPG is redundant for EMS-induced point mutations but may play a role in EMS-induced clastogenicity. Interestingly, Zair and others [85] also showed the upregulation of MPG mRNA and other proteins of the BER cascade following EMS treatment. Such an event has been observed in the adaptive response to alkylation damage but this was not investigated. Whether genotoxicant-induced gene induction is important for PoDs remains to be seen and would open up hypotheses of the involvement of response proteins and transcription factors and their potential involvement in mutation PoDs.

On the other hand, MGMT may be implicated in protecting against EMS-induced mutations. *Salmonella typhimurium* Ames tester strains differing in their *Ogt* and *Ada* proficiencies, two alkyltransferase homologs equivalent to human MGMT, showed drastically different levels of tolerance, and therefore, shapes of dose–response curves [86,87].

Mechanistic Evidence Supporting a PoD for ENU

ENU is considered to be more mutagenic than EMS because it induces a higher proportion of mutagenic O^6 adducts [5]. While the evidence for nonlinear mutagenesis by EMS was accumulating, the same test systems initially showed linear dose-responses for ENU for both mutations and micronuclei [20,81,82]. However, more advanced statistical analysis showed a BPD of 0.32 µg/mL ENU in AHH-1 cells in the HPRT assay [88]. This is supported by evidence of a nonlinear dose-response of ENU with a BPD of approximately 0.9 mg/kg in the murine *pig-a* assay [83]. Similarly, BPDs were found in two independent in vitro TK6 micronucleus experiments, at approximately 3 and 6 mg/kg [84]. Recently, a study [89] examined low-dose mutagenicity of ENU at the *lacZ* locus in spermatogonial stem cells in Mutamouse to provide a comment on the possibility of transgenerational mutagenicity of acute and chronic low-dose treatments. BPDs were found for both treatment regimens at 0.5 and 51.7 mg/kg, respectively. The difference in BPDs is not known but may involve DNA repair akin to the adaptive response [90].

Although MPG may play a role in protecting against EMS-induced chromosome breaks but not mutations, in the test system used [85], the opposite appears true for ENU. Knockdown of MPG did not alter the PoD for ENU-induced chromosome breaks in the micronucleus assay. However, the PoD for HPRT mutants increased from 0.3 to 1.0 µg/mL in MPG knockdown AHH-1 cells. This suggests that the tolerance toward ENU actually improves upon inhibition of MPG-mediated accumulation of AP sites. However, it is likely that this is an artifact and a direct comparison between the repair proficiencies cannot be made due to the differences in background mutant frequencies. The situation is particularly confused with ENU because it induces comparatively high levels of lesser understood adducts such as ethyl adducts on the exocyclic oxygens of cytosine (O^2C) and thymine (O^2T and O^4T). Further study of these adducts, their propensity to insult the genome, and opposing repair mechanisms need to be conducted in order to fully assess the low-dose mutagenicity of ENU. However, given the high proportion of O^6G adducts within the mutation spectra it is likely that MGMT may be involved [41]. This has been substantiated in Ames bacterial systems differing in their repair efficiencies that show a complete abrogation of a BPD and a significantly reduced PoD (from 51 to 0.6 µg/plate) in *Ogt/Ada*-deficient bacteria [87]. Incidentally, cells differing in NER capabilities show no difference in ENU susceptibility suggesting that NER is not involved in protecting against ENU-induced damage [41].

Mechanistic Evidence Supporting a PoD for MMS

MMS is possibly the least studied alkylating agent at low doses. MMS is very similar to its ethylating equivalent, although MMS has a slightly higher s value and therefore alkylates O^6G to a comparatively lower amount [5]. However, inexplicably, this difference is not reflected in the PoDs between the G4 compounds in AHH-1 cells for HPRT mutation and micronuclei [20]. Nevertheless, MMS is perhaps the least mutagenic of the alkylating agents. It is therefore not surprising that studies have reported PoDs for MMS-induced mutations in AHH-1 cells through the HPRT assay [20] and at the thymidine kinase (TK) locus in L5178Y mouse lymphoma cells [91]. PoDs are several-fold lower than those for MNU, a much more potent point mutagen. Nonlinear curves are also reported for MMS-induced chromosome breaks in AHH-1 cells at $0.8\,\mu g/mL$ [20] and TK6 cells at 0.8 and $0.7\,\mu g/mL$ [85], slightly lower than those for the other G4 compounds due to the very high proportions of N-alkylpurines adducts (N3MeA and N7MeG) [92] in the adduct spectra of MMS. It is logical to implicate MPG in the tolerance to low-dose MMS-induced clastogenicity although this needs substantiation. Evidence exists to implicate alkyltransferase in tolerance against MMS-induced mutations at low doses, which depicts a complete loss of BPD and a severely reduced PoD in Ogt- and Adt-deficient bacteria [88].

Mechanistic Evidence Supporting a PoD for MNU

Initial evidence suggests that MNU, like ENU, is linear at the low doses tested for mutation and chromosome breaks [20,88]. For a while, this was accepted given their much higher mutagenic potencies than the alkyl alkanesulfonates [21]. However, within the same test system (the HPRT assay in AHH-1 cells), lower doses of MNU have a PoD for mutation at $0.0075\,\mu g/mL$ [93]. This is in agreement with data generated from a variety of test systems that shows nonlinear mutation induction curves at the Pig-a locus in vivo in rat reticulocytes [94], a PoD in mouse lymphoma cells at 71 ng/mL [93] and a BPD at $125\,\mu g/plate$ in the bacteria-based Ames assay [87]. In addition, PoDs have been found for MNU-induced chromosome breaks in the micronucleus assay in TK6 cells at 0.4 and $0.3\,\mu g/mL$ [84]. The nonlinear induction of MNU-induced mutations has been attributed to the protective role of MGMT [89,93]. Detailed sequencing analysis of HPRT mutants following treatment has shown the dramatic increase in GC to AT transitions only at a dose above the PoD [93]. At a dose below the PoD, the GC to AT transitions are slightly lower compared to the solvent (DMSO) control. This implicates MGMT in preventing MNU-induced GC to AT transitions at low doses, which has been substantiated by MGMT inactivation through O^6-benzylguanine (O^6BG), a competitive MGMT inhibitor and alkyltransferase-deficient Ames tester strains [87]. In AHH-1 cells pretreated with O^6BG, the PoD is 10-fold lower [93]. Interestingly, the mutation spectra are different between the low dose (below PoD) and the solvent control. This suggests that MNU is having an effect at doses below the PoD and may not be genotoxically inert. One explanation could be that at these low doses, O^6alkG adducts are repaired by MGMT but other mutagenic adducts, which are less abundant, become the predominant mutagenic lesions and cause a change in mutation spectra.

Concluding Remarks

While our exposure to alkylating agents needs to be controlled to limit human cancer risk, it is becoming clear that acceptable exposure levels can be defined for human populations [95,96]. Understanding the mechanisms of low-dose tolerance is particularly important for regulatory purposes. As a result, a huge effort is underway to characterize the mutagenic potential and opposing cellular resistance mechanisms to low doses of alkylating agents.

Many assays have reported nonlinear metrics for alkylating agent–induced mutations and chromosome breaks. The differences in the numerical value of the metrics can be attributed to the differences in assay sensitivities, statistical power, and chemical treatment in vitro and in vivo. Nevertheless, such evidence contributes to a WOE in support of nonlinear mutation induction for the G4 alkylating agents discussed here.

Evidence is mounting that substantiates the role of DNA repair in preventing mutagenicity at low doses of carcinogenic alkylating agents, thereby causing a nonlinear dose-response. If we take MGMT as an example, its stoichiometric mode of action means that the PoD for mutation induction by O^6 alkylating agents may be dependent upon the expression level, which dictates the maximum level of repair. For traditional enzymes, the PoD may be dependent on the V_{max}. However, the question remains whether this nonlinearity extends to cancer endpoints and whether DNA repair is the main protective factor responsible.

For investigations of DNA repair in low-dose protection, the relevant cytoprotective mechanism will depend upon the mechanism of action of the alkylating agent, that is, the reaction with DNA and the resulting adduct spectra. For mutations, O^6alkG and MGMT become important. For chromosome aberrations the $N7$alkG and $N3$alkA adducts along with MPG and BER repair pathways will be important. The use of repair knockdown isogenic clones or pharmacological inhibitors is a very effective method to assess the role of DNA repair in nonlinear dose-responses to alkylating agents and other direct genotoxic carcinogens.

References

[1] Johnson GE, Soeteman-Hernandez LG, Gollapudi BB, Bodger OG, Dearfield KL, Heflich RH, et al. Derivation of pot of departure (PoD) estimates in genetic toxicology studies and their potential applications in risk assessment. Environ Mol Mutagen 2014;55:609–23.
[2] Lutz WK, Lutz RW. Statistical model to estimate a threshold dose and its confidence limits for the analysis of sublinear dose-response relationships, exemplified for mutagenicity data. Mutat Res 2009;678:118–22.

[3] Gollapudi BB, Johnson GE, Hernandez LG, Pottenger LH, Dearfield KL, Jeffrey AM, et al. Quantitative approaches for assessing dose-response relationships in genetic toxicology studies. Environ Mol Mutagen 2013;54:8–18.

[4] Speit G, Autrup H, Crebelli R, Henderson L, Kirsch-Volders M, Madle S, et al. Thresholds in genetic toxicology-concluding remarks. Mutat Res 2000;464:149–53.

[5] Jenkins GJS, Doak SH, Johnson GE, Quick E, Water EM, Parry JM. Do dose response thresholds exist for genotoxic alkylating agents? Mutagenesis 2005;20(6):389–98.

[6] Thomas AD, Johnson GE, Kaina B. Theoretical considerations for thresholds in chemical carcinogenesis. Mutat Res Rev 2015;765:56–67.

[7] Gerber C, Toelle H-G. What happened: the chemistry side of the incident with EMS contamination in Viracept tablets. Toxicol Lett 2009;190:248–53.

[8] Muller L, Singer T. EMS in Viracept: the course of events in 2007 and 2008 from the non-clinical safety point of view. Toxicol Lett 2009;190:243–7.

[9] Guerard M, Baum M, Bitsch A, Eisenbrand G, Elhajouji A, Epe B, et al. Assessment of mechanisms driving non-linear dose-response relationships in genotoxicity testing. Mutat Res Rev Mutat Res 2015;763:181–201.

[10] Larson K, Sahm J, Shenkar R, Strauss B. Methylation-induced blocks to in vitro DNA replication. Mutat Res 1985;150:77–84.

[11] Fronza G, Gold B. The biological effects of N3-methyladenine. J Cell Biochem 2004;91:250–7.

[12] Kaina B, Fritz G, Coquerelle T. Contribution of O^6-alkylguanine and N-alkylpurines to the formation of sister chromatid exchanges, chromosomal aberrations and gene mutations: new insights gained from studies of genetically engineered mammalian cell lines. Envrion Mol Mutagen 2002;22:283–92.

[13] Bignami M, O'Driscoll M, Aquilina G, Karran P. Unmasking a killer: O^6-methylguanine and the cytotoxicity of methylating agents. Mutat Res 2000;462:71–82.

[14] Fu D, Calvo JA, Samson LD. Balancing repair and tolerance of DNA damage caused by alkylating agents. Nat Rev Cancer 2012;12(2):104–20.

[15] Zhang J, Stevens MFG, Bradshaw TD. Temozolomide: mechanisms of action, repair and resistance. Curr Mol Pharmacol 2012;5:102–14.

[16] Helleday T, Petermann E, Lundin C, Hodgson B, Sharma RA. DNA repair pathways as targets for cancer therapy. Nat Rev Cancer 2008;8(3):193–204.

[17] Jenssen D, Ramel C. Relationship between chemical damage of DNA and mutations in mammalian cells I. Dose-response curves for the induction of 6-thioguanine-resistant mutants by low doses of monofunctional alkylating agents, X-rays and UV radiation in V79 Chinese hamster cells. Mutat Res 1980;73:339–47.

[18] Jenssen D. Elimination of MNU-induced mutational lesions in V79 Chinese hamster cells. Mutat Res 1982;106:291–6.

[19] Kaina B. The interrelationship between SCE induction, cell survival, mutagenesis, aberration formation and DNA synthesis inhibition in V79 cells treated with N-methyl-N-nitrosourea or N-methyl-N'-nitro-N-nitrosoguanidine. Mutat Res 1985;142:49–54.

[20] Doak SH, Jenkins GJS, Johnson GE, Quick E, Parry EM, Parry JM. Mechanistic influences for mutation induction curves after exposure to DNA-reactive carcinogens. Cancer Res 2007;67:3904–11.

[21] Donovan P, Smith G. Mutagenicity of N-ethyl-N-nitrosourea, N-methyl-N-nitrosourea, methyl methanesulfonate and ethyl methylsulfonate in the developing Syrian hamster fetus. Mutat Res 2010;699:55–7.

[22] Beranek T. Distribution of methyl and ethyl adducts following alkylation with monofunctional alkylating agents. Mutat Res 1990;231:11–30.

[23] Warwick G. The mechanism of action of alkylating agents. Cancer Res 1963;23:1315–33.

[24] Singer B. In vivo formation and persistence of modified nucleoside analogues resulting from alkylating agents. Environ Health Perspect 1985;62:41–8.

[25] Suter W, Brennand J, McMillan S, Fox M. Relative mutagenicity of antineoplastic drugs and other alkylating agents in V79 Chinese hamster cells, independence of cytotoxic and mutagenic responses. Mutat Res 1980;73:171–81.

[26] Swann PF. Why do O^6-alkylguanine and O^4-alkylthymine miscode? The relationship between the structure of DNA containing O^6-alkylguanine and O^4-alkylthymine and the mutagenic properties of these bases. Mutat Res 1990;233(1–2):81–94.

[27] Loveless A. Possible relevance of O^6-alkylation of deoxyguanosine to the mutagenicity and carcinogenicity of nitrosamines. Nature 1969;223:206–7.

[28] Bos J.L. Ras oncogenes in human cancer: a review. Cancer Res 1989;49:4682-4689.

[29] Jacoby RF, Alexander RJ, Raicht RF, Brasitus TA. K-ras oncogene mutations in rat colon tumors induced by *N-methyl-N*-nitrosourea. Carcinogenesis 1992;13(1):45–9.

[30] Pfeiffer P, Goedecke W, Obe G. Mechanisms of DNA double-strand break repair and their potential to induce chromosomal aberrations. Mutagenesis 2000;15(4):289–302.

[31] Liu Y, Prased R, Beard WA, Kedar PS, Hou EW, Shock DD, et al. Coordination of steps in single-nucleotide base excision repair mediated by apurinic/apyrmidinic endonuclease 1 and DNA polymerase β. J. Biol Chem 2007;282(18):13532–41.

[32] Ensminger M, Iloff L, Ebel C, Nikolova T, Kaina B, Loebrich M. DNA breaks and chromosomal aberrations arise when replication meets base excision repair. J Cell Biol 2014;206(1):29–43.

[33] Ide H, Murayama H, Sakamoto S, Makino K, Honda K, Nakamuta H, et al. On the mechanism of preferential incorporation of dAMP at abasic sites in translesional DNA synthesis. Role of proofreading activity of DNA polymerase and thermodynamic characterization of model template-primers containing an abasic site. Nucleic Acids Res 1995;23:123–9.

[34] Boiteux S, Guillet M. Abasic sites in DNA: repair and biological consequences in *Saccharomyces cerevisiae*. DNA Repair (Amst) 2004;3:1–12.

[35] Boysen G, Pachkowski BF, Nakamura J, Swenberg JA. The formation and biological significance of *N*7-guanine adducts. Mutat Res 2009;678(2):76–96.

[36] Sharma V, Collins LB, Clement JM, Zhang Z, Nakamura J, Swenberg JA. Molecular dosimetry of endogenous and exogenous O^6-methyl-dG and *N*7-methyl-G adducts following low dose [D₃]-Methylnitrosourea exposures in cultured human cells. Chem Res Toxicol 2014;27(4):480–2.

[37] Swenberg JA, Fryar-Tita E, Joeng YC, Boysen G, Starr T, Walker VE, et al. Biomarkers in toxicology and risk assessment: informing critical dose-response relationships. Chem Res Toxicol 2008;21(1):253–65.

[38] Pegg AE, Dolan ME, Scicchitano D, Morimoto K. Studies of the repair of O^6-alkylguanine and O^4-alkylthymine in DNA by alkyltransferase from mammalian cells and bacteria. Environ Health Perspect 1985;62:109–14.

[39] Sassanfar M, Dosanjh MK, Essigmann JM, Samson L. Relative efficiencies of the bacterial, yeast and human DNA methyltransferase for the repair of O^6-methylguanine and O^4-methylthymine. J Biol Chem 1991;266(5):1767–71.

[40] Kaina B, Fritz G, Mitra S, Coquerele T. Transfection and expression of human O^6-methylguanine-DNA methyltransferase (MGMT) cDNA in Chinese hamster cells: the role of MGMT in protection against the genotoxic effects of alkylating agents. Carcinogenesis 1991;12(10):1857–67.

[41] Bronstein SM, Cochrane JE, Craft TR, Swenberg JA, Skopek TR. Toxicity, mutagenicity and mutational spectra of *N*-ethyl-*N*-nitrosourea in human cell lines with different DNA repair phenotypes. Cancer Res 1991;51:5188–97.

[42] Xu-Welliver M, Pegg AE. Degradation of the alkylated form of the DNA repair protein, O(6)-alkylguanine-DNA alkyltransferase. Carcinogenesis 2002;23:823–30.

[43] Mushina Y, Duguid EM, He C. Direct reversal of DNA alkylation damage. Chem Rev 2006;106(2):215–32.

[44] Srivenugopal KS, Yuan XH, Friedman HS, Ali-Osman F. Ubiquitination-dependent proteolysis of O^6-methylguanine-DNA methyltransferase in human and murine tumor cells following inactivation with O^6-benzylguanine or 1,3-bis(2-chloroethyl)-1-nitrosourea. Biochemistry 1996;35:1328–34.

[45] Liu L, Schwartz S, Davis BM, Gerson SL. Chemotherapy-induced O(6)-benzylguanine-resistant alkyltransferase mutations in mismatch-deficient colon cancer. Cancer Res 2002;62:3070–6.

[46] Glickman MH, Ciechanover A. The ubiquitin-proteasome proteolytic pathway: destruction for the sake of construction. Physiol Rev 2002;82:373–428.

[47] Kaina B, Fritz G, Ochs K, Simone H, Grombacher T, Dosch J, et al. Transgenic systems in studies on genotoxicity of alkylating agents: critical lesions, thresholds and defense mechanism. Mutat Res 1998;405:179–91.

[48] Zaidi NH, Pretlow TP, O'Riordan MA, Dumenco LL, Allay E, Gerson SL. Transgenic expression of human MGMT protects against azoxymethane-iduced aberrant crypt foci and G to A mutations in the K-ras oncogene of mouse colon. Carcinogenesis 1995;16(3):451–6.

[49] Gerson S. MGMT: its role in cancer aetiology and cancer therapeutics. Nat Rev Cancer 2004;4:296–307.

[50] Dumenco LL, Allay E, Norton K, Gerson SL. The prevention of thymic lymphomas in transgenic mice by human O^6-alkylguanine-DNA alkyltransferase. Science 1993;259(5092):219–22.

[51] Becker K, Dosch J, Gregel CM, Martin BA, Kaina B. Targeted expression of human O^6-methylguanine-DNA methyltransferase (MGMT) in transgenic mice protects against tumor initiation in two-stage skin carcinogenesis. Cancer Res 1996;56:3244–9.

[52] Becker K, Gregel C, Fricke C, Komitowski D, Dosch J, Kaina B. DNA repair protein MGMT protects against N-methyl-N-nitrosourea-induced conversion of benign into malignant tumors. Carcinogenesis 2003;24(3):541–6.

[53] Becker K, Thomas AD, Kaina B. Does increase in DNA repair allow "tolerance-to-insult" in chemical carcinogenesis? Experiments with MGMT-overexpressing mice. Environ Mol Mutagen 2014;55:145–50.

[54] Zhou Z-Q, Manguino D, Kewitt K, Intano GW, McMahan CA, Herbert DC, et al. Spontaneous hepatocellular carcinoma is reduced in transgenic mice overexpressing human O^6-methylguanine-DNA methyltransferase. Proc Natl Acad Sci USA 2001;98:12566–71.

[55] Sakumi K, Shiraishi A, Shimizu S, Tsuzuki T, Ishikawa T, Sekiguchi M. Methylnitrosourea-induced tumorigenesis in MGMT gene knockout mice. Cancer Res 1997;57:2415–25.

[56] Wirtz S, Nagel G, Eshkind L, Neurath MF, Samson LD, Kaina B. Both base excision repair and O^6 methylguanine-DNA methyltransferase protect against methylation-induced colon carcinogenesis. Carcinogenesis 2010;31(12):2111–7.

[57] Svrcek M, Buhard O, Colas C, Coulet F, Dumont S, Massaoudi I, et al. Methylation tolerance due to an O^6-methylguanine DNA methyltransferase (MGMT) field defect in the colonic mucosa: an initiating step in the development of mismatch repair-deficient colorectal cancers. Gut 2010;59:1516–26.

[58] Christmann M, Kaina B. Transcriptional regulation of human DNA repair genes following genotoxic stress: trigger mechanisms, inducible reponses and genotoxic adaptation. Nucleic Acids Res 2013;41(18):8403–20.

[59] Cao X, Mittelstaedt RA, Pearce MG, Allen BC, Soeteman-Hernandez LG, Johnson GE, et al. Quantitative dose-response analysis of ethyl methanesulfonate genotoxicity in adult *gpt*-delta transgenic mice. Environ Mol Mutagen 2014;55:385–99.

[60] Kaina B, Christmass M, Naumann S, Roos WP. MGMT: key node in the battle against genotoxicity, carcinogenicity and apoptosis induced by alkylating agents. DNA Repair 2007;6:1079–99.

[61] Feitsma H, Akay A, Cuppen E. Alkylation damage causes MMR-dependent chromosomal instability in vertebrate embryos. Nucleic Acids Res 2008;36(12):4047–56.

[62] Kaina B. DNA damage-triggered apoptosis: critical role of DNA repair, double-strand breaks, cell proliferation and signaling. Biochem Pharmacol 2003;66:1547–54.

[63] O'Brien V, Brown R. Signalling cell cycle arrest and cell death through the MMR system. Carcinogenesis 2006;27(4):682–92.

[64] Yoshioka K-I, Yoshioka Y, Hseih P. ATR kinase activation mediated by MutSα and MutLα in response to cytotoxic O^6-methylguanine adducts. Mol Cell 2006;22(4):5001–10.

[65] Dianov GL, Hubscher U. Mammalian base excision repair: the forgotten archangel. Nucleic Acids Res 2013;41(6):3483–90.

[66] Sobol RW, Watson DE, Nakamura J, Yakes FM, Hou E, Horton JK, et al. Mutations associated with base excision repair and methylation-induced genotoxic stress. Proc. Natl. Acad. Sci. USA 2002;99(10):6860–5.

[67] Robertson AB, Klungland Am Rognes T, Leiros I. Base excision repair: the long and short of it. Cell Mol Life Sci 2009;66:981–93.

[68]   Coquerelle D, Dosch J, Kaina B. Overexpression of *N*-methylpurine-DNA glycosylase in Chinese hamster ovary cells renders them more sensitive to the production of chromosomal aberrations by methylating agents-a case of imbalanced DNA repair. Mutat Res 1995;336:9–17.

[69]   Roth RB, Samson LD. 3-Methyladenine DNA glycosylase-deficient *Aag* null mice display unexpected bone marrow alkylation resistance. Cancer Res 2002;62:656–60.

[70]   Li X, Heyer W-D. Homologous recombination in DNA repair and DNA damage tolerance. Cell Res 2008;18:99–113.

[71]   Weterings E, Chen DJ. The endless tale of non-homologous end-joining. Cell Res 2008;18:114–24.

[72]   Kastan MB, Onyekwere O, Sidransky D, Vogelstein B, Craig RW. Participation of p53 protein in the cellular response to DNA damage. Cancer Res 1991;51:6304–11.

[73]   Smith J, Tho LM, Xu N, Gillespie DA. The ATM-Chk2 and ATR-Chk1 pathways in DNA damage signaling and cancer. Adv Cancer Res 2010;10:73–112.

[74]   Roos WP, Kaina B. DNA damage-induced cell death by apoptosis. Trends Mol Med 2006;12(9):440–50.

[75]   Margison GP, Santibanez Koref MF, Povey AC. Mechanisms of carcinogenicity/chemotherapy by O^6-methylguanine. Mutagenesis 2002;17(6):483–7.

[76]   Tubiana M, Feinendegen LE, Yang C, Kaminski JM. The linear no-threshold relationship is inconsistent with radiation biologic and experimental data. Radiology 2009;251(1):13–22.

[77]   Nikolova T, Ensminger M, Lobrich M, Kaina B. Homologous recombination protects mammalian cells from recombination-associated DNA double-strand breaks arising in response to methyl methanesulfonate. DNA Repair 2010;9:1050–63.

[78]   Nowosielska A, Smith SA, Engelward BP, Marinus MG. Homologous recombination prevents methylation-induced toxicity in *Escherichia coli*. Nucleic Acids Res 2006;34(8):2258–68.

[79]   de Laat WL, Jaspers NGJ, Hoeijmakers JHJ. Molecular mechanism of nucleotide excision repair. Gene Dev 1999;13:768–85.

[80]   Kondo N, Takahashi A, Ono K, Ohnishi T. DNA damage induced by alkylating agents and repair pathways. J. Nucleic Acids 2010:543531.

[81]   Gocke E, Ballantyne M, Whitwell J, Muller L. MNT and MutaMouse studies to define the in vivo dose response relations of the genotoxicity of EMS and ENU. Toxicol Lett 2009;190:286–97.

[82]   Gocke E, Muller L. In vivo studies in the mouse to define a threshold for the genotoxicity of EMS and ENU. Mutat Res 2009;678:101–7.

[83]   Dobo KL, Fiedler RD, Gunther WC, Thiffeault CJ, Cammerer Z, Coffing SL, et al. Defining EMS and ENU dose-response relationships using the *Pig-a* mutation assay in rats. Mutat Res 2011;725:13–21.

[84]   Bryce SM, Avlasevich SL, Bemis JC, Phonethepswath S, Dertinger SD. Miniaturized flow cytometric in vitro micronucleus assay represents an efficient tool for comprehensively characterizing genotoxicity dose-response relationships. Mutat Res 2010;703:191–9.

[85]   Zair ZM, Jenkins GJ, Doak SH, Singh R, Brown K, Johnson GE. *N*-methylpurine DNA glycosylase plays a pivotal role in the threshold response of ethyl methane sulfonate-induced chromosome damage. Toxicol Sci 2011;119(2):346–58.

[86]   Gocke E, Tang L, Singer T. Exposure to alkylating agents: where do the thresholds for mutagenic/ clastogenic effects arise? Gene Environ 2012;34(4):171–8.

[87]   Tang L, Guerard M, Zeller A. Quantitative analysis of the dose-response of alkylating agents in DNA repair proficient and deficient Ames tester strains. Environ Mol Mutagen 2014;55:15–23.

[88]   Johnson GE, Doak SH, Griffiths SM, Quick EL, Skibinski DOF, Zair ZM, et al. Non-linear dose-response of DNA-reactive genotoxins: recommendations for data analysis. Mutat Res 2009;678:95–100.

[89]   O'Brien JM, Walker M, Sivathayalan A, Douglas GR, Yauk CL, Marchetti F. Sublinear response in *lacZ* mutant frequency of Mutamouse spermatogonial stem cells after low dose subchronic exposure to *N*-ethyl-*N*-nitrosourea. Environ Mol Mutagen 2014 http://dx.doi.org/10.1002/em.21932.

[90]   Volkert MR. Adaptive response of *Escherichia coli* to alkylation damage. Environ Mol Mutagen 1988;11:241–55.

[91] Pottenger LH, Schisler MR, Zhang F, Bartels MJ, Fontaine DD, McFadden LG, et al. Dose-response and operational thresholds/NOAELs for in vitro mutagenic effects from DNA-reactive mutagens, MMS and MNU. Mutat Res 2009;678:138–47.

[92] Monti P, Foggetti G, Menichini P, Inga A, Gold G, Fronza G. Comparison of the biological effects of MMS and Me-lex, a minor groove methylating agent: clarifying the role of *N*3-methyladenine. Mutat Res 2014;759:45–51.

[93] Thomas AD, Jenkins GJS, Kaina B, Bodger OG, Tomaszowski K-H, Lewis PD, et al. Influence of DNA repair on nonlinear dose-responses for mutation. Toxicol Sci 2013;132(1):87–95.

[94] Lynch AM, Giddings A, Custer L, Gleason C, Henwood A, Aylott M, et al. International *Pig-a* gene mutation assay trial (stage III): results with *N*-methyl-*N*-nitrosourea. Environ Mol Mutagen 2010;52:699–720.

[95] MacGregor JT, Froetschl R, White PA, Crump KS, Eastmond DA, Fukushima S, et al. IWGT report on quantitative approaches to genotoxicity risk assessment I. Methods and metrics for defining exposure-response relationships and points of departure (PoDs). Mutat Res 2014 http://dx.doi.org/10.1016/j.mrgentox.2014.09.011.

[96] Jenkins GJS, Zair Z, Johnson GE, Doak SH. Genotoxic thresholds, DNA repair, and susceptibility in human populations. Toxicology 2010;278:305–10.

CHAPTER 6

The Role of Endogenous Versus Exogenous DNA Damage in Risk Assessment

James Swenberg[1], Yongquan Lai[1], Rui Yu[1], Vyom Sharma[1],
Benjamin C. Moeller[1,2], Hadley Hartwell[1], Jacqueline Gibson[1] and
Jun Nakamura[1]

[1]Department of Environmental Sciences and Engineering, University of North Carolina, Chapel Hill, NC, United States [2]Lovelace Respiratory Research Institute, Albuquerque, NM, United States

Chapter Outline

Introduction   83
Aldehydes   84
Alkylating Agents   88
Oxidative Stress   90
Ionizing Radiation   92
Quantifying Complex Dose–Response Relationships to Support Risk Assessments   92
    Approach 1: Threshold Models   93
    Approach 2: Bottom-Up Method   93
    Approach 3: Distributional Method   94
    Approach 4: Bayesian Belief Networks   95
Conclusion   98
References   98

Introduction

New scientific approaches and ultrasensitive instrumentation have greatly improved our understanding of both endogenous and exogenous DNA damage. Presently, it is well known that our DNA is not pristine, having ~40,000 lesions in every cell in our body [1–9]. Yet, linear extrapolations of risk down to zero remain the most common default approach used by regulators, in spite of the fact that Dr Crump, the major proponent of the Linearized Multistage Model (LMS) stated "that the LMS is 'biological,' only to the extent that the true biological dose response is linear at low dose and that low-dose slope is reflected in the experimental data" [10]. "If the true dose response is nonlinear, the LMS upper bound may overestimate the true risk by many orders of magnitude." This chapter will summarize

Thresholds of Genotoxic Carcinogens.
DOI: http://dx.doi.org/10.1016/B978-0-12-801663-3.00006-6

numerous examples of recent studies that review high-quality studies that demonstrate that nonlinear responses are very common and that linear extrapolations are clearly exaggerating risks associated with low exogenous exposures. The chapter will then present several possible mathematical frameworks that could be used to account for low-dose nonlinearities and endogenous DNA damage in cancer risk assessments.

Aldehydes

Formaldehyde and acetaldehyde are classified as known human and animal carcinogens according to the International Agency for Research on Cancer (IARC) [11,12]. Their well-known toxicity and carcinogenicity, coupled with widespread human exposure, has raised long-standing public concerns over their safety. Formaldehyde is a by-product of fires, cigarette smoke, automotive exhaust, and as a metabolite of various environmental compounds, such as demethylation reactions in the metabolism of nitrosamines, methanol, and so on [13]. Likewise, a variety of potential human exposures of acetaldehyde range from occupational activities, consumer products, lifestyle choices (food, alcohol, cigarette consumption, etc.), and environmental sources [14,15]. Acetaldehyde is also a metabolite of vinyl acetate, a common industrial chemical used in the manufacturing of a variety of consumer and industrial products.

Exposure to formaldehyde and acetaldehyde results in DNA damage. Both aldehydes can covalently bind to DNA, proteins, and other cellular nucleophiles, forming DNA adducts [13,16–19], DNA–DNA cross-links, DNA–protein cross-links (DPCs) [20–26], and/or DNA–glutathione adducts [27] that, if not repaired or hydrolyzed, can lead to mutagenesis and carcinogenesis. The primary DNA adducts are N^2-hydroxymethyl-dG and N^6-hydroxymethyl-dA formed by formaldehyde [28], and N^2-ethylidene-dG, and $1,N^2$-propano-dG formed by acetaldehyde [29,30]. However, the primary genotoxic effects from formaldehyde exposure are due to the formation of DPCs, which represent a potentially useful biomarker of exposure and genotoxicity. The carcinogenic mode of action is based on synergism of the formation of DNA monoadducts, DPCs, and increased cell proliferation which, collectively, lead to mutations [13].

What is often not realized is that formaldehyde and acetaldehyde can also be formed as products of normal cellular metabolism and as building blocks of all living cells [1]. The endogenous presence and the high concentrations normally found in cells also result in the formation of identical DNA adducts and cross-links to those caused by exogenous aldehydes. Epidemiologic associations have been reported between formaldehyde exposure and the induction of leukemia [31]. However, whether or not inhaled formaldehyde exposure causes leukemia remains debatable, since previous experimental results have not supported the induction of leukemia [28], and epidemiological reports have been inconsistent across different studies [31,32]. K.J. Patel's laboratory has recently reported that mice deficient in both acetaldehyde catabolism (ALDH2$^{-/-}$) and the Fanconi anemia (FA) DNA repair pathway (FANCD2$^{-/-}$), spontaneously develop severe bone marrow toxicity and acute leukemia [33,34]. Moreover, they have shown endogenous formaldehyde to be both more abundant and genotoxic than acetaldehyde [35], demonstrating that endogenous aldehydes are sufficient to cause DNA damage and induce leukemia in the presence of deficiencies in dehydrogenases and DNA repair.

The primary genotoxic effects of formaldehyde are thought to result from the formation of DPCs. Due to their significant biological consequences, DPCs have been widely used as a biomarker for exposure to formaldehyde. Increased DPCs were detected in nasal mucosa of rats exposed to formaldehyde by inhalation at concentrations greater than 2 ppm [36]. However, there were no detectable DPCs in the bone marrow of normal rats exposed to formaldehyde at concentrations as high as 15 ppm. Similarly, DPCs were found in the nasal turbinates and anterior lateral wall/septum of nonhuman primates (NHPs) following inhalation exposure to as little as 0.7 ppm formaldehyde, while no DPCs were detected in the bone marrow at concentrations as high as 6 ppm [37]. Further studies indicate that protein adducts and DPCs were not detected in the bone marrow of rats exposed to formaldehyde at concentrations as high as 10 ppm, even when the degradation of formaldehyde was inhibited by glutathione depletion [20]. On the contrary, some studies indicate increased DPCs were found in several remote tissues, such as bone marrow, liver, kidney, and testes of mice exposed to inhaled formaldehyde [38]. The debate on the formation of formaldehyde-induced DPCs in the animal tissues distant to initial contact may be due to the use of nonspecific DPC assays, such as potassium–SDS precipitation or chloroform/*iso*-amyl alcohol/phenol extraction. These nonspecific measurements are not only unable to differentiate formaldehyde DPCs from DPCs induced by other cross-linking chemicals, but are also easily interfered with by incomplete separation of noncovalent DNA–protein complexes. Moreover, the inability to distinguish between exogenous and endogenous formaldehyde-associated DNA damage is another clear shortcoming for all previous studies measuring the formation of formaldehyde-induced DPCs. To this end, our laboratory developed an ultrasensitive measurement that can distinguish between endogenous and exogenous formaldehyde-induced DPCs [38a]. In our method, formaldehyde-induced DPCs are digested to specific cross-links consisting of dG and cysteine (dG-Me-Cys), followed by detection using nanoliquid chromatography–tandem mass spectrometry (nano-LC-MS/MS). Using this specific method, endogenous and exogenous DPCs, specifically dG-Me-Cys and $^{13}CD_2$-dG-Me-Cys, were quantified in rats and NHPs exposed to 15 or 6 ppm [$^{13}CD_2$]-formaldehyde, respectively (6 h/day). Consistent results from primate and rat studies clearly demonstrated that exogenous DPCs were only found in nasal respiratory epithelium. However, endogenous DPCs were present in all examined tissues including peripheral blood mononuclear cells, bone marrow, and liver.

In a study of formaldehyde-DPCs formed between deoxyribose nucleosides and amino acids or their oligos, we found that dG-lysine was the most abundant cross-link formed, but that it very rapidly (2–5 min) underwent hydrolysis [39]. The second most abundant cross-link was dG-cysteine. This cross-link was also shown to be the most stable. We have now evaluated the dG-cysteine, dG-glutathione, and a peptide from O^6-alkyguanine DNA methyltransferase (MGMT) that also forms a dG-cysteine cross-link for hydrolytic degradation. We found that N^2-hydroxymethyl-dG was the dominant product [34]. This demonstrates that N^2-hydroxymethyl-dG represents an excellent biomarker for both spontaneous DPC hydrolysis and direct adduction of inhaled formaldehyde to DNA.

Similar to the specific DPC measurement, our laboratory has employed stable isotope-labeled formaldehyde and acetaldehyde exposures to afford the ability to differentiate between formaldehyde- and acetaldehyde-induced DNA adducts of endogenous and inhaled exogenous origin. DNA adducts induced by exposure to stable isotope-labeled aldehydes and the associated endogenous aldehydes can readily be measured using nanoultra-performance liquid chromatography–tandem mass spectrometry (nanoUPLC-MS-MS) [28,40,41]. The limit of detection is 0.5 attomoles of the N^2-hydroxymethyl-dG adducts formed from formaldehyde and 0.25 attomoles of the N^2-ethylidene-dG adducts formed from acetaldehyde [42]. These DNA adducts caused by formaldehyde and acetaldehyde are chemically unstable, and must be reduced to a more stable form using the reducing agent, cyanoborohydride, prior to analysis [28].

In studies using inhalation exposure, we clearly demonstrated that exposures to labeled [$^{13}CD_2$]-formaldehyde induced [$^{13}CD_2$]-N^2-hydroxymethyl-dG adducts in nasal respiratory epithelium of rats and monkeys; however, these adducts were not detected in tissues distant to the site of contact, including lung, liver, spleen, mononuclear white blood cells, or bone marrow [28,40,41]. In contrast, endogenous N^2-hydroxymethyl-dG and N^6-hydroxymethyl-dA adducts were readily detected in all tissues examined [28]. When [$^{13}CD_4$]-methanol was administered orally to rats, [$^{13}CD_4$]-N^2-hydroxymethyl-dG and [$^{13}CD_4$]-N^6-hydroxymethyl-dA adducts were formed in the kidney and bone marrow [43], suggesting that the N^6-hydroxymethyl-dA adducts are only formed when methanol is metabolized to formaldehyde within a cell.

Our most recent study that exposed rats to 2-ppm [$^{13}CD_2$]-formaldehyde for up to 28 consecutive days further demonstrated [$^{13}CD_2$]-N^2-hydroxymethyl-dG accumulation, with 28 days being the approximate time to reach steady-state concentration, and the $t_{1/2}$ for the repair/loss of [$^{13}CD_2$]-N^2-hydroxymethyl-dG in vivo being ~171 h (7.125 days) [42]. As with our previous studies [28,40,41], endogenous formaldehyde-induced N^2-hydroxymethyl-dG adducts were observed in all tissues analyzed; however, exogenous formaldehyde-induced [$^{13}CD_2$]-N^2-hydroxymethyl-dG adducts were only detected in the nasal respiratory epithelium DNA of rats exposed to [$^{13}CD_2$]-formaldehyde by inhalation, providing compelling evidence that inhaled formaldehyde does not reach tissues distant to the sites of initial contact in an active form. An NHP study consisting of 6 ppm [$^{13}CD_2$]-formaldehyde exposures for 2 days

(6h/day) had the ability to detect one $[^{13}CD_2]$-N^2-hydroxymethyl-dG adduct in 10 billion unmodified dG, but no exogenous adducts were found in bone marrow, mononuclear white blood cells, lung, or trachea [41,42]. A similar sensitivity was used to evaluate mononuclear white blood cells in the 28-day rat study, and comparably no exogenous adducts were found. This raises important questions regarding how inhaled formaldehyde could cause leukemia.

By conducting studies at durations ranging from a single 6-h exposure [40], to 5 days (6h/day) [28], and up to 28 consecutive days (6h/day) [42], our evidence clearly shows that exogenous N^2-hydroxymethyl-dG adducts do not reach steady-state concentrations until ~4 weeks of inhalation exposure, while endogenous N^2-hydroxymethyl-dG adducts are at steady-state concentrations due to continuous intracellular formation of formaldehyde through normal metabolic pathways. When the National Research Council reviewed the 2010 EPA Integrated Risk Information System Cancer Risk Assessment [44], they pointed out that understanding what exposures to formaldehyde increased the intracellular amounts of total formaldehyde above the endogenous represented critical data for risk assessment.

Similar to the N^2-hydroxymethyl-dG adduct from formaldehyde, N^2-ethylidene-dG is unstable ($t_{1/2}$=20min) at the nucleoside level [45]. Our recent data reporting N^2-ethylidene-dG adduct formation in TK6 cells exposed to a $[^{13}CD_2]$-acetaldehyde concentration range ≥4.5 orders of magnitude greater than control cells illustrated several key points [45]. Using the stable isotope approach, the endogenous adducts remained relatively constant across the dose range (~2–3 adducts/10^7dG), with similar results to what has been observed in our $[^{13}CD_2]$-formaldehyde and stable isotope-labeled N-methyl-N-nitrosourea ($[D_3]$-MNU) studies [28,40,41]. At low exogenous exposure conditions (≤10µM), the amount of endogenous N^2-ethylidene-dG adducts dominates over much smaller numbers of exogenous adducts [45]. At high exposure conditions (≥250µM), exogenous adducts were significantly greater than endogenous adducts [45]. The stable isotope exposures allowed for a 50 × difference in the lowest concentration (1µM), with observable formation of exogenous DNA adducts over the sum (endogenous + exogenous) of the adducts at 50µM [45]. Importantly, the exogenous adducts had a linear dose-response across the dose range, while the sum of the adducts showed a nonlinear response that demonstrated a threshold in DNA adduct formation at 50µM and below [45]. This nonlinearity was also observed for micronucleus (MN) formation rates and cell survival, with statistically significant increases over background occurring at 1mM. A more in-depth study investigating the chromosomal and gene level effects of acetaldehyde using 4 and 24h exposures showed a nonlinear dose-response for MN formation and the induction of mutations at the thymidine kinase ($TK^{-/-}$) loci between 50 and 100µM in TK6 cells [46].

In summary, the use of stable isotope-labeled formaldehyde and acetaldehyde exposures has provided new insight and tools for science-based risk assessment, which support the hypothesis that endogenously produced reactive species, including acetaldehyde, formaldehyde, and lipid peroxidation (LPO) are always present, and constitute a majority of the observed background DNA damage following low exposures to these compounds. The data generated in these studies provide pivotal information for understanding the genotoxicity and carcinogenicity of formaldehyde and acetaldehyde, as well as negate the biological plausibility of leukemia induction following inhalation exposure to formaldehyde.

Alkylating Agents

There is accumulating experimental evidence indicating the existence of thresholds of genotoxic effects caused by alkylating agents [47–49]. The mechanism of this dose-response appears to be derived partly from the elimination of reactive agents and DNA repair, but also from background levels of mutagenic and clastogenic events. Methyl methanesulfonate (MMS) and ethyl methanesulfonate (EMS) are S_N2 and S_N1/S_N2 alkylating agents, respectively. They have a high Swain–Scott constant and preferentially alkylate $N7$-G and $N3$-A, leading to the formation of $N7$-methylguanine ($N7$-mG) and $N3$-methyladenine ($N3$-mA) [50,51]. In contrast to O^6-methylguanine (O^6-mG), $N7$-mG and $N3$-mA are not mutagenic base lesions; however, these adducts cause mutations through abasic site formation either by spontaneous depurination or by DNA glycosylase activity (methylpurine DNA glycosylase). In addition to exogenous alkylating agents, cells have an endogenous source of a S_N2 methylating agent, *S*-adenosylmethionine (SAM), which serves as a one-carbon donor involved in many metabolic reactions including histone and cytosine methylation in the presence of methyltransferase [52,53]. SAM also weakly alkylates DNA in a nonenzymatic manner [2]. When human lymphoblastoid AHH1 cells were exposed to either MMS or EMS, MN and hypoxanthine phosphoribosyl transferase (HPRT) mutation frequencies showed a clear hockey-stick dose–response relationship [47]. DT40 chicken B lymphocytes also showed a hockey stick–like dose–response in MMS-induced *PIG-O* mutations [49]. The *PIG-O* mutational spectrum analysis revealed that MMS predominantly causes transversion mutations and frame-shift/deletion mutations without any G to A transition mutations. These results strongly suggest that S_N2 methylating agents, such as MMS, cause mutations through base excision repair (BER) intermediates derived from $N7$-mG and $N3$-mA if MGMT and mismatch repair (MMR) are proficient. Based on our results combined with the published literature, the threshold of mutations caused by MMS and EMS appears to be significantly modulated by the status of repair pathways including BER, MMR, and MGMT [54,55] in cultured cells. This is also the case in vivo. Muta[tm] mice treated with a single high dose of EMS showed a significant increase in lacZ mutations, but the same cumulative dose of EMS treatment over 28 days caused no increase in lacZ mutations in the mice [56]. These results suggest that low-dose repeated treatment may allow mice to repair DNA lesions and maintain alkylated DNA lesions at low levels that do not increase mutations over spontaneous levels of mutation frequency.

Compared to S_N2 alkylation agents, S_N1 compounds, such as MNU and *N*-ethyl-*N*-nitrosourea (ENU), preferentially alkylate O^6-G and O^2- and O^4-T, resulting in mutagenic base adducts. Although O^6-alkylguanine (O^6-AG) accounts for only a small percentage (6–8%) of the total DNA adducts formed, they are potent mutagenic lesions and cause MMR-mediated cytotoxicity [57,58]. Cells use a repair pathway for directly eliminating alkyl group from O^6-AG through a constitutively expressed MGMT [59]. If O^6-AG escapes MGMT-mediated direct DNA repair, this DNA lesion efficiently mispairs with thymine without DNA replication inhibition during the first round of DNA replication. This O^6-AG:T mismatch is then recognized by MutSα (MSH2/MSH6) leading to a futile MMR cycle of excision repair of newly synthesized DNA segments containing thymines opposite the O^6-AG site of the parent strand, resulting in severe toxicity [58]. In the absence of proficient MMR, therefore, alkylating agents markedly increase G to A transition mutations [60]. While MNU and ENU failed to demonstrate the threshold of mutagenesis [47], the same research group later successfully showed a hockey stick–like dose-response in mutation frequency caused by MNU at much lower concentrations in AHH1 cells [48]. Similar to the S_N2 compounds, the threshold of mutations induced by S_N1 alkylating agents is at a lower dose if either MGMT or MutSα is deficient.

In addition to DNA repair, spontaneous mutations and chromosome aberrations derived from endogenous DNA lesions, as well as polymerase errors, contribute to the threshold of genotoxicity of exogenous genotoxic agents. Such data challenge the linear risk assessment and demonstrate scientific evidence that explains the mechanism of the threshold for mutations caused by alkylating agents. The number of endogenous and exogenous levels of $N7$-mG and O^6-mG was quantitated in AHH1 cells exposed to low concentrations of [D3]-MNU (0.0075–2.5 μM) for 1 h [61]. We utilized a similar dose range, the same cell line and the same cell density to the MNU mutagenesis study [48] to compare the effects of exposure. We shortened the exposure time from 24 to 1 h. Due to the very short half-life of MNU under neutral pH, MNU exposure over 1 h does not cause major alkylation events in AHH1 cells. Endogenous $N7$-mG and O^6-mG levels were 232 and 0.30 adducts/10^8 G, respectively. While the amounts of each endogenous adduct were constant across different concentrations of MNU exposure, both exogenous adducts were linearly elevated with increasing concentrations of MNU. Exogenous $N7$-mG exceeded corresponding endogenous adducts by [D3]-MNU at 2.5 μM; on the other hand, exogenous O^6-mG increased over corresponding endogenous adducts at 0.025 μM. The total (endogenous and exogenous) number of each $N7$-mG and O^6-mG adduct significantly increased compared to corresponding endogenous adducts by [D3]-MNU at 0.75 and 0.025 μM, respectively. Taken together, with the lowest observed genotoxic effect level of ~0.1 μM of MNU [48], O^6-mG likely plays important roles in MNU-induced mutagenesis in MGMT-deficient AHH1 cells.

Ethylene oxide (EO) represents another alkylating agent that is classified as a human carcinogen, yet it is also formed endogenously. In studies examining *Hprt* mutations in mice exposed to ethylene, the data were clearly not linear at low exposures, but mutations were clearly present at high doses [3]. Marsden et al. [4] demonstrated that high exposures to ^{14}C-EO caused increases in endogenous *N*7-hydroxyguanine adducts as a result of oxidative stress. In both cases, low exposures did not cause increases in endogenous DNA damage and nonlinear responses were clearly defined. Our understanding of EO mutagenesis and carcinogenesis could be improved by using $[^{13}C_2]$-EO inhalation exposures so that endogenous and exogenous EO DNA adducts could be determined.

Oxidative Stress

The human body encounters a variety of exogenous and endogenous sources of reactive oxygen species (ROS) in everyday life. Exogenous sources include ionizing irradiation, air pollutants, cigarette smoke, industrial contaminants. In addition, many pharmaceuticals, xenobiotics, and industrial chemicals produce ROS as a by-product of their metabolism in vivo. Apart from exogenous sources, multiple mechanisms in the intra- and intercellular environment lead to endogenous production of ROS. Although exposure to ROS is extremely high from exogenous sources, the exposure from endogenous sources is more important and extensive, due to its continuous process over the life span of every cell [62]. Endogenous ROS-induced DNA adducts are constantly produced in genomic DNA owing to different mechanisms. In fact, abasic sites, which are a major product of oxidative DNA damage, are the most abundant endogenous DNA lesions existing in the human body [5]. To counter this oxidative DNA damage, mammalian cells possess efficient DNA-repair systems that serve to remove any ROS-induced damage, thus maintaining a cellular homeostasis. It has been suggested that compounds producing ROS are expected to show a threshold effect due to the presence of high amounts of endogenous DNA lesions and protective repair processes [63,64].

One of the most common and most studied endogenous oxidative-stress-related oxidants is hydrogen peroxide (H_2O_2). There is sufficient evidence available in the literature that H_2O_2 is a physiological constituent of living cells that is constantly produced as well as quenched in the cells [6]. The foremost oxidative DNA lesion formed by H_2O_2 is 8-oxo-2'-deoxyguanosine (8-*oxo*-dG), which serves as a popular biomarker for oxidative DNA damage. A background level of 60 8-*oxo*-dG/10^8 dG has been shown to exist in cultured human cells [5]. Seager et al. have shown that H_2O_2 and potassium bromate ($KBrO_3$) display threshold responses in the HPRT mutation assay and MN induction in human B-lymphocyte AHH1 cells, exhibiting a range of nongenotoxic low doses. Furthermore, the H_2O_2 dose–response curve was shifted by modulating the antioxidant glutathione. They concluded that the genotoxic tolerance to low levels of prooxidant chemicals appears to be due, in part, to basal BER of DNA, plus the protective capacity of antioxidants against DNA damage [64]. On similar lines, Platel et al. have shown in human TK6 lymphoblastoid cells, that DNA-oxidizing agents ($KBrO_3$, bleomycin, and H_2O_2) produced nonlinear dose-responses in the in vitro MN test, comet assay, and thymidine kinase (TK) mutation assay, thus allowing the determination of no-observed genotoxic effect levels [65,66].

LPO-induced etheno and malondialdehyde-deoxyguanosine (M1dG) adducts represent another class of endogenous and exogenous ROS-induced DNA adducts. ROS attack on polyunsaturated fatty acids (eg, cell membrane) leads to the generation of α,β-unsaturated aldehydes, such as 4-oxo-2-nonenal, 4-hydroxy-2-nonenal, malondialdehyde, and acrolein [7]. Such aldehydes then react with DNA to form M1dG and ethano adducts. Etheno DNA adducts are also formed exogenously as a consequence of exposure to the human carcinogen vinyl chloride [7]. Vinyl chloride produces the formation of four different kinds of adducts: 7-(2-oxoethyl)guanine (7-OEG), N^2,3-ethenoguanine, 1,N^6-ethenodeoxyadenosine, and 3,N^4-ethenodeoxycytosine. However, endogenous 7-OEG, N^2,3-ethenoguanine, 1,N^6-ethenodeoxyadenosine, and 3,N^4-ethenodeoxycytosine adducts have been shown to be present in unexposed rodent populations [5,67,68]. An earlier study from our group has demonstrated the formation of $[^{13}C_2]$-7-OEG from the reaction of calf thymus DNA with $[^{13}C_{18}]$-ethyl linoleate under peroxidizing conditions, thus confirming the endogenous formation of 7-OEG from LPO [7].

Previous studies from our lab have also shown that oxidative DNA damage plays a key role in toxicity and carcinogenicity following chronic polychlorinated biphenyl (PCB) exposure [69]. Rats exposed to PCB 126 for 1 year demonstrated an increase in M1dG adduct accumulation in the liver. Coadministration of PCB 126 and PCB 152 enhanced the adduct accumulation in a dose-dependent manner [69].

Based on the above evidence, it is clear that oxidative stress makes a significant contribution in causing carcinogenicity and/or cellular toxicity by many nongenotoxic environmental chemicals. The nongenotoxic carcinogens present major problems for risk assessment, since at low exposures the biology driving the induction of mutations may be derived from endogenous sources. This nonzero background causes uncertainty when regulatory agencies are required to extrapolate risks for hazardous chemicals that are thought to produce ROS as an important mode of action for toxicity and/or carcinogenicity. Genetic polymorphism, differences in DNA repair capacity, and inflammatory status may all contribute to the variations in the endogenous oxidative DNA damage in human populations [6]. More sensitive methods and data are needed to explore the dose–response relationships for oxidative stress and to understand where the biomarkers of *exposure* and *effect* are increased over background and where they are driven by endogenous biological processes.

As one of our approaches to address mechanisms of nonlinear dose–response curves in mutations, we chose H_2O_2 as a model compound [5]. We conducted TK gene mutation and 8-*oxo*-dG assays in human lymphoblastoid (TK6) cells exposed to H_2O_2 at concentrations ranging from 1 to 56.6 μM. H_2O_2 induced a hockey-stick dose-response in the mutation assay indicative of a threshold. This suggests that H_2O_2 increases the frequency of mutations when oxidative DNA lesions are increased above spontaneous oxidative DNA damage.

Ionizing Radiation

Ionizing radiation (X- and γ-rays) is classified as a known human and animal carcinogen according to the IARC [70]. The deleterious effects of ionizing radiation, particularly at high doses, are well-recognized by both public and scientific communities. However, the risk assessment associated with low-dose exposures and their possible carcinogenic potentials is controversial and more challenging to address from a regulatory perspective [71]. As with the other sources of DNA damage discussed above, there is a naturally occurring background level of radiation and thus constant exposure to all biological organisms. There is a large amount of literature available on the biological effects of radiation exposures that are summarized by other sources [70,71] and are outside the scope of this chapter. Instead, we will focus on recent publications investigating the genotoxicity of low-level radiation exposures and the observed dose–response relationships.

Ionizing radiation may directly damage DNA, or may do so indirectly through reactive species [70]. Detection of DNA damage resulting from ionizing radiation has been accomplished using a number of biomarkers: DNA adducts, MN formation, double-strand breaks (DSBs), and transcriptional changes in DNA repair genes. A recent example by Olipitz et al. [72] assessed a number of these markers (DNA adducts (hypoxanthine, 8-oxo-dG, 1,N^6-ethnoadenine, 3,N^4-ethnocytosine), MN formation, DSBs, and transcriptional changes) following continuous low-dose exposures at 0.00017 cGy/min (~400-fold higher than background) and showed no changes in any of the measured outcomes. In contrast, an acute dose at an equivalent total delivered dose of ~10 cGy induced MN formation and changes in gene expression. Olipitiz and colleagues showed that at exposures ~200-fold higher than the maximum permissible amounts did not induce DNA damage or cause changes in DNA-repair pathways. These data are supported by other studies that also suggest nonlinearity in DNA damage may occur at low doses of radiation [73,74]. The use of highly sensitive biomarkers of effect, such as the MN and COMET assays, have allowed for a better understanding of potential thresholds in the dose–response relationship [75]. It should be noted, however, that others have argued that low-dose ionizing radiation exposures may cause a hormetic dose–response relationship [76]. The data discussed above and others, challenge the linear-no-dose threshold hypothesis that has been the central dogma for regulation of radiation exposures [77].

Quantifying Complex Dose–Response Relationships to Support Risk Assessments

This chapter has provided substantial evidence of the potential for nonlinear (hockey stick–shaped) dose–response relationships arising from multiple mechanisms, including endogenous DNA damage. However, risk assessments conducted to support the development of US environmental regulations have long assumed and continue to assume that dose–response relationships for carcinogens are linear. Furthermore, regulatory policy requires that the origin of these linear models be set at zero, based on the assumption that no level of exposure to a carcinogen can be considered safe. Such linear dose–response models continue to be used to establish regulations on carcinogenic chemicals under all the major US environmental regulations, from the Safe Drinking Water Act to the Clean Air Act. Yet, the linear model is based on a long-disproven theory from radiation genetics [78], and it provides no means by which to incorporate the kinds of research on endogenously produced chemicals and threshold effects described in this chapter. As such, reliance on these linear models could result in a substantial misallocation of funds spent to protect public health from environmental exposure risks. By assuming the dose–response relationship is always linear, this approach fails to prioritize investment in chemicals that may pose supralinear risks over those with sublinear risks or having high thresholds between exposure and risk of disease.

Several potential mathematical approaches could be used to incorporate new knowledge on endogenous DNA damage into regulatory risk assessments of carcinogens. Here, we present four alternatives in order of increasing mathematical sophistication.

Approach 1: Threshold Models

The simplest approach to accounting for the type of hockey stick–shaped dose–response effects observed in this study is to use dose–response models that reflect zero additional cancer risk unless the exposure or associated exposure biomarker rises above an observed threshold level (the bend in the hockey stick). Such an approach has long been suggested, but has been rejected by the EPA due to its policy to adopt conservative approaches to ensure health protection in the face of scientific uncertainty [79]. In addition to being unlikely to be accepted by regulators due to the longstanding objections to using a threshold model [79], this approach fails to account for the increasing evidence on modes of action for carcinogens. In addition, it does not account for the possibility that different studies could suggest different possible thresholds.

Approach 2: Bottom-Up Method

A second, slightly more complex approach to estimating low-dose cancer risks while also accounting for endogenous DNA damage could involve computing slope factors from measured endogenous exposure levels combined with information on background cancer risks. That is, if one assumes that some portion of cancers in individuals not exposed to chemicals exogenously are attributable to endogenous exposures, and if one can measure these endogenous exposure levels, then the probability of cancer at low exposure levels can be estimated without having to use high-dose exposure experiments in animals or estimates from high occupational exposures in humans. Starr and Swenberg recently illustrated how such an approach, which they call the "bottom-up" method, could be applied to estimating risks from exposure to low doses of formaldehyde [80]. They used measurements of endogenous formaldehyde–DNA adducts, denoted as C_0, to estimate the adduct concentration corresponding to background cancer risks, denoted as P_0. Then, a cancer slope factor, q, can be computed from

$$q = \frac{P_0}{C_0} \times \frac{C_{x-SS}}{x} \tag{1}$$

where C_{x-SS} is the concentration of formaldehyde–DNA adducts due to exogenous formaldehyde exposure concentration x. C_{x-SS} can be measured in experiments that expose animals to $^{13}CD_2$-labeled formaldehyde.

While the bottom-up approach overcomes some of the problems of both low-dose extrapolation and failure to account for identical endogenous DNA damage, as Starr and Swenberg note, it still has limitations. Chiefly, like traditional regulatory risk assessment methods, the bottom-up approach assumes cancer risk is a linear function of dose (in this case, the dose of DNA adducts). In addition, it assumes that all background cancers are caused by endogenous DNA adducts; if multiple mechanisms are involved, the bottom-up approach therefore will overestimate the risk. A related limitation is that the method does not account for nongenotoxic modes of action or for uncertainty in cross-species extrapolation. Starr and Swenberg conclude, "The bottom-up approach may not be appropriate for developing 'best' or central estimates of low-dose human cancer risks which, at least in our view, can best be accomplished through a comprehensive and deep mechanistic understanding of how chemical exposures give rise to human cancer."

Approach 3: Distributional Method

Multiple authors have proposed a third potential method, the "distributional approach," that could be used to estimate low-dose cancer risks, accounting for endogenous exposure and nonlinearities [81–83]. As described by Small [83], this approach represents each uncertain assumption in a dose–response model as a probability distribution (hence the title "distributional approach"). It then considers all possible combinations of outcomes of these uncertain assumptions, resulting in probability distributions for both the maximum likelihood and upper confidence level estimates of cancer risk for a given dose. For example, Small illustrates the use of the distributional approach for predicting risks of low-dose formaldehyde exposure accounting for uncertainties in which tissues are vulnerable, mode of action, dose scale, dose–response model shape, best experimental data set, and interspecies extrapolation (Table 6.1). In all, there are 432 possible combinations of the plausible assumptions underlying these variables (from Table 6.1; $2 \times 3 \times 3 \times 4 \times 2 \times 3$). The resulting probability

Table 6.1 Variables represented in Small's assessment of low-dose formaldehyde exposure risks using a distributional approach.

Uncertain Variable/Assumption	Possible Outcomes
Formaldehyde is carcinogenic to target tissue	1. Yes 2. No
Mode of action	1. Cell proliferation only 2. Genotoxicity only 3. Both cell proliferation and genotoxicity
Dose scale	1. Inhaled concentration (ppm) 2. Total daily intake 3. DNA–protein cross-links
Dose–response model	1. Probit nonlinear threshold 2. Five-stage sublinear 3. Five-stage linear 4. One-stage linear
Experimental data set	1. Malignant squamous cell carcinoma (MSCC) 2. MSCC or benign polypoid adenoma
Interspecies extrapolation	1. Human same as rat 2. Body-weight ratio to three-fourths power 3. Body-weight ratio to two-thirds power

distribution of the cancer risk associated with one lifetime exposure to 1 ppb of formaldehyde has a mean value of 2×10^{-6} but is highly right-skewed, with an 83% probability that formaldehyde poses zero cancer risk at this dose. Small's distributional model includes the possibility of a threshold dose, such as could arise from endogenous exposures (see "dose–response model" variable in Table 6.1).

Approach 4: Bayesian Belief Networks

All of the above three approaches fall short of a full, mechanistic representation of the biological and biochemical sequences of events leading from exposure to disease. In addition, the first two approaches cannot account for data drawn from multiple studies, studies at different organismal levels (eg, chemical, cellular, tissue, organ), or studies in multiple species. To overcome these limitations, new research in mapping adverse outcome pathways (AOPs) could be combined with Bayesian belief network (BBN) modeling to develop dose–response models that reflect a modern mechanistic understanding of the processes leading from chemical exposure to disease. Formally, a BBN is a directed, acyclic graph in which the nodes represent variables (eg, the expression of a particular gene) and the edges represent probabilistic dependencies among the variables (eg, the probability of the proliferation of mutated cells given the presence of promutation DNA adducts). Use of BBNs to guide reasoning when faced with complex systems having multiple uncertainties has emerged in a wide variety of applications since Judea Pearl developed the first algorithms for solving such networks in 1989 [84]. Applications have ranged from internet security and large engineering project risk analyses to medical diagnostics [85–88]. Several examples of BBNs for use in ecological risk assessment have been published [89]. However, the BBN concept has not yet been extended to assessment of human health risks from environmental carcinogens.

Over the past several years, toxicologists have increasingly emphasized the concept of developing AOP models as a means of representing the mechanisms leading from chemical exposure to disease. BBNs provide an ideal quantitative tool for developing mechanistic dose–response functions that represent the steps in AOPs, which could account for endogenous exposures and other causes of nonlinearities in dose–response functions. As an example, consider how a BBN could be developed to support the hypothetical AOP presented in a recent review by Villeneuve et al. (Fig. 6.1) [90]. The hypothetical AOP in Fig. 6.1 shows how two separate molecular initiating events (MIEs) (assumed to result directly or indirectly from environmental chemical exposures) lead through a chain of key events (KEs) to three different adverse health outcomes. For example, an MIE might be the formation of an exogenously

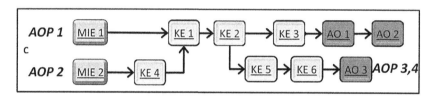

Figure 6.1

Hypothetical adverse outcome pathway diagram showing how molecular initiating events (MIEs), perhaps triggered by exposure to an environmental toxin, induce a chain reaction of key events (KEs) that may lead to an adverse health outcome (AO). Each event (node) in this sequence can be viewed as a Bernoulli random variable (ie, the event either occurs or it does not occur). The occurrence probability of each event is influenced by the upstream nodes.
Source: Villeneuve DL, Crump D, Garcia-Reyero N, Hecker M, Hutchinson TH, LaLone CA, et al. Adverse outcome pathway (AOP) development I: strategies and principles. Toxicol Sci 2014;142:312–20.

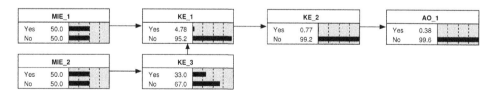

Figure 6.2

Bayesian belief network version of the adverse outcome pathway model in Fig. 6.1 with hypothetical event probabilities. The event probabilities and underlying conditional probabilities were developed by simulating a random sequence of these events that leads to the overall dose–response function shown in Fig. 6.3. The probabilities shown here correspond to a hypothetical dose level of 10 in Fig. 6.3.

induced DNA adduct, and a KE could represent an increase in the adduct concentration significantly above endogenous levels. Fig. 6.2 shows a version of part of this AOP diagram with hypothetical conditional probability tables reflecting relationships among the events in the AOPs. This diagram was created using Netica (Norsys, Vancouver, BC, Canada) (other software packages are available). The conditional probabilities underlying the nodes were determined from the simulated, noisy dose–response model in Fig. 6.3; relationships among nodes in the AOP were simulated with arbitrary functions and then converted to conditional probability tables for a dose equal to 10. If this BBN were developed to represent an actual AOP, then these conditional probability tables could be developed, for example, through review of existing literature (including previous animal testing and high-throughput studies), through new experiments, and/or through expert elicitation. As Figs. 6.2 and 6.3 show, this type of network model can be used effectively to model dose–response function in which there is a sequence of random events occurring along the pathway from exposure to response.

Overall, BBNs have great potential as the basis for developing modern, sophisticated dose–response models due to their ability to combine qualitative or semiquantitative understanding of pathways leading from environmental exposure to disease with probabilistic modeling, traditional toxicological data from animal studies, human epidemiologic studies, and modern high-throughput toxicity data. BBNs could serve as the tool through which quantitative risk estimates are developed from AOP models. BBNs can be used to update prior assumptions (eg, the level of certainty about the association of a particular pathway with subsequent onset of cancer) based on new empirical evidence (eg, new high-throughput data or new epidemiologic studies) [91]. In addition to supporting population-level risk assessments, such models could be used to create personalized risk assessment information for vulnerable individuals. Indeed, BBNs already have been developed for personalizing medical treatments (such as for colon cancer) to individual patients [92].

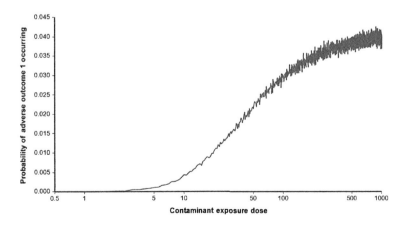

Figure 6.3
Simulated dose–response model corresponding to the adverse outcome pathway model in Fig. 6.2.

In order for BBNs to achieve their potential for quantifying AOPs in support of the development of nonlinear dose–response models, several steps are needed. First, prototype BBNs for already-established AOPs should be developed. As a starting point, the AOP models provided in the Collaborative AOP Wiki (https://aopkb.org/aopwiki/index.php/Main_Page) could be parameterized. Ideally, these prototype BBNs then would be validated against epidemiologic data. User-friendly versions of these BBN models then could be developed to support regulatory decisions. For example, Stojadinovic et al. describe user-friendly BBNs for use by physicians in developing treatment plans for treating colon cancer patients [92]. The growing use of BBNs in medical diagnostics shows the potential for this tool to gain wide use in environmental regulatory practice, if the underlying models are built. In the future, these mechanistic BBNs could replace the reliance on simplistic linear dose–response models.

Conclusion

The example agents discussed above all share the commonality of being both toxic and mutagenic at high enough doses, but are all constantly present due to their ubiquitous existence. Accordingly, the dose–response relationship between exposures of toxic agents that can be formed endogenously is complex and requires additional consideration when evaluating the potential impacts on human health. The observed dose–response curves from exogenous exposures of these compounds are highly dependent upon the selected doses and the sensitivity of the biomarker or experimental endpoint. The use of stable isotope exposures for compounds such as formaldehyde or acetaldehyde and the measurement of endogenous and exogenous DNA adducts has allowed a better understanding of the dose–response relationship from these exposures. For endpoints (biomarkers) that can allow for differentiation between endogenous and exogenous agents, a linear through zero relationship can be observed due to the ability to have highly sensitive and selective markers. These considerations must then be translated and addressed by the proper regulatory authorities to protect public health while reflecting the tremendous gains in toxicology research on environmental contaminants that have occurred over the past several decades. BBNs can serve as a vehicle for incorporating these complex dose–response considerations into the regulatory process.

References

[1]   Swenberg JA, Lu K, Moeller BC, Gao L, Upton PB, Nakamura J, et al. Endogenous versus exogenous DNA adducts: their role in carcinogenesis, epidemiology, and risk assessment. Toxicol Sci 2011;120(Suppl. 1): S130–45.

[2]   Rydberg B, Lindahl T. Nonenzymatic methylation of DNA by the intracellular methyl group donor *S*-adenosyl-L-methionine is a potentially mutagenic reaction. EMBO J 1982;1:211–6.

[3]   Swenberg JA, Fryar-Tita E, Jeong Y-C, Boysen G, Starr T, Walker VE, et al. Biomarkers in toxicology and risk assessment: informing critical dose–response relationships. Chem Res Toxicol 2008;21:253–65.

[4]   Marsden DA, Jones DJL, Britton RG, Ognibene T, Ubick E, Johnson GE, et al. Dose-response relationships for *N*7-(2-Hydroxyethyl)guanine induced by low-dose [^{14}C]ethylene oxide: evidence for a novel mechanism of endogenous adduct formation. Cancer Res 2009;69:3052–9.

[5] Nakamura J, Mutlu E, Sharma V, Collins L, Bodnar W, Yu R, et al. The endogenous exposome. DNA Repair 2014;19:3–13.

[6] Bolt HM. Enzymatic detoxification of endogenously produced mutagenic carcinogens maintaining cellular homeostasis. In: Greim H, Albertini RJ, editors. The cellular response to the genotoxic insult: the question of threshold for genotoxic carcinogens. Cambridge, UK: RSC Publishing 2012; p. 65–91.

[7] Mutlu E, Jeong YC, Collins LB, Ham AJ, Upton PB, Hatch G, et al. A new LC-MS/MS method for the quantification of endogenous and vinyl chloride-induced 7-(2-oxoethyl)guanine in Sprague-Dawley rats. Chem Res Toxicol 2012;25:391–9.

[8] De Bont R, van Larebeke N. Endogenous DNA damage in humans: a review of quantitative data. Mutagenesis 2004;19:169–85.

[9] Farmer PB, Shuker DE. What is the significance of increases in background levels of carcinogen-derived protein and DNA adducts? Some considerations for incremental risk assessment. Mutat Res 1999;424:275–86.

[10] Crump K. The linearized multistage model and the future of quantitative risk assessment. Hum Exp Toxicol 1996;15:787–98.

[11] IARC. Formaldehyde, a review of human carcinogens. Part F: chemical agents and related occupations. IARC monographs on the evaluation of carcinogenic risks to human. Lyon, France: World Health Organization; 2012.401.35

[12] IARC. Alcohol consumption and ethyl carbamate. IARC monographs on the evaluation of carcinogenic risks to human. Lyon, France: World Health Organization; 2010.

[13] IARC. Formaldehyde, 2-butoxyethanol and 1-*tert*-butoxypropan-2-ol. IARC monographs on the evaluation of carcinogenic risks to human. Lyon, France: World Health Organization; 2006. p. 1–287.

[14] O'Brien PJ, Siraki AG, Shangari N. Aldehyde sources, metabolism, molecular toxicity mechanisms, and possible effects on human health. Crit Rev Toxicol 2005;35:609–62.

[15] Shin HW, Umber BJ, Meinardi S, Leu SY, Zaldivar F, Blake DR, et al. Acetaldehyde and hexanaldehyde from cultured white cells. J Transl Med 2009;7:31.

[16] McGhee JD, von Hippel PH. Formaldehyde as a probe of DNA structure. I. Reaction with exocyclic amino groups of DNA bases. Biochemistry 1975;14:1281–96.

[17] McGhee JD, von Hippel PH. Formaldehyde as a probe of DNA structure. II. Reaction with endocyclic imino groups of DNA bases. Biochemistry 1975;14:1297–303.

[18] McGhee JD, von Hippel PH. Formaldehyde as a probe of DNA structure. 3. Equilibrium denaturation of DNA and synthetic polynucleotides. Biochemistry 1977;16:3267–76.

[19] McGhee JD, von Hippel PH. Formaldehyde as a probe of DNA structure. r. Mechanism of the initial reaction of Formaldehyde with DNA. Biochemistry 1977;16:3276–93.

[20] Casanova M, Heck Hd A. Further studies of the metabolic incorporation and covalent binding of inhaled [3H]- and [14C]formaldehyde in Fischer-344 rats: effects of glutathione depletion. Toxicol Appl Pharmacol 1987;89:105–21.

[21] Heck Hd A, Casanova M. Isotope effects and their implications for the covalent binding of inhaled [3H]- and [14C]formaldehyde in the rat nasal mucosa. Toxicol Appl Pharmacol 1987;89:122–34.

[22] Merk O, Speit G. Significance of formaldehyde-induced DNA-protein crosslinks for mutagenesis. Environ Mol Mutagen 1998;32:260–8.

[23] Merk O, Speit G. Detection of crosslinks with the comet assay in relationship to genotoxicity and cytotoxicity. Environ Mol Mutagen 1999;33:167–72.

[24] Quievryn G, Zhitkovich A. Loss of DNA-protein crosslinks from formaldehyde-exposed cells occurs through spontaneous hydrolysis and an active repair process linked to proteasome function. Carcinogenesis 2000;21:1573–80.

[25] Solomon MJ, Varshavsky A. Formaldehyde-mediated DNA-protein crosslinking: a probe for in vivo chromatin structures. Proc Natl Acad Sci USA 1985;82:6470–4.

[26] Solomon MJ, Larsen PL, Varshavsky A. Mapping protein-DNA interactions in vivo with formaldehyde: evidence that histone H4 is retained on a highly transcribed gene. Cell 1988;53:937–47.

[27] Lu K, Ye W, Gold A, Ball LM, Swenberg JA. Formation of *S*-[1-(*N*2-deoxyguanosinyl)methyl]glutathione between glutathione and DNA induced by formaldehyde. J Am Chem Soc 2009;131:3414–5.

[28] Lu K, Collins LB, Ru H, Bermudez E, Swenberg JA. Distribution of DNA adducts caused by inhaled formaldehyde is consistent with induction of nasal carcinoma but not leukemia. Toxicol Sci 2010;116:441–51.

[29] Hecht SS, McIntee EJ, Wang M. New DNA adducts of crotonaldehyde and acetaldehyde. Toxicology 2001;166:31–6.

[30] Garcia CC, Angeli JP, Freitas FP, Gomes OF, de Oliveira TF, Loureiro AP, et al. [13C2]-Acetaldehyde promotes unequivocal formation of 1,N2-propano-2'-deoxyguanosine in human cells. J Am Chem Soc 2011;133:9140–3.

[31] Beane Freeman LE, Blair A, Lubin JH, Stewart PA, Hayes RB, Hoover RN, et al. Mortality from lymphohematopoietic malignancies among workers in formaldehyde industries: the National Cancer Institute Cohort. J Natl Cancer Inst 2009;101:751–61.

[32] Coggon D, Ntani G, Harris EC, Palmer KT. Upper airway cancer, myeloid leukemia, and other cancers in a cohort of British chemical workers exposed to formaldehyde. Am J Epidemiol 2014;179:1301–11.

[33] Langevin F, Crossan GP, Rosado IV Arends MJ, Patel KJ. Fancd2 counteracts the toxic effects of naturally produced aldehydes in mice. Nature 2011;475:53–8.

[34] Garaycoechea JI, Crossan GP, Langevin F, Daly M, Arends MJ, Patel KJ. Genotoxic consequences of endogenous aldehydes on mouse haematopoietic stem cell function. Nature 2012;489:571–5.

[35] Rosado IV Langevin F, Crossan GP, Takata M, Patel KJ. Formaldehyde catabolism is essential in cells deficient for the Fanconi anemia DNA-repair pathway. Nat Struct Mol Biol 2011;18:1432–4.

[36] Casanova-Schmitz M, Starr TB, Heck HD. Differentiation between metabolic incorporation and covalent binding in the labeling of macromolecules in the rat nasal mucosa and bone marrow by inhaled [14C]- and [3H]formaldehyde. Toxicol Appl Pharmacol 1984;76:26–44.

[37] Casanova M, Morgan KT, Steinhagen WH, Everitt JI, Popp JA, Heck HD. Covalent binding of inhaled formaldehyde to DNA in the respiratory tract of rhesus monkeys: pharmacokinetics, rat-to-monkey interspecies scaling, and extrapolation to man. Fundam Appl Toxicol 1991;17:409–28.

[38] Ye X, Ji Z, Wei C, McHale CM, Ding S, Thomas R, et al. Inhaled formaldehyde induces DNA-protein crosslinks and oxidative stress in bone marrow and other distant organs of exposed mice. Environ Mol Mutagen 2013;54:705–18.

[38a] Lai Y, Yu R, Hartwell H, Moeller B, Bodnar W, Swenberg J. Distribution of Endogenous and Exogenous Formaldehyde-Induced DNA-Protein Crosslinks. Cancer Res. 2016.

[39] Lu K, Ye W, Zhou L, Collins LB, Chen X, Gold A, et al. Structural characterization of formaldehyde-induced cross-links between amino acids and deoxynucleosides and their oligomers. J Am Chem Soc 2010;132:3388–99.

[40] Lu K, Moeller B, Doyle-Eisele M, McDonald J, Swenberg JA. Molecular dosimetry of N2-hydroxymethyl-dG DNA adducts in rats exposed to formaldehyde. Chem Res Toxicol 2011;24:159–61.

[41] Moeller BC, Lu K, Doyle-Eisele M, McDonald J, Gigliotti A, Swenberg JA. Determination of N2-hydroxymethyl-dG adducts in the nasal epithelium and bone marrow of nonhuman primates following 13CD2-formaldehyde inhalation exposure. Chem Res Toxicol 2011;24:162–4.

[42] Yu R, Lai Y, Hartwell HJ, Moeller BC, Doyle-Eisele M, Kracko D, et al. Formation, accumulation and hydrolysis of endogenous and exogenous formaldehyde induced DNA damage. Toxicol Sci 2015;146:170–82.

[43] Lu K, Gul H, Upton PB, Moeller BC, Swenberg JA. Formation of hydroxymethyl DNA adducts in rats orally exposed to stable isotope labeled methanol. Toxicol Sci 2012;126:28–38.

[44] Formaldehyde CtRCsDIAo. Review of the environmental protection agency's draft IRIS assessment of formaldehyde. Washington, DC: The National Academies Press; 2011.

[45] Moeller BC, Recio L, Green A, Sun W, Wright FA, Bodnar WM, et al. Biomarkers of exposure and effect in human lymphoblastoid TK6 cells following [13C2]-acetaldehyde exposure. Toxicol Sci 2013;133:1–12.

[46] Budinsky R, Gollapudi B, Albertini RJ, Valentine R, Stavanja M, Teeguarden J, et al. Nonlinear responses for chromosome and gene level effects induced by vinyl acetate monomer and its metabolite, acetaldehyde in TK6 cells. Environ Mol Mutagen 2013;54:755–68.

[47] Doak SH, Jenkins GJ, Johnson GE, Quick E, Parry EM, Parry JM. Mechanistic influences for mutation induction curves after exposure to DNA-reactive carcinogens. Cancer Res 2007;67:3904–11.

[48] Thomas AD, Jenkins GJ, Kaina B, Bodger OG, Tomaszowski KH, Lewis PD, et al. Influence of DNA repair on nonlinear dose-responses for mutation. Toxicol Sci 2013;132:87–95.

[49] Nakamura J, Gul H, Tian X, Bultman SJ, Swenberg JA. Detection of PIGO-deficient cells using proaerolysin: a valuable tool to investigate mechanisms of mutagenesis in the DT40 cell system. PLoS One 2012;7:e33563.

[50] Singer B, Grunberger D. Molecular biology of mutagens and carcinogens. New York, NY: Plenum Press; 1983.

[51] Gates KS, Nooner T, Dutta S. Biologically relevant chemical reactions of *N*7-alkylguanine residues in DNA. Chem Res Toxicol 2004;17:839–56.

[52] Suzuki MM, Bird A. DNA methylation landscapes: provocative insights from epigenomics. Nat Rev Genet 2008;9:465–76.

[53] Xiao B, Jing C, Wilson JR, Walker PA, Vasisht N, Kelly G, et al. Structure and catalytic mechanism of the human histone methyltransferase SET7/9. Nature 2003;421:652–6.

[54] Klungland A, Laake K, Hoff E, Seeberg E. Spectrum of mutations induced by methyl and ethyl methanesulfonate at the HPRT locus of normal and tag expressing Chinese hamster fibroblasts. Carcinogenesis 1995;16:1281–5.

[55] Kaina B, Ochs K, Grosch S, Fritz G, Lips J, Tomicic M, et al. BER, MGMT, and MMR in defense against alkylation-induced genotoxicity and apoptosis. Prog Nucleic Acid Res Mol Biol 2001;68:41–54.

[56] Gocke E, Muller L. In vivo studies in the mouse to define a threshold for the genotoxicity of EMS and ENU. Mutat Res 2009;678:101–7.

[57] Parthasarathy R, Fridey SM. Conformation of *O*6-alkylguanosines: molecular mechanism of mutagenesis. Carcinogenesis 1986;7:221–7.

[58] Hickman MJ, Samson LD. Apoptotic signaling in response to a single type of DNA lesion, *O*(6)-methylguanine. Mol Cell 2004;14:105–16.

[59] Tano K, Shiota S, Collier J, Foote RS, Mitra S. Isolation and structural characterization of a cDNA clone encoding the human DNA repair protein for *O*6-alkylguanine. Proc Natl Acad Sci USA 1990;87:686–90.

[60] Engelbergs J, Thomale J, Galhoff A, Rajewsky MF. Fast repair of *O*6-ethylguanine, but not *O*6-methylguanine, in transcribed genes prevents mutation of H-ras in rat mammary tumorigenesis induced by ethylnitrosourea in place of methylnitrosourea. Proc Natl Acad Sci USA 1998;95:1635–40.

[61] Sharma V, Collins LB, Clement JM, Zhang Z, Nakamura J, Swenberg JA. Molecular dosimetry of endogenous and exogenous *O*(6)-methyl-dG and *N*7-methyl-G adducts following low dose [D3]-methylnitrosourea exposures in cultured human cells. Chem Res Toxicol 2014;27:480–2.

[62] Kohen R, Nyska A. Oxidation of biological systems: oxidative stress phenomena, antioxidants, redox reactions, and methods for their quantification. Toxicol Pathol 2002;30:620–50.

[63] Jenkins GJ, Zair Z, Johnson GE, Doak SH. Genotoxic thresholds, DNA repair, and susceptibility in human populations. Toxicology 2010;278:305–10.

[64] Seager AL, Shah UK, Mikhail JM, Nelson BC, Marquis BJ, Doak SH, et al. Pro-oxidant induced DNA damage in human lymphoblastoid cells: homeostatic mechanisms of genotoxic tolerance. Toxicol Sci 2012;128:387–97.

[65] Platel A, Nesslany F, Gervais V, Claude N, Marzin D. Study of oxidative DNA damage in TK6 human lymphoblastoid cells by use of the thymidine kinase gene-mutation assay and the in vitro modified comet assay: determination of no-observed-genotoxic-effect-levels. Mutat Res 2011;726:151–9.

[66] Platel A, Nesslany F, Gervais V, Marzin D. Study of oxidative DNA damage in TK6 human lymphoblastoid cells by use of the in vitro micronucleus test: determination of no-observed-effect levels. Mutat Res 2009;678:30–7.

[67] Morinello EJ, Ham AJ, Ranasinghe A, Nakamura J, Upton PB, Swenberg JA. Molecular dosimetry and repair of *N*(2),3-ethenoguanine in rats exposed to vinyl chloride. Cancer Res 2002;62:5189–95.

[68] Mutlu E, Collins LB, Stout MD, Upton PB, Daye LR, Winsett D, et al. Development and application of an LC-MS/MS method for the detection of the vinyl chloride-induced DNA adduct N(2),3-ethenoguanine in tissues of adult and weanling rats following exposure to [(13)C(2)]-VC. Chem Res Toxicol 2010;23:1485–91.

[69] Jeong YC, Walker NJ, Burgin DE, Kissling G, Gupta M, Kupper L, et al. Accumulation of M1dG DNA adducts after chronic exposure to PCBs, but not from acute exposure to polychlorinated aromatic hydrocarbons. Free Radic Biol Med 2008;45:585–91.

[70] IARC. Radiation. IARC monographs on the evaluation of carcinogenic risks to human. Lyon, France: World Health Organization; 2012. p. 103–230.

[71] Council NR. Health risks from exposure to low levels of ionizing radiation: BEIR VII phase 2. Washington, DC: The National Academies Press; 2006.

[72] Olipitz W, Wiktor-Brown D, Shuga J, Pang B, McFaline J, Lonkar P, et al. Integrated molecular analysis indicates undetectable change in DNA damage in mice after continuous irradiation at ~400-fold natural background radiation. Environ Health Perspect 2012;120:1130–6.

[73] Osipov AN, Klokov DY, Elakov AL, Rozanova OM, Zaichkina SI, Aptikaeva GF, et al. Comparison in vivo study of genotoxic action of high- versus very low dose-rate gamma-irradiation. Nonlinearity Biol Toxicol Med 2004;2:223–32.

[74] Velegzhaninov IO, Shadrin DM, Pylina YI, Ermakova AV, Shostal OA, Belykh ES, et al. Differential molecular stress responses to low compared to high doses of ionizing radiation in normal human fibroblasts. Dose-Response 2015;13:1–22.

[75] Elhajouji A, Lukamowicz M, Cammerer Z, Kirsch-Volders M. Potential thresholds for genotoxic effects by micronucleus scoring. Mutagenesis 2011;26:199–204.

[76] Calabrese EJ. Key studies used to support cancer risk assessment questioned. Environ Mol Mutagen 2011;52:595–606.

[77] Pollycove M, Feinendegen LE. Radiation-induced versus endogenous DNA damage: possible effect of inducible protective responses in mitigating endogenous damage. Hum Exp Toxicol 2003;22:290–306. discussion 7, 15–7, 19–23.

[78] Calabrese EJ. Origin of the linearity no threshold (LNT) dose-response concept. Arch Toxicol 2013;87:1621–33.

[79] Lynn FM. The interplay of science and values in assessing and regulating environmental risks. Sci Technol Hum Val 1986;11:40–50.

[80] Starr TB, Swenberg JA. A novel bottom-up approach to bounding low-dose human cancer risks from chemical exposures. Regul Toxicol Pharmacol 2013;65:311–5.

[81] Evans JS, Graham JD, Gray GM, Sielken Jr. RL. A distributional approach to characterizing low-dose cancer risk. Risk Anal 1994;14:25–34.

[82] Evans JS, Gray GM, Sielken Jr. RL, Smith AE, Valdez-Flores C, Graham JD. Use of probabilistic expert judgment in uncertainty analysis of carcinogenic potency. Regul Toxicol Pharmacol 1994;20:15–36.

[83] Small MJ. Methods for assessing uncertainty in fundamental assumptions and associated models for cancer risk assessment. Risk Anal 2008;28:1289–308.

[84] Pearl J. Probabilistic reasoning in intelligent systems: networks of plausible inference. San Francisco, CA: Morgan Kaufmann Publishers, Inc.; 1988.

[85] Weber P, Medina-Oliva G, Simon C, Iung B. Overview on Bayesian networks applications for dependability, risk analysis and maintenance areas. Eng Appl Artif Intel 2012;25:671–82.

[86] Poolsappasit N, Dewri R, Ray I. Dynamic security risk management using Bayesian attack graphs. IEEE Trans Depend Secure Comput 2012;9:61–674.

[87] Zheng B, Ramalingam P, Hariharan H, Leader JK, Gur D. Prediction of near-term breast cancer risk using a Bayesian belief network. In: Abbey CK, Mello-Thoms CR, editors. Medical Imaging 2013: Image Perception, Observer Performance, and Technology Assessment. SPIE; 2013. p. 86731F-F-7.

[88] Liao Y, Wang J, Guo Y, Zheng X. Risk assessment of human neural tube defects using a Bayesian belief network. Stoch Environ Res Risk Assess 2010;24:93–100.

[89] McCann RK, Marcot BG, Ellis R. Bayesian belief networks: applications in ecology and natural resource management. Can J For Res 2006;36:3053–62.

[90] Villeneuve DL, Crump D, Garcia-Reyero N, Hecker M, Hutchinson TH, LaLone CA, et al. Adverse outcome pathway (AOP) development I: strategies and principles. Toxicol Sci 2014;142:312–20.

[91] Gat-Viks I, Tanay A, Raijman D, Shamir R. A probabilistic methodology for integrating knowledge and experiments on biological networks. J Comput Biol 2006;13:165–81.

[92] Stojadinovic A, Nissan A, Eberhardt J, Chua TC, Pelz JO, Esquivel J. Development of a Bayesian Belief Network Model for personalized prognostic risk assessment in colon carcinomatosis. Am Surg 2011;77:221–30.

CHAPTER 7

Thresholds of Toxicological Concern for Genotoxic Impurities in Pharmaceuticals

Masamitsu Honma

Division of Genetics and Mutagenesis, National Institute of Health Sciences, Tokyo, Japan

Chapter Outline

Introduction   103
Genotoxic and Nongenotoxic Carcinogens   104
Thresholds of Chemical Genotoxicity   105
Risk Management for Genotoxic Carcinogens   107
Risk Assessment and Control of Genotoxic Impurities in Pharmaceuticals   109
    Principles for Assessment and Control of Genotoxic Impurities in Pharmaceuticals   109
    Less-Than-Lifetime TTC   112
    Compound-Specific TTC   112
Conclusion   114
References   114

Introduction

Food safety is a common concern among people and is assessed in terms of the health effects of trace amounts of chemical substances such as residual pesticides and food additives. Moreover, potential risks of various substances have been assessed using a dose–response model that determines a safety threshold; acceptable daily intakes (ADIs) are calculated from thresholds below which no adverse effects are observed [1]. These procedures are, however, problematic for assessments of potential genotoxicity, because, unlike other toxicities, thresholds cannot be established for genotoxicity. Therefore, ADI cannot be determined, and health risks cannot be ruled out for any nonzero intake of genotoxic substances.

The term "genotoxicity" is broad and ambiguous. Genotoxic agents damage DNA and/or the cellular components that regulate genome integrity. In contrast, mutagenic substances induce permanent transmissible changes comprising numerical or structural alterations of DNA or chromosomes [2]. Therefore, mutagenicity is a consequence of DNA or chromosome

Thresholds of Genotoxic Carcinogens.
DOI: http://dx.doi.org/10.1016/B978-0-12-801663-3.00007-8

damage (mutations), whereas genotoxicity, in addition, manifests as transient changes in DNA or chromosome structures. However, unlike other toxicities, such as hepatotoxicity and neurotoxicity, the consequences of genotoxicity are not physiologically recognized and do not often manifest as lesions or symptoms. Nonetheless, genotoxicity is a primary etiological factor in the development of cancers and various genetic disorders, and a genotoxicity test reveals the genotoxic potential of chemical substances.

Because DNA is the primary genetic material in all organisms, various species, ranging from bacteria to mammals, have been used to develop genotoxicity tests. Endpoints of these tests include DNA damage, gene mutations, and changes in the structure or number of chromosomes. These tests include the Ames test, chromosomal aberration test, and in vivo micronucleus assays and are obligatory for the safety assessments of various chemicals, including pharmaceuticals, industrial and agricultural chemicals, and food additives [3–6]. Genotoxicity tests are generally qualitative, and results are often presented as positive or negative [7]. Because toxicity generally depends on the degree of exposure, dichotomous and categorical variables fail to offer thresholds for genotoxicity.

Genotoxic and Nongenotoxic Carcinogens

Although genotoxicity tests are often used to screen potentially carcinogenic chemicals, these do not necessarily indicate carcinogenicity. The correlation between genotoxicity and rodent carcinogenicity ranged from 60% to 80% depending on the test system [8]. Although genotoxicity tests have been designed to detect as many carcinogens as possible, some carcinogens do not elicit a positive genotoxic effect and are classified as nongenotoxic carcinogens. Although cancer is always associated with genetic changes, nongenotoxic carcinogens may promote carcinogenesis through alternative nongenetic mechanisms such as accelerating the growth of naturally occurring precarcinogenic cells.

Highly genotoxic chemicals include the known potent carcinogens benzo(a)pyrene, aflatoxin B_1, N-nitroso compounds, and various alkylating agents that directly act on DNA, causing breakage and cross-linking, and the formation of DNA adducts, abasic sites, oxidative damage, alkylation, and various other DNA lesions [9]. These chemicals generate mutations and chromosome alterations with high probability, whereas other genotoxic chemicals shown below do not directly act on DNA. For example, colchicine inhibits tubulin polymerization and results in numerical chromosome aberrations during cell division [10]. Chemicals that inhibit DNA repair, suppress apoptosis, or disrupt the cell cycle by targeting specific proteins may also show positive effects in genotoxicity tests and are defined as non-DNA-damaging genotoxic chemicals. Moreover, genotoxic mechanisms are unknown for various chemicals with demonstrated in vitro genotoxicity. Therefore, the positive genotoxicity may reflect secondary effects, such as severe cytotoxicity, high osmotic pressure, formation of precipitates, or nonphysiological pH [11], warranting careful performance of these tests.

Identification of genotoxic chemical substances requires multiple assessments using different tests with consideration of test conditions and degrees of response.

Thresholds of Chemical Genotoxicity

A genotoxic chemical reacts with DNA, inducing a gene mutation. A single mutation may initiate carcinogenesis, if it occurs on specific genes that are important for malignant transformation, such as oncogenes and tumor suppressor genes. Mutations are stochastic, and because mutation frequencies can never be reduced to zero, the possibility of carcinogenesis can never be eliminated. Therefore, it is theoretically impossible to establish an absolute threshold for genotoxic carcinogens [12].

Nongenotoxic carcinogens generally act on proteins. In contrast to the presence of only one or two copies of genes in cells, protein molecules are present in large numbers in cells, and thus high concentrations of nongenotoxic carcinogens elicit effects through interactions with many protein molecules. At low concentrations, they react with only a few key protein molecules, not resulting in carcinogenicity. This mechanistic idea suggests that theoretical thresholds are relevant to nongenotoxic carcinogens that act through proteins.

Thresholds for carcinogenicity, genotoxicity, and the formation of DNA adducts following exposure to genotoxic carcinogens have been investigated in various animal models. In particular, administration of aflatoxin B_1 or benzo(a)pyrene to animals led to dose-dependent formation of DNA adducts in liver. Moreover, recent advances in mass spectrometric technology allow detection of DNA adducts at one one-hundredth of their normal human exposures, and dose-dependent DNA adduct responses are evident even at an extremely low doses [13]. Because DNA adducts are formed in chemical reactions, no threshold can be applied, and DNA adducts occur at any concentration of DNA-reactive chemical. However, genotoxicity refers to a biological effect, and corresponding thresholds can only be identified in animal models following stepwise reductions of effective doses until no effect is observed. Similarly, thresholds of gene mutation are demonstrated at doses that do not increase the mutation frequency above spontaneous levels. These experiments are performed using dilutions of doses ranging from 1000- to 100,000-fold, and the data are often expressed logarithmically. Fig. 7.1 illustrates a linear dose-response ($y = ax + b$) and its corresponding logarithmic plot. Although no threshold is present in either of the graphs, the appearance of the logarithmic plot leads to misinterpretation of the actual shape of the response [14], particularly in the low-dose range where dose increments do not result in significant differences in biological responses. At these levels, low statistical power, detection limits, and variability of spontaneous mutation rates preclude identification of responses and obscure thresholds. Practical thresholds that are established in this way often reflect the sensitivity of the experimental tests rather than biological effects. Hence, thresholds are not demonstrable by the absence of detectable genotoxicity.

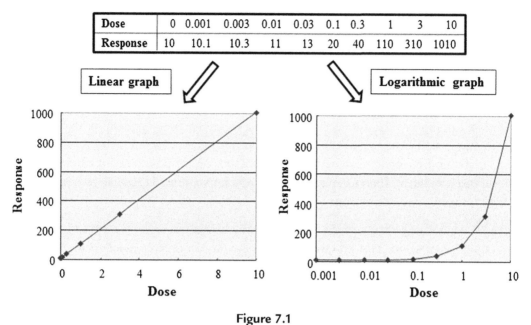

Dose	0	0.001	0.003	0.01	0.03	0.1	0.3	1	3	10
Response	10	10.1	10.3	11	13	20	40	110	310	1010

Figure 7.1

Linear and logarithmic plots of a linear dose-response ($y = ax + b$); although no threshold is present in either graph, the appearance of the logarithmic plot is suggestive of a threshold.

Another line of logic demonstrating the existence of genotoxic thresholds is as follows: genotoxic responses observed at extremely low-dose ranges cannot be linearly extrapolated from those at higher doses because of the efficacy of defense mechanisms at lower doses. Although the defense mechanisms such as DNA repair, metabolic detoxification, and scavenging of oxygen radicals [15] can reduce genotoxicity, however, their actions may not be considered evidence of absolute thresholds. Base excision repair removes small DNA adducts with high integrity, whereas mutations causing errors occur at a rate of 10^{-6}. Accordingly, Yasui et al. have developed a targeted mutagenesis system for tracing DNA adducts and investigated consequences of the 8-*oxo*-7,8-dihydroguanine (8-*oxo*-G) adduct, which is a typical product of oxidative DNA damage in human genomes [16]. These experiments demonstrated that single 8-*oxo*-G adducts invariably induce GT transversions, and mutation frequencies were not reduced to zero following overexpression of MutY homologs that prevent transversions by performing base excision repair [17]. These observations indicate that only single 8-*oxo*-G adducts produce high-probability gene mutations in the human genome, but that DNA repair mechanisms do not establish a threshold of genotoxicity through 8-*oxo*-G.

Similarly, there is no evidence that metabolic detoxification or scavenger mechanisms always function at 100% efficiency. Thus, it is impossible to determine absolute thresholds for demonstrably genotoxic carcinogens, particularly when assessed in target tissues. Thus, no ADI can currently be established for genotoxic carcinogens.

Risk Management for Genotoxic Carcinogens

In the United States in 1958, sales of processed foods containing residual amounts of agricultural chemicals that were carcinogenic to animals were prohibited by the Delaney Clause, which stated that the Secretary of the Food and Drug Administration (FDA) "shall not approve for use in food any chemical additive found to induce cancer in man, or, after tests, found to induce cancer in animals." The Delaney Clause was later extended to cover colorants, animal drugs, and feed. However, the ensuing concept of zero risk was later contradicted by (1) advances in analytical technologies that have systematically lowered detection limits and thereby safety levels. Moreover, (2) because carcinogenicity was considered in isolation, potentially useful compounds with low toxicity were banned because of weak carcinogenicity. In addition, (3) only manufactured chemicals were assessed for carcinogenicity, and naturally occurring carcinogens were neglected. (4) The carcinogenicity test results in high-dose animal experiments were not in complete agreement with those in humans exposed at environmental or occupational levels. To focus limited resources on issues of tangible concern, the FDA changed the policy in 1995 and introduced a "Threshold of Regulation" policy for food contact materials. Accordingly, the agency developed an approach to set a threshold for food packaging applications that was intended to protect against all types of toxicity including carcinogenicity and promised that below-threshold exposure to an individual chemical came "with reasonable certainty of no harm." Finally, the Delaney Clause was abolished in favor of the Food Quality Protection Act of 1996.

In contrast to risk management using zero-risk thresholds, concentrations of carcinogenic chemicals can be sufficiently low, regardless of genotoxicity, to ensure very low potential carcinogenicity of products. A substance can be regarded as virtually safe if the risk level is socially acceptable, giving rise to the "virtually safe dose" (VSD) for which risk is described as "negligible" or "acceptable" [7]. Accordingly, a one in a million (10^{-6}) lifetime risk of cancer may be acceptable, because in a population of 10^8 individuals with a life expectancy of 80 years (as is the case in Japan), this increment of risk is associated with $10^8 \times 1/80 \times 10^{-6}$ (1.25) cancer-related deaths per year. Cancer is now the leading cause of mortality in developed countries, with 350,000 cancer-related deaths per year in Japan. Hence, a one in a million increment of risk can be considered negligible and acceptable. VSDs are generally calculated using multistage models or by linear extrapolation from doses that cause cancer in 50% of test animals (TD_{50}; Fig. 7.2A). Gold et al. have compiled a carcinogenic potency database (CPDB) of nearly 700 chemical carcinogens that had been tested in animals using lifetime exposures [18]. Subsequently, TD_{50} distributions were transformed by sliding the curve to the left, and exposures that represented an estimated lifetime cancer risk of one in a million were calculated to determine VSDs (Fig. 7.2B).

Assuming that risks in animals are representative of those in humans, the distribution of carcinogenic potencies can be used to estimate a dietary concentration that is associated with less than a one in a million lifetime cancer risk for most carcinogens. In a study by

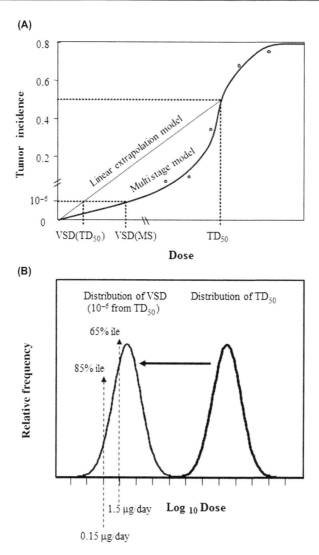

Figure 7.2

(A) Calculation of the virtually safety dose (VSD) by extrapolation from the chronic dose that induces tumors in 50% of test animals (TD_{50}). This calculation could be performed with either linear extrapolation or multistage models. The VSD causing a one in a million (10^{-6}) lifetime risk of cancer could be acceptable and is calculated as follows: $VSD = TD_{50}/50{,}000 \times 50\,kg$. The weight adjustment assumes an arbitrary adult human body weight for either sex of 50 kg. (B) Distributions of TD_{50}s and dietary concentrations for 709 carcinogens at the one in one million risk level.

Cheeseman et al., this exposure level was estimated at 0.5 μg/kg of diet [19] or 1.5 μg/day assuming that carcinogenic chemicals are present at constant concentrations and that the daily dietary intake per person is 3 kg (1.5 kg of food and 1.5 kg of fluids daily; [20]). This indicates that most chemicals, including carcinogens, are unlikely to be injurious to human health when the daily intake is below 1.5 µg/day. This comprehensive threshold is termed the "threshold of toxicological concern" (TTC; [21]).

The TTC can be applied to numerous chemicals of known and unknown toxicity, and, in Japan, a positive list system for agricultural chemical residues was enforced in 2006 according to the Food Sanitation Act. Under this system, a limit of 0.01 ppm was stipulated for agricultural chemical residues for which standard residual limits had not been established. This value is based on both the TTC (1.5 µg/day) and a national nutrition survey showing that the daily intake of any agricultural or livestock product, excluding rice, does not exceed 150 g (1.5/150 = 0.01). The TTC is also used by the FDA to manage risks associated with chemicals leached from plastic containers (indirect additives; [22]) and was applied to food-flavoring agents by the Joint FAO/WHO Expert Committee on Food Additives [23]. However, the TTC may not be appropriate for all classes of genotoxic carcinogens. Kroes et al. have compared more than 700 carcinogenic chemicals and suggested that some genotoxic chemicals with suspect structures posed a high carcinogenic risk at 1.5 µg/day [24]. Subsequently, it was recommended that the TTC for genotoxic compounds be reduced by one-tenth to 0.15 µg/day with a lifetime risk of 10^{-6}. Moreover, aflatoxins, azoxy compounds, and nitroso compounds were identified as extremely potent genotoxic carcinogens for which the TTC is not applicable. These compounds have since been included in the "cohort of concern" (COC) and require individual toxicity data and risk management strategies [19].

Risk Assessment and Control of Genotoxic Impurities in Pharmaceuticals

Principles for Assessment and Control of Genotoxic Impurities in Pharmaceuticals

Residual impurities from manufacturing and formulation processes or degradation of active pharmaceutical ingredients are often present in synthetic pharmaceutical products. Some of these impurities are potentially genotoxic and pose additional safety concerns. The International Conference on Harmonization (ICH) of Technical Requirements for Registration of Pharmaceuticals for Human Use guideline on impurity evaluation (Q3A/B) provides guidance on how to identify genotoxic impurities but does not indicate acceptable levels. Accordingly, guidelines for the management of genotoxic impurities in pharmaceuticals from the European Medicines Agency in 2006 and the US-FDA in 2008 [25,26] widely acknowledged deficiencies of the impurity assessments in Q3A/B and development of the new ICH guidance was initiated. Subsequently, the new guideline (ICH-M7), entitled *Assessment and Control of DNA-Reactive (Mutagenic) Impurities in Pharmaceuticals to Limit Potential Carcinogenic Risk*, was finalized in Jun. 2014. It addresses various methods for characterizing mutagenic hazards of impurities in pharmaceuticals, and gives risk assessment considering potential lifetime cancer risks that are associated with patient exposures to genotoxic impurities during clinical development and after approval [27].

The ICH-M7 guideline focuses on substances that have the potential to directly damage DNA when present at low levels and usually invokes the Ames mutagenicity. On the other hand, nonmutagenic chemicals without Ames mutagenicity are out of the focus, because they have threshold mechanisms and usually do not pose carcinogenic risks in humans at the level ordinarily present as impurities. Computational toxicology assessments using quantitative structure–activity relationship (QSAR) methodologies may be predictive of Ames mutagenicity outcomes based on established knowledge.

The ICH-M7 guideline also uses the TTC to define acceptable intakes of unassessed pharmaceutical impurities that pose negligible risks of carcinogenicity or other toxic effects. Accordingly, the acceptable limit of mutagenic impurities in drug substances and drug products was set at 1.5 µg/day and corresponds to a theoretical 10^{-5} excess lifetime risk of cancer, which is 10× higher than that for genotoxic chemicals in foods. The higher exposure limits for pharmaceuticals are justified by their benefits, and by the fact that exposure is intentional and is unusually sustained for a lifetime. Given the lifetime risk of cancer in populations of developed countries, this TTC remains highly conservative. However, structural classes of mutagens with extremely high carcinogenic potency (COC), such as aflatoxin-, N-nitroso-, and alkyl-azoxy-like structures, require significantly lower acceptable intakes than the default TTC level.

Although mutagenic impurities must be reduced to less than the TTC or to an appropriate acceptable level, further hazard assessments may be warranted, and it is recommended that impurities are tested using in vivo gene mutation assays to confirm the relevance of bacterial mutagenicity under in vivo conditions. Such in vivo studies should be designed with consideration of existing ICH genotoxicity guidelines (S2R1).

In Fig. 7.3, a decision tree for hazard assessment and control of mutagenic impurities in pharmaceuticals is presented according to the ICH-M7 guideline. In this scheme, hazard assessments are initiated as database and literature searches for carcinogenicity and Ames mutagenicity data. Subsequently, impurities are classified into five categories according to Table 7.1, and known mutagenic carcinogens (Class 1) and mutagens (Class 2) require control below TTC levels or compound-specific acceptable levels. If a lack of mutagenic or carcinogenic activities of impurities is demonstrated with sufficient data (Class 5) or is indicated by mutagenicity tests of structure-related compounds (Class 4), the chemical can be treated as a nonmutagenic impurity. If data for such a classification are not available (Class 3), impurities should be controlled as Class 1 and 2 chemicals, or QSAR assessments should be conducted for predicting Ames mutagenicity. When negative predictions of two QSAR methodologies (expert rule-based and statistical) are sufficient to conclude that the impurity is of no mutagenic concern, no further testing is recommended (Class 5). Potential mutagenicity indicated by QSAR analyses is followed up using Ames mutagenicity assays, and QSAR concerns can be considered negligible after negative Ames mutagenicity assays.

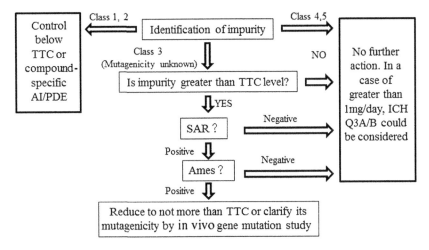

Figure 7.3

Decision tree for hazard assessment and control of mutagenic impurities of pharmaceuticals according to the ICH-M7 guideline.

Table 7.1 Impurities classification with respect to mutagenic and carcinogenic potential and resulting control actions.

Class	Definition	Proposed Action for Control (details in Section 7 and 8)
1	Known mutagenic carcinogens	Control at or below compound-specific acceptable limit
2	Known mutagens with unknown carcinogenic potential (bacterial mutagenicity positive[a], no rodent carcinogenicity data)	Control at or below acceptable limits (appropriate TTC)
3	Alerting structure, unrelated to the structure of the drug substance; nonmutagenicity data	Control at or below acceptable limits (appropriate TTC) or conduct bacterial mutagenicity assay If nonmutagenic = Class 5 If mutagenic = Class 2
4	Alerting structure, same alert in drug substance or compounds related to the drug substance (eg, process intermediates) which have been tested and are nonmutagenic	Treat as nonmutagenic impurity
5	No structural alerts, or alerting structure with sufficient data to demonstrate lack of mutagenicity or carcinogenicity	Treat as nonmutagenic impurity

[a]Or other relevant positive mutagenicity data indicative of DNA reactivity–related induction of gene mutations (eg, positive findings in in vivo gene mutation studies).

In contrast, Ames mutagenicity assays indicate the need for control of impurities as Class 2 chemicals, or warrant further in vivo hazard assessment. For nonmutagenic impurities (Classes 4 and 5) that are present at less than 1 mg, no further genotoxicity testing is required regardless of other qualification thresholds. However, for impurities that are present in excess of 1 mg in daily doses for chronic administration, evaluation of genotoxic potential should be performed as recommended in ICH Q3A/B.

Less-Than-Lifetime TTC

The TTC of 1.5 μg/day for mutagenic impurities in pharmaceuticals was established assuming lifetime exposure and lacks relevance to short-term exposures. Hence, a less-than-lifetime (LTL) TTC concept for mutagenic impurities in pharmaceuticals was originally developed as a series of staged TTC limits for clinical development [28]. Accordingly, the ICH-M7 guideline was expanded to advise on LTL-TTC for pharmaceuticals under clinical development and for marketed products.

Standard risk assessments of known carcinogens assume that cancer risk increases as a function of cumulative doses. Hence, LTL-TTC values are calculated according to Haber's rule (dose × duration = cumulative dose), which is a fundamental concept in carcinogenesis [29]. For constant cumulative doses, the carcinogenic effect is equal based on the dose and duration of exposure, and the acceptable cumulative lifetime dose (1.5 μg/day × 25,550 days = 38.3 mg) is uniformly distributed over the total number of LTL exposure days (Fig. 7.4). The dashed step-shaped curve in Fig. 7.4 represents measured daily intake levels adjusted to LTL exposure, as recommended by the ICH-M7 guideline for agents under clinical development and for marketed products. These proposed levels are generally significantly lower than calculated values, thus providing safety margins that increase with shorter treatment durations (Table 7.2). The proposed accepted daily intakes are also in compliance with a 10^{-6} cancer risk level for treatment durations of <6 months and are therefore relevant to early clinical trials in which benefits have not yet been established. However, under these conditions, the safety factors shown in the upper graph of Fig. 7.4 would be reduced by a factor of 10 to allow higher daily intakes of mutagenic impurities than for lifetime exposures but with comparable risk levels for daily and nondaily treatment regimens.

Compound-Specific TTC

Compound-specific calculations of acceptable intakes can be performed without carcinogenicity data for mutagens with structural similarities to chemically defined classes of known carcinogens. In a recent study, chemicals with structural alerts for mutagenicity during drug synthesis were compared with mutagenic carcinogens in the CPDB, and structural classifications with lower carcinogenic potency than those used to derive the TTC were confirmed. Hence, ADIs that are higher than the default TTC level (1.5 μg/day) can be

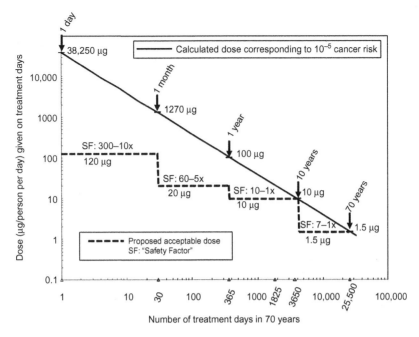

Figure 7.4

Illustration of calculated daily doses of mutagenic impurities corresponding to a theoretical 1 in 10^{-5} cancer risk as a function of treatment duration compared with acceptable intake levels. The solid line represents the linear relationship between the daily intake of a mutagenic impurity that corresponds to a 1 in 10^{-5} cancer risk and the number of treatment days. The dashed step-shaped curve represents measured daily intake levels adjusted to less-than-lifetime exposures as recommended in the ICH-M7 guideline (Table 7.2).

Table 7.2 Acceptable intakes for an individual impurity.

Duration of Treatment	≤1 Month	>1–12 Months	>1–10 Years	>10 Years to Lifetime
Daily intake (µg/day)	120	20	10	1.5

established for many structural classes [30]. For example, monofunctional alkyl chlorides are commonly used in drug synthesis and have comparatively low TD_{50} values of 36–1810 mg/kg per day [31]. A TD_{50} value of 36 mg/kg per day remains a conservative class-specific potency reference point for calculation of acceptable intakes of monofunctional alkyl chlorides and is at least 10-fold lower than the TD_{50} of 1.25 mg/kg per day that corresponds with the default lifetime TTC of 1.5 µg/day. Hence, lifetime and LTL daily intakes of monofunctional alkyl chlorides could be 10-fold greater than default values without consequence.

Conclusion

Residual impurities from manufacture and formulation or from degradation of active pharmaceutical ingredients may be present in synthetic pharmaceutical products. Because of the potential carcinogenicity of some impurities, additional safety concerns have been addressed in the ICH-M7 guideline, which prescribes methods for identifying mutagenic hazards and assessing cancer risks of pharmaceutical impurities. The guideline focuses on DNA reactive impurities that can be detected using Ames mutagenicity assays. Other types of genotoxic agents have threshold mechanisms that limit carcinogenic risks at the concentrations ordinarily present as impurities in pharmaceuticals. The TTC of 1.5 µg per day is currently the accepted criterion for control of mutagenic impurities, and exposures to most nonthreshold direct-acting mutagens at this level are considered safe. The ICH-M7 guidance also allows the excesses of TTC levels for mutagenic impurities with LTL exposures and of certain chemical classes. Considering the relationships between mutagenicity, genotoxicity, and carcinogenicity, these approaches are appropriate for the management of genotoxic carcinogens and operate on negligible or low-level risks that are publically acceptable rather than thresholds and concepts of zero risk.

References

[1] Lu FC, Sielken Jr RL. Assessment of safety/risk of chemicals: inception and evolution of the ADI and dose-response modeling procedures. Toxicol Lett 1991;59(1–3):5–40.

[2] Eastmond DA, Hartwig A, Anderson D, Anwar WA, Cimino MC, Dobrev I, et al. Mutagenicity testing for chemical risk assessment: update of the WHO/IPCS Harmonized Scheme. Mutagenesis 2009;24(4):341–9.

[3] Muller L, Kikuchi Y, Probst G, Schechtman L, Shimada H, Sofuni T, et al. ICH-harmonised guidances on genotoxicity testing of pharmaceuticals: evolution, reasoning and impact. Mutat Res 1999;436(3):195–225.

[4] Gollapudi BB, Krishna G. Practical aspects of mutagenicity testing strategy: an industrial perspective. Mutat Res 2000;455(1–2):21–8.

[5] Dearfield KL, Thybaud V, Cimino MC, Custer L, Czich A, Harvey JS, et al. Follow-up actions from positive results of in vitro genetic toxicity testing. Environ Mol Mutagen 2011;52(3):177–204.

[6] ICH. International conference on harmonisation of technical requirements for registration of pharmaceuticals for human use, S2A guideline. Guidance on genotoxicity testing and data interpretation for pharmaceuticals intended for human use, step 4; 1995.

[7] Rulis A. De Minimis and the threshold of regulation. In: Felix C, editor. Food protection technology. Chelsea, MI: Lewis Publishers Inc; 1986. p. 29–37.

[8] Kirkland D, Aardema M, Henderson L, Muller L. Evaluation of the ability of a battery of three in vitro genotoxicity tests to discriminate rodent carcinogens and noncarcinogens. I. Sensitivity, specificity and relative predictivity. Mutat Res 2005;584(1–2):1–256.

[9] Wogan GN, Hecht SS, Felton JS, Conney AH, Loeb LA. Environmental and chemical carcinogenesis. Semin Cancer Biol 2004;14(6):473–86.

[10] Honma M, Momose M, Sakamoto H, Sofuni T, Hayashi M. Spindle poisons induce allelic loss in mouse lymphoma cells through mitotic nondisjunction. Mutat Res 2001;493(1–2):101–14.

[11] Scott D, Galloway SM, Marshall RR, Ishidate Jr M, Brusick D, Ashby J, et al. International commission for protection against environmental mutagens and carcinogens. Genotoxicity under extreme culture conditions. A report from ICPEMC Task Group 9. Mutat Res 1991;257(2):147–205.

[12] Neumann HG. Risk assessment of chemical carcinogens and thresholds. Crit Rev Toxicol 2009;39(6):449–61.

[13] Kanaly RA, Matsui S, Hanaoka T, Matsuda T. Application of the adductome approach to assess intertissue DNA damage variations in human lung and esophagus. Mutat Res 2007;625(1–2):83–93.

[14] Gollapudi BB, Johnson GE, Hernandez LG, Pottenger LH, Dearfield KL, Jeffrey AM, et al. Quantitative approaches for assessing dose-response relationships in genetic toxicology studies. Environ Mol Mutagen 2013;54(1):8–18.

[15] Guerard M, Baum M, Bitsch A, Eisenbrand G, Elhajouji A, Epe B, et al. Assessment of mechanisms driving nonlinear dose-response relationships in genotoxicity testing. Mutat Res Rev Mutat Res 2015;763:181–201.

[16] Yasui M, Kanemaru Y, Kamoshita N, Suzuki T, Arakawa T, Honma M. Tracing the fates of site-specifically introduced DNA adducts in the human genome. DNA Repair (Amst) 2014;15:11–20.

[17] Ohtsubo T, Nishioka K, Imaiso Y, Iwai S, Shimokawa H, Oda H, et al. Identification of human MutY homolog (hMYH) as a repair enzyme for 2-hydroxyadenine in DNA and detection of multiple forms of hMYH located in nuclei and mitochondria. Nucleic Acids Res 2000;28(6):1355–64.

[18] Gold LS, Manley NB, Slone TH, Garfinkel GB, Ames BN, Rohrbach L, et al. Sixth plot of the carcinogenic potency database: results of animal bioassays published in the General Literature 1989 to 1990 and by the National Toxicology Program 1990 to 1993. Environ Health Perspect 1995;103(Suppl. 8):3–122.

[19] Cheeseman MA, Machuga EJ, Bailey AB. A tiered approach to threshold of regulation. Food Chem Toxicol 1999;37(4):387–412.

[20] EFSA. Scientific opinion on exploring options for providing advice about possible human health risks based on the concept of Threshold of Toxicological Concern (TTC). EFSA J 2012;10:2750.

[21] Munro IC. Safety assessment procedures for indirect food additives: an overview. Report of a workshop. Regul Toxicol Pharmacol 1990;12(1):2–12.

[22] FDA. Food additives; threshold of regulation for substances used in food-contact articles. Fed Regist 1995;60:36582–96.

[23] EFSA. Outcome of the public consultation on the draft EFSA opinion on exploring options for providing preliminary advice about possible human health risks based on the concept of Threshold of Toxicological Concern (TTC). EFSA J 2012.

[24] Kroes R, Renwick AG, Cheeseman M, Kleiner J, Mangelsdorf I, Piersma A, et al. European branch of the International Life Sciences I. Structure-based Thresholds of Toxicological Concern (TTC): guidance for application to substances present at low levels in the diet. Food Chem Toxicol 2004;42(1):65–83.

[25] EMEA. Evaluation of medicines for human use: guideline on the limits of genotoxic impurities, vol. CPMP/SWP/5199, 251344; 2006.

[26] FDA. Guidance for industry genotoxic and carcinogenic impurities in drug substances and products: recommended approaches. In: U.S. Department of Health and Human Services, F. a. D. A., Center for Drug Evaluation and Research (CDER), editors; 2008.

[27] ICH. Assessment and control of DNA-reactive (Mutagenic) impurities in pharmaceuticals to limit potential carcinogenic risk; M7 Step 4. In: International conference on harmonisation of technical requirements for registration of pharmaceuticals for human use; 2014.

[28] Muller L, Mauthe RJ, Riley CM, Andino MM, Antonis DD, Beels C, et al. A rationale for determining, testing, and controlling specific impurities in pharmaceuticals that possess potential for genotoxicity. Regul Toxicol Pharmacol 2006;44(3):198–211.

[29] Miller FJ, Schlosser PM, Janszen DB. Haber's rule: a special case in a family of curves relating concentration and duration of exposure to a fixed level of response for a given endpoint. Toxicology 2000;149(1):21–34.

[30] Galloway SM, Vijayaraj Reddy M, McGettigan K, Gealy R, Bercu J. Potentially mutagenic impurities: analysis of structural classes and carcinogenic potencies of chemical intermediates in pharmaceutical syntheses supports alternative methods to the default TTC for calculating safe levels of impurities. Regul Toxicol Pharmacol 2013;66(3):326–35.

[31] Brigo A, Müller L. Development of the threshold of toxicological concern concept and its relationship to duration of exposure. In: Teasdale A, editor. Genotoxic impurities. Hoboken, NJ: John Wiley & Sons, Inc.; 2010. p. 27–63.

Practical Thresholds in the Derivation of Occupational Exposure Limits (OELs) for Carcinogens

Hermann M. Bolt

Leibniz Research Centre for Working Environment and Human Factors, TU Dortmund, Dortmund, Germany

Chapter Outline

Introduction 117
Derivation of Occupational Exposure Limits for Carcinogenic Substances 118
Concept of the German DFG (MAK (Maximale Arbeitsstoffkonzentration) Commission) 118
Discourse and Further Development in Europe 120
The Concept of SCOEL 121
Recent Examples of Carcinogens With a Practical Threshold Assigned by SCOEL 122
  Propylene Oxide 122
  Naphthalene 123
  Nickel 124
  Cadmium 125
Conclusions 126
Abbreviations 126
References 126

Introduction

The thesis that no thresholds can be identified for carcinogens has been challenged by research into the mechanisms of chemically induced cancer [1]. Although scientific development in this field is rapid, regulatory concepts change only slowly and are lagging behind.

There has been growing scientific recognition and consensus that carcinogenic risk extrapolation to/from high/low doses, a key step in setting standards for carcinogenic

Thresholds of Genotoxic Carcinogens.
DOI: http://dx.doi.org/10.1016/B978-0-12-801663-3.00008-X

substances, must consider the respective mode of action [2]. This has been accepted by a number of official bodies. Examples are a joint opinion of scientific committees of the EU Directorate-General for Health & Consumer Protection [3] and Guidelines for Carcinogenic Risk Assessment of the US Environmental Protection Agency, which indicate that even direct, DNA-reactive carcinogens might act via a nonlinear mode of action [4]. Overviews of existing systems for the classification of carcinogenic compounds are available [5,6].

Derivation of Occupational Exposure Limits for Carcinogenic Substances

Until the mid-1990s the general dogma held valid that no health-based occupational exposure limits (OELs) (and biological limit values (BLVs)) can be derived for carcinogenic compounds. This referred to all carcinogens, as evidenced by either human epidemiology or animal experimentation, equivalent to the carcinogen categories 1A and 1B of the Globally Harmonized System [7].

In the differentiation of occupational carcinogens, different concepts exist internationally. Thus, the American Conference of Governmental Hygienists (ACGIH) follows mostly the classical system used by IARC and distinguishes between the categories: *A1, confirmed human carcinogen; A2, suspected human carcinogen; A3, confirmed animal carcinogen with unknown relevance to humans; A4, not classifiable as a human carcinogen; A5, not suspected as a human carcinogen* [8]. The ACGIH system is used, officially or semiofficially, by many countries. It does not address the problem of different modes of action and associated different dose–response patterns of carcinogens.

Concept of the German DFG (MAK (Maximale Arbeitsstoffkonzentration) Commission)

The classical dogma of no thresholds for occupational carcinogens was first challenged by Neumann et al. [9], when proposing to differentiate not only between genotoxic and nongenotoxic carcinogens, but also to consider health-based OELs for "genotoxic chemicals for which low carcinogenic potency can be expected on the basis of dose–response relationships and toxicokinetics, and for which the risk at low doses can be assessed." This was the first time to consider what has later been called a "practical threshold" for a group of (genotoxic) occupational carcinogens. This idea has been adopted and further developed by the Deutsche Forschungsgemeinschaft (DFG) in its list of MAK values (OELs) and BAT (Biologischer Arbeitsstoff-Toleranzwert) values (BLVs). After several revisions, the DFG now distinguishes between the following categories of carcinogens: [10]

1. *Substances that cause cancer in man and can be assumed to contribute to cancer risk. Epidemiological studies provide adequate evidence of a positive correlation between the exposure of humans and the occurrence of cancer. Limited epidemiological data can be*

substantiated by evidence that the substance causes cancer by a mode of action that is relevant to man.

2. *Substances that are considered to be carcinogenic for man because sufficient data from long-term animal studies or limited evidence from animal studies substantiated by evidence from epidemiological studies indicate that they can contribute to cancer risk. Limited data from animal studies can be supported by evidence that the substance causes cancer by a mode of action that is relevant to man and by results of in vitro tests and short-term animal studies.*

   For substances in categories 1 and 2, no health-based MAK/BAT values (ie, OELs/BLVs) are assigned.

3. *Substances that cause concern that they could be carcinogenic for man but cannot be assessed conclusively because of lack of data. The classification in category 3 is provisional.*

   3A. *Substances that cause cancer in humans or animals or that are considered to be carcinogenic for humans, for which the criteria for classification in category 4 or 5 are in principle fulfilled. However, the database for these substances is insufficient for the establishment of an MAK/BAT value (OELs/BLVs).*

   3B. *Substances for which in vitro or animal studies have yielded evidence of carcinogenic effects that are not sufficient for classification of the substance in one of the other categories. Further studies are required before a final decision can be made. A MAK/BAT value (OEL/BLV) can be established provided no genotoxic effects have been detected.*

4. *Substances that cause cancer in humans or animals or that are considered to be carcinogenic for humans and for which an MAK/BAT value (OEL/BLV) can be derived. A non-genotoxic mode of action is of prime importance and genotoxic effects play no or at most a minor part provided the MAK/BAT values (OEL/BLV) are observed. Under these conditions no contribution to human cancer risk is expected. The classification is supported especially by evidence that, for example, increases in cellular proliferation, inhibition of apoptosis or disturbances in cellular differentiation are important in the modes of action. The classification and the MAK/BAT values (OEL/BLV) take into consideration the manifold mechanisms contributing to carcinogenesis and their characteristic dose–time–response relationships.*

   Thus, category 4 of this system comprises on the one hand nongenotoxic carcinogens, and on the other hand carcinogens for which genotoxicity plays only a minor role, compared to a higher impact of mechanisms such as chronic cell proliferation. Examples in this category are aniline, chlorinated biphenyls, DEHP, formaldehyde, chloroform, and carbon tetrachloride.

5. *Substances that cause cancer in humans or animals or that are considered to be carcinogenic for humans and for which an MAK/BAT value (OEL/BLV) value can be derived. A genotoxic mode of action is of prime importance but is considered to contribute*

only very slightly to human cancer risk, provided the MAK/BAT values (OELs/BLVs) are observed. The classification and the MAK and BAT values (OELs/BLVs) are supported by information on the mode of action, dose-dependence, and toxicokinetic data.

In the 2014 MAK list, category 5 comprises five compounds (acetaldehyde, dichloromethane, ethanol, isoprene, and styrene).

In essence, in this system category 4 addresses nongenotoxic carcinogens, but also genotoxic carcinogens with a practical threshold. Category 5 also comprises an additional set of genotoxic carcinogens with a practical threshold.

Discourse and Further Development in Europe

An independent discourse was initiated by the *European Academy Bad Neuenahr-Ahrweiler*, which convened an international panel (from 2001 to 2003), to discuss matters of dose–effect relationships and risk evaluation, focused on carcinogenic agents [11]. The panel covered the disciplines of radiation, toxicology, epidemiology, mathematical modeling, ethics, and environmental law and arrived at the following statements: (1) Environmental standard setting has to be based on reliable, sound scientific data. (2) The distinction of harmful agents into two groups, those that act with a threshold and those that act without a threshold should be maintained. (3) When a threshold dose can be verified on the basis of scientific data, regulatory standards should be set below the threshold level. Safety factors should be used in these cases to acknowledge uncertainties in the evaluation procedures and individual differences in susceptibility. (4) For mutagens and most genotoxic carcinogens, for example, ionizing radiation, where there is no evidence for a threshold dose, the LNT (linear-nonthreshold) model remains the most appropriate convention for risk evaluation by extrapolation into the low-dose range and for the control of carcinogens. Its simplicity for risk assessment is advantageous. Its application is therefore recommended for risk estimates of genotoxic agents. (The LNT model is a linear extrapolation of the dose-response from high to low exposure/dose levels. It does not imply a threshold; consequently, any dose that is different from zero will exert an effect also different from zero.) (5) One can distinguish between "group 1" (genotoxic carcinogens without a threshold, where a LNT extrapolation model should be applied), "group 2" (genotoxic substances, where sufficient data, concerning the underlying mechanisms, suggest existence of a *practical threshold*), "group 3" (nongenotoxic carcinogens: compounds displaying a clear threshold of carcinogenicity, and health-based exposure limits may be established by starting from the "no observed adverse effect level" (NOAEL) and the introduction of a safety/uncertainty factor, if this is applicable). (6) Further research of mechanisms in the multistep process of carcinogenesis is needed to reduce existing uncertainties [11].

This discourse was immediately taken up and further implemented by the EUROTOX Speciality Section Carcinogenesis [12] and was decisive for the acceptance of the concept of "practical thresholds" in the derivation of OELs and BLVs for carcinogenic substances by the Scientific Committee on Occupational Exposure Limits (SCOEL) of the European Union [2]. The SCOEL system basically distinguishes between "perfect" and "practical" thresholds [13]. "Perfect" thresholds were assigned to nongenotoxic carcinogens, and "practical thresholds" (equivalent to "apparent" thresholds, as previously proposed by Kirsch-Volders et al. [14]), were assigned to genotoxic carcinogens for with the mode of action suggests a thresholded nonlinear dose-response.

The Concept of SCOEL

Details of the concept of SCOEL have been explained previously [13], and the concept at large is part of the official "Key Documentation" of SCOEL [15]. This documentation states a growing recognition of the fact that carcinogenic risk extrapolation to low doses (and standard setting) must consider the mode of action of a given chemical. For genotoxic carcinogens, case studies of chemicals point to an array of possibilities. For instance, positive data of chromosomal effects only, in the absence of mutagenicity, support the characterization of a compound that produces carcinogenic effects only at high, toxic doses. Also for non-DNA reactive genotoxicants, such as aneugens, thresholds should be defined. Specific mechanisms of clastogenicity have also been addressed as also having thresholds, such as topoisomerase II poisons or inducers of reactive oxygen species.

These and other mechanistic arguments, taken together, led to the distinction of the following four main groups of carcinogens and mutagens in relation to setting of OELs (see also Fig. 8.1):

> *Group A: Non-threshold genotoxic carcinogens; for low-dose risk assessment the linear non-threshold (LNT) model appears appropriate.*
> *Group B: Genotoxic carcinogens, for which the existence of a threshold cannot be sufficiently supported at present. In these cases the LNT model may be used as a default assumption, based on the scientific uncertainty.*
> *Group C: Genotoxic carcinogens for which a practical threshold is supported.*
> *Group D: Non-genotoxic carcinogens and non-DNA reactive carcinogens; for these compounds a true ("perfect") threshold is associated with a clearly founded NOAEL.*

Health-based OELs are derived by SCOEL for carcinogens of groups C and D. If the dataset allows, SCOEL performs a quantitative risk assessment for carcinogens placed in categories A and B. In such cases, the corresponding SCOEL recommendation will state that a carcinogenic risk assessment has been carried out. Typical examples of compounds for each group (A–D) have been presented earlier [12].

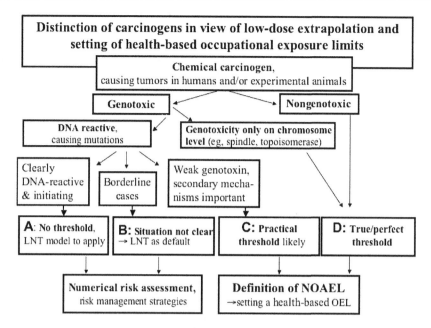

Figure 8.1

The SCOEL concept. *Source: Adapted from the SCOEL Key Documentation, European Commission Adapted from European Commission. Methodology for the derivation of occupational exposure limits. Scientific Committee on Occupational Exposure Limits (SCOEL). Key documentation, version 7. Luxemburg: DG Employment, Social Affairs & Inclusion; June 2013. Available via <http:// ec.europa.eu/social/keyDocuments.jsp?type=0&policyArea=82&subCategory=153&country =0&year=0&advSearchKey=recommendation&mode=advancedSubmit&langId=en>.*

Recent Examples of Carcinogens With a Practical Threshold Assigned by SCOEL

SCOEL recognized that locally active carcinogens, for which local irritancy and consecutive cell proliferation are an indispensible prerequisite for carcinogenicity, have a practical threshold. Therefore, avoidance of irritancy will allow to derive a health-based OEL. Classical examples are formaldehyde and vinyl acetate [13], but there was further development when discussing specific compounds. The following gives essentials from the respective SCOEL recommendations.

Propylene Oxide

Propylene oxide is a weakly DNA-reactive genotoxic agent. When administered by oral gavage to rats, it produced tumors of the forestomach, mainly squamous-cell carcinomas. In mice exposed by inhalation, propylene oxide produced hemangiomas/hemangiosarcomas of the nasal cavity and a few malignant nasal epithelial tumors. In rats exposed by inhalation, papillary adenomas of the nasal cavity were observed. Thus, propylene oxide induces tumors in rodents, although at high concentrations and mainly confined to the portals of entry [16].

Since the 1990s, there have been efforts to elucidate modes of action of rodent nasal carcinogens in general and of propylene oxide in particular. The overall weight of evidence for propylene oxide indicates that this is genotoxic, but that its potency as a DNA-reactive mutagen is weak (much weaker than that of ethylene oxide) [17,18]. Aspects of target tissue toxicity appear relevant, namely with attention to concentration-dependent glutathione (GSH) depletion, cell proliferation, cell death, and necrosis at the nasal tissue target. Toxic tissue responses occur in the same anatomical regions in rodents as do the tumors. Some of these tissue toxicities may produce effects that either augment the DNA-reactive mutagenicity or are genotoxic by themselves. Taking these arguments together, the DNA reactivity of propylene oxide appears to be connected with its genotoxicity, and to contribute to its carcinogenicity in rodents. However, this genotoxicity increment alone seems not to be sufficient for cancer induction. Compound-associated tissue toxicities, which are rate-limiting, appear as major quantitative determinants [19]. Since the latter are threshold effects, a practical threshold for the overall cancer outcomes has been inferred [17,18]. Consequently, propylene oxide was assigned to the SCOEL carcinogen group C.

Considering a LOAEL for local changes at the rat nasal epithelium at 30 ppm and a minimal local glutathione depletion in the nasal tissue of the rats at 5 ppm, SCOEL concluded that a health-based OEL should be well below 5 ppm. A species scaling with regard to humans is not required in this case, as it is generally accepted that the nasal epithelium of rodents is more susceptible to irritation and irritation-based carcinogenicity than that of humans. Therefore, SCOEL proposed a health-based OEL for propylene oxide of 1 ppm, in order to remain below the indicator infect of a beginning local glutathione depletion. This also took into account results of no observed sister chromatid exchange effects in blood cells of exposed workers below 2 ppm exposure [20].

Naphthalene

In lifetime studies, naphthalene was carcinogenic towards the nasal epithelium in rats. In principle, these tumors were considered of relevance for human health. Naphthalene appears not to express genotoxic activity under relevant exposure conditions in vivo. The mode of action of the experimental tumor formation by naphthalene has been a matter for an expert panel [21]. The panel pointed to critical areas of uncertainty: Cytotoxic naphthalene metabolites, their modes of cytotoxic action, and detailed low-dose dose–response patterns needed to be clarified, including primate and human tissues, and neonatal tissues. Mouse, rat, and monkey inhalation studies were needed to better define in vivo naphthalene uptake and metabolism in the upper respiratory tract. In vivo validation studies were needed for a PBPK (physiologically based pharmacokinetic) model for monkeys exposed to naphthalene by inhalation, coupled to cytotoxicity studies referred to above; and in vivo studies are needed to validate a human PBPK model for naphthalene.

In order to eliminate these uncertainties related to the mode of action [21], the following investigations were initiated.

(1) A PBPK model for naphthalene in rats and humans was developed that incorporated a hybrid computational fluid dynamics (CFD)-PBPK description of the upper respiratory tract to support cross-species dosimetry comparisons of naphthalene concentrations and tissue-normalized rates of metabolism in the nasal respiratory and olfactory epithelium, lung, and liver. In vitro measurements of metabolic rates from microsomal incubations published for rat and monkey (as a surrogate for human) were scaled to the specific tissue based on the tissue microsomal content and volume of tissue. The model reproduced time courses for naphthalene blood concentrations from intravenous and inhalation exposures in rats and upper respiratory tract extraction data in both naïve rats and rats pretreated to inhibit nasal metabolism. This naphthalene model was applied to estimate human-equivalent inhalation concentrations corresponding to NOAECs or LOAECs for the noncancer effects of naphthalene in rats. Also, approaches for cross-species extrapolation were compared [22].

(2) Male and female F344 rats were subchronically exposed to naphthalene vapors up to 30 ppm for 6 h/day, 5 days/week. The nature of responses supported a mode of action involving oxidative stress, inflammation, and proliferation. The results were consistent with a dose-dependent transition in the mode of action for naphthalene toxicity/carcinogenicity between 1.0 and 10 ppm in the rat [23]. Using the new PBPK model to estimate target tissue doses (total naphthalene metabolism per gram nasal tissue) relevant to the proposed mode of action [22] the lowest transcriptional benchmark dose limits from this analysis equated to a human continuous naphthalene exposure at approximately 0.3 ppm. On this basis, it was considered unlikely that significant effects of naphthalene or its metabolites will occur at exposures below this concentration [23].

Therefore, and considering that humans appear to be less sensitive that rats (which are obligatory nose-breathers), SCOEL finally considered naphthalene as a carcinogen with a practical threshold (group C) and proposed an OEL (8-h TWA) of 0.1 ppm.

Nickel

The carcinogenicity of nickel compounds has been clearly demonstrated in epidemiological studies. With respect to animal studies in rats, mice, or hamsters, long-term inhalation studies revealed carcinogenicity in the lung for poorly soluble nickel compounds (nickel oxide: 1.0 mg Ni/m^3; nickel subsulfide: >0.11 mg Ni/m^3).

From a mechanistic point of view, nickel and nickel compounds are not directly mutagenic. Based on cellular investigations, at low concentrations nickel ions do not directly interact with DNA but rather exert indirect genotoxic effects, such as interference with DNA repair systems and DNA methylation patterns, which lead to clastogenicity and an increased genomic instability. These effects are mediated by nickel ions, even though it cannot be excluded that on conditions of particle overload chronic inflammation may contribute to the carcinogenicity. Therefore, nickel was considered a carcinogen with a practical threshold (group C). With respect to quantitative estimates on the carcinogenicity in humans, the International Committee on Nickel Carcinogenicity in Man [24] concluded that the increase in cancers of the nasal cavity (ethmoid) and lungs (bronchi, etc.) among workers in nickel refineries is associated with a minimum exposure of $1\,mg/m^3$ for water-soluble salts and $10\,mg/m^3$ for insoluble compounds (sulfides, oxide, etc.) of nickel. However, a Finnish epidemiological study [25] revealed an excess of bronchial cancer and two cancers of the sinuses (nasal cavity) among workers exposed to concentrations of about $0.25\,mg/m^3$ water-soluble nickel salts (sulfate). Concerning a particular cohort (Kristiansand), a significant increase in cancer incidence for water-soluble nickel was observed at a cumulative exposure of $1.6\,mg/m^3 \times$ years, equivalent to $0.04\,mg\,Ni/m^3$ when calculated for 40 years exposure [26]. This was seen by SCOEL as a conservative estimate, since current evidence strongly suggests indirect mechanisms with sublinear dose–response relationships in the low concentration range.

Therefore, to protect from nickel-induced carcinogenicity, an OEL of $0.01\,mg\,Ni/m^3$ was proposed by SCOEL for the inhalable fraction of water-soluble as well as poorly water-soluble nickel compounds. Metallic nickel was excluded, since neither animal data nor epidemiological data point toward a carcinogenic action of nickel metal. The proposed value should also protect against nickel-induced indirect genotoxicity, including chromosomal damage. As far as biological monitoring is concerned, nickel levels in plasma and urine at the proposed OEL of $0.01\,mg/m^3$ would be around 80 and $10\,\mu g/L$, respectively, which is well below DNA repair inhibitory concentrations in experimental systems in vitro.

Cadmium

The kidneys represent the most sensitive targets of systemic Cd toxicity and carcinogenicity upon occupational exposure. Owing to its strong binding to metallothionein, Cd is a highly cumulative toxicant; the systemic manifestations associated with chronic exposure are related to the body burden of the element.

It appears that Cd nephrotoxicity is highly connected with its nephrocarcinogenicity. On this basis, the following considerations by SCOEL led to deriving an acceptable occupational exposure level for Cd and its inorganic compounds. There is an abundant database on the health effects of Cd and its compounds. The mechanisms of the systemic toxicity of Cd are well understood, and the dose–effect/response data characterizing have been extensively and reliably documented in human studies. Mean urinary Cd levels in European individuals with no occupational exposure to Cd or living in an area with no specific Cd pollution are generally below 1 µg/g creatinine. The critical systemic effect selected to define the point of departure in epidemiological studies (urinary excretion of low-molecular-weight proteins reflecting tubular dysfunction) is an early sign occurring before the onset of overt clinical manifestations of kidney disease.

Cd and its compounds were considered as group C carcinogens (with a practical threshold), because prolonged (renal) tissue toxicity appears essential for tumor formation. Under these provisions it seems prudent, in view of the cumulative nature of Cd, to recommend limiting the body burden of the working force to a strict minimum. Therefore a BLV of 2 µg Cd/g creatinine was recommended, in addition to the recommendation of an OEL of 4 µg/m^3 (respirable fraction). The OEL was primarily based on noncancer respiratory effects, to protect workers against local respiratory effects of Cd exposure.

Conclusions

The concept of "practical thresholds" in the derivation of OELs and BLVs has been advanced by the SCOEL of the European Union. This concept is being applied for genotoxic carcinogens with well-investigated modes of action. In such cases genotoxicity needs further steps for cancer development, notably chronic tissue damage and cell proliferation. The concept of "practical thresholds" is also applied for carcinogens with secondary genotoxicity, based on excess generation of reactive oxygen species at high doses. Particularly important is the concept for metals and inorganic metal compounds.

Abbreviations

OEL occupational exposure limit (maximum exposure concentration for the workplace)
BLV biological limit value (recommended exposure limits for biological monitoring)
MAK *Maximale Arbeitsstoffkonzentration* (OEL in Germany)
BAT *Biologischer Arbeitsstoff-Toleranzwert* (BLV in Germany)

References

[1] Greim H, Albertini RJ. Cellular response to the genotoxic insult: the question of threshold for genotoxic carcinogens. Toxicol Res R Soc Chem 2015;4:36–45. http://dx.doi.org/10.1039/c4tx00078a.
[2] Bolt HM, Huici-Montagud A. Strategy of the Scientific Committee on Occupational Exposure Limits (SCOEL) in the derivation of occupational exposure limits for carcinogens and mutagens. Arch Toxicol 2008;82:61–4.

[3] European Commission. Risk assessment methodologies and approaches for mutagenic and carcinogenic substances. Preliminary report agreed by written procedure by SCHER, SCCP and SCENIHS on 24 October 2008. Brussels: Health & Consumer Protection Directorate-General; 2008. Available via <http://ec.europa.eu/health/archive/ph_risk/committees/04_scher/docs/scher_o_107.pdf>.

[4] EPA [US Environmental Protection Agency]. Guidelines for carcinogen risk assessment. Risk assessment forum. EPA/630/P-03/001F. Washington DC: US Environmental Protection Agency; March 2005. Available online via <http://www.epa.gov/raf/publications/pdfs/CANCER_GUIDELINES_FINAL_3-25-05.PDF>.

[5] Seeley MR, Tonner-Navarro LE, Beck BD, Deskin R, Feron VJ, Johanson G, et al. Procedures for health risk assessment in Europe. Regul Toxicol Pharmacol. 2001;34(2):153–69.

[6] DECOS [Dutch Expert Committee on Occupational Safety, Health Council of the Netherlands]. Guideline to the classification of carcinogenic compounds. Publication no. A10/07E. The Hague: Health Council of the Netherlands; 2010. Available online via <http://www.gezondheidsraad.nl/default/files/A1007_0.pdf>.

[7] United Nations. Globally harmonized system of classification and labelling of chemicals (GHS). Fourth revised edition. New York and Geneva: United Nations; 2011. Available via <http://www.unece.org/fileadmin/DAM/trans/danger/publi/ghs/ghs_rev04/English/ST-SG-AC10-30-Rev4e.pdf>.

[8] ACGIH [American Conference of Governmental Industrial Hygienists]. TLVs and BEIs based on the documentation of the threshold limit values for chemical substances and physical agents & biological exposure indices. Cincinnati, OH: ACGIH Signature Publications; 2014.

[9] Neumann HG, Vamvakas D, Thielmann HW, Gelbke H-P, Filser JG, Reuter U, et al. Changes in the classification of carcinogenic chemicals in the work area. Int Arch Occup Environ Health 1998;71:566–74.

[10] DFG [Deutsche Forschungsgemeinschaft]. MAK- und BAT-Werte-Liste 2014. Senatskommission zur Prüfung gesundheitsschädlicher Arbeitsstoffe. Mitteilung 50. Weinheim, Germany: WILEY-VCH; 2014. Available online via <http://onlinelibrary.wiley.com/book/10.1002/9783527682010>.

[11] Streffer C, Bolt HM, Føllesdal D, Hall P, Hengstler JG, Jakob P, et al. Low dose exposures in the environment. dose-effect relations and risk evaluation. New York, NY: Springer Berlin-Heidelberg; 2004.

[12] Bolt HM, Degen GH. Human carcinogenic risk evaluation, part II: contributions of the EUROTOX speciality section for carcinogenesis. Toxicol Sci 2004;81:3–6.

[13] Bolt HM. The concept of "practical thresholds" in the derivation of occupational exposure limits for carcinogens by the Scientific Committee on Occupational Exposure Limits (SCOEL) of the European Union. Gene Environ 2008;30(4):114–9.

[14] Kirsch-Volders M, Aardema M, Elhajouji A. Concept of threshold in mutagenesis and carcinogenesis. Mutat Res 2000;464:3–11.

[15] European Commission. Methodology for the derivation of occupational exposure limits. Scientific Committee on Occupational Exposure Limits (SCOEL). Key documentation, version 7. Luxemburg: DG Employment, Social Affairs & Inclusion; June 2013. Available via <http://ec.europa.eu/social/keyDocuments.jsp?type=0&policyArea=82&subCategory=153&country=0&year=0&advSearchKey=recommendation&mode=advancedSubmit&langId=en>.

[16] IARC. Propylene oxide. In: IARC monographs on the evaluation of carcinogenic risk of chemicals to man, vol. 60. Lyon; 1994. p. 191–9.

[17] Albertini RJ, Sweeney LM. Propylene oxide: genotoxicity profile of a rodent nasal carcinogen. Crit Rev Toxicol 2007;37:489–520.

[18] Sweeney LM, Kirman CR, Albertini RJ, Tan YM, Clewell HJ, Filser JG, et al. Derivation of inhalation toxicity reference values for propylene oxide using mode of action analysis: examples of a threshold carcinogen. Crit Rev Toxicol 2009;39(6):462–86.

[19] Ríos-Blanco MN, Plna K, Faller T, Kessler W, Håkansson K, Kreuzer PE, et al. Propylene oxide: mutagenesis, carcinogenesis and molecular dose. Mutat Res 1997;380:179–97.

[20] Czene K, Osterman-Golkar S, Yun X, Li G, Zhao F, Perez HL, et al. Analysis of DNA and hemoglobin adducts and sister chromatid exchanges in a human population occupationally exposed to propylene oxide: a pilot study. Cancer Epidemiol Biomarkers Prev 2002;11:315–8.

[21] Bogen KT, Benson JM, Yost GS, Morris JB, Dahl AR, Clewell HJ, et al. Naphthalene metabolism in relation to target tissue anatomy, physiology, cytotoxicity and tumorigenic mechanism of action. Regul Toxicol Pharmacol 2008;51(Suppl. 2):S27–36.

[22] Campbell JL, Andersen ME, Clewell HJ. A hybrid CFD-PBPK model for naphthalene in rat and human with IVIVE for nasal tissue metabolism and cross-species dosimetry. Inhal Toxicol 2014;26:333–44.

[23] Clewell HJ, Efremenko A, Campbell JL, Dodd DE, Thomas RS. Transcriptional responses in the nasal epithelium following subchronic inhalation of naphthalene vapour. Toxicol Appl Pharmacol 2014;280:78–85.

[24] ICNCM (International Committee on Nickel Carcinogenicity in Man). Report of the international committee on nickel carcinogenesis in man. Scand J Work Environ Health 1990;16:1–84.

[25] Anttila A, Pukkala E, Aitio A, Rantanen T, Karjalainen S. Update of cancer incidence among workers at a copper/nickel smelter and nickel refinery. Int Arch Occup Environ Health 1998;71:245–50.

[26] Grimsrud TK, Berge SR, Haldorsen T, Andersen A. Exposure to different forms of nickel and risk of lung cancer. Am J Epidemiol 2002;156:1123–32.

Experimental Design and Statistical Analysis of Threshold Studies

David P. Lovell

Institute of Medical and Biomedical Education (IMBE), St George's, University of London, London, United Kingdom

Chapter Outline

Introduction   129
Definitions of Thresholds   131
Dose–Response Modeling in Radiation (The No Safe Dose of Radiation Concept)   132
Linear and Nonlinear   132
Experimental Designs for Dose–Response Modeling   133
No-Observed Genotoxic Effect Level   138
Dose–Response Modeling   139
Interpolation and Extrapolations   143
Goodness of Fit Issues: Acceptance and Rejection of Models   143
BMD Approach   145
Mathematical Modeling for the BMD   146
Software   146
    BMDS   147
    PROAST   147
    Drsmooth   147
    Other R Packages   148
    GraphPad PRISM   148
Conclusions   149
Acronyms   149
References   150

Introduction

This chapter aims to give an introduction to issues related to the design and analysis of studies carried out to investigate possible thresholds related to exposures to agents with genotoxic potential. It discusses methods for identifying and using points of departure (PODs) in the subsequent interpretation of genotoxicity studies.

Thresholds of Genotoxic Carcinogens.
DOI: http://dx.doi.org/10.1016/B978-0-12-801663-3.00009-1

The determination of a dose–response relationship is central to the quantification of toxicology and to the subsequent regulatory discussion on the quantitative assessments of risks. The identification of thresholds in experimental systems has been particularly problematic because of the difficulties of experimentation at low doses and the philosophical and semantic problems associated with the definitions of thresholds.

In this context, genotoxic chemicals have had a special place in the regulations associated with carcinogenicity but are also of interest in their own right [1]. The concept that genotoxic chemicals induce DNA damage at any level of exposure and that there is no threshold in the dose–response relationship has for a long time been almost axiomatic [2,3]. An in vivo genotoxin has been considered effectively, in the absence of other evidence, to be a genotoxic carcinogen where the default is that the dose–response relationship is considered to be low-dose linear and nonthresholded. The UK Committee on Mutagenicity, for instance, concluded in 2010 that it "… reaffirmed the default position that for *in vivo* mutagens, in the absence of mechanistic data to infer a threshold, it is prudent to assume that there is no threshold for mutagenicity" [4].

The linear no-threshold dose model of cancer has, in effect, been the default approach to cancer risk assessment for a long time [5]. This is in contrast to the concept of a threshold for many other toxicological endpoints where there is considered to be a dose below which no adverse event occurs [6].

This has led to different approaches to risk assessment and management. Firstly, the "threshold/no safe dose" concept, where risk management takes the form of approaches such as ALARA (as low as reasonably attainable) or ALARP (as low as reasonably practical) for genotoxic agents. Secondly, the threshold/reference dose approach where no-observed effect levels (NOELs) (or at least no-observed adverse effect levels (NOAELs)) are identified and followed by the application of uncertainty factors (UFs) (formerly safety factors (SFs)) to derive acceptable daily intakes (ADIs), tolerable daily intakes (TDIs), or comparable permitted daily exposures (PDEs) [7,8].

Genetic damage can take a number of forms: gene mutation, chromosomal loss (aneuploidy), and chromosomal damage (clastogenicity). A number of regulatory guidelines suggest that a battery or combination of short-term genotoxicity (or mutagenicity) tests (STTs) should be used to identify chemicals with genotoxic potential [9]. Some areas of genotoxicity such as aneuploidy have increasingly been considered to be thresholded based upon a (putative) mechanism or mode of action such as redundancy of targets (such as spindle protein) [10,11].

There is an important difference between genotoxicity and mutation. The former is a surrogate/biomarker of quantitative damage. The latter is a qualitative (and rare spontaneous event of the order of one in a million divisions) event. In this context it is important to realize that mutagenic risk (as opposed to carcinogenicity) is an important endpoint in its own right [12].

There is, though, a movement to unify the methods for assessing risk between the different toxicological endpoints [13]. One development is the benchmark dose (BMD) approach suggested for both cancer and noncancer endpoints in preference to the traditional curve-fitting and NOEL/SF approaches. Traditionally the use of STTs to detect genotoxicity potential is a qualitative hazard identification stage and quantification has not been a major component (perhaps because early work showed a lack of a strong correlation between mutagenic and cancer potency [14]).

Some nongenotoxic carcinogens (such as clastogens) are now recognized as having a threshold while the BMD methodology is being promoted for genotoxicity in general [15] in preference to the no-observed genotoxic effect level (NOGEL) approach [16]. Approaches based upon the margin of exposure (MoE) [17] and the threshold of toxicological concern (TTC) [18] are also of increasing interest in the regulatory arena. The MoE is the ratio of the point of departure (POD) to the human exposure and is used as a guide for risk management. Both the European Food Safety Authority (EFSA) and Joint FAO/WHO Expert Committee on Food Additives (JECFA) [19] have proposed using the $BMDL_{10}$ (benchmark dose lower bound) as the reference point (RP) of POD. The EFSA [20] has suggested MoEs >10,000 indicate low concern while MoEs <10,000 "may be of concern" [21]. The TTC approach has been used in developing approaches to the control of genotoxic impurities in pharmaceuticals [22].

Definitions of Thresholds

There has been considerable debate over the inconsistencies in the terminology of dose–response relationships and the definition of a threshold [23]. The terminology used is complicated [24]. A variety of terms such as "absolute," "real or biological," "apparent," and "statistical" have been added to "threshold" to surmount some of the problems of definition [11,25]. Crump has pointed out that the use of these terms can be misleading because they are imprecise and imply value judgement about just how large a risk is considered acceptable [26].

The no-threshold model is based upon the possibility that, firstly, there is a finite (but possibly vanishingly small) probability that a single molecule could cause an irreversible change to DNA which could ultimately lead to a cancer and that, secondly, given the distribution of individual susceptibilities (tolerances) there is also a finite (but possibly vanishingly) small probability of an individual having extreme susceptibility (the "infinite sensitivity of the population") argument. Boobis et al. have produced counterarguments to these suppositions [27].

A mechanistic argument is that a threshold is not possible when the mechanism producing the effect is also contributing to the background level so that even the smallest exposure can act additively to the background level [28]. They argued that low-dose linearity will occur because the smallest dose is capable of adding an increment to the background level of DNA damage if the same mechanism applies to both the background and the additional damage.

The US National Research Council's "Toxicology in the 21st Century" makes the case for quantification, modeling, and in vitro and in silico experimentation [29]. Zhang et al. have suggested that the technology now exists to be able to identify the mechanistic basis of thresholds at the cellular level [30]. They provide an overview of the development of methods for the identification of a mechanistic basis for in vitro thresholds based upon, for instance, an analysis of molecular signaling network motifs.

Various "quasi" threshold approaches have been used within the regulatory arena to try to provide practical management approaches. These include the use of concepts such as MoEs or ALARA/ALARP and virtually safe doses (VSDs). In part, these are attempts to resolve practical problems and have led to the idea of developing quantitative risk assessment (QRA) approaches for genetic toxicology endpoints [31,32].

Dose–Response Modeling in Radiation (The No Safe Dose of Radiation Concept)

Many of the concepts associated with low-dose modeling come from radiation biology and its linear nonthreshold (LNT) model with the associated statement of "no safe dose of radiation" [33]. This model, while widely used by many international organizations, is contentious and is a continuing area of debate and experimental studies [34,35].[1] A recent review assessed the evidence for transgenerational effects following exposure to ionizing radiation and chemotherapy and concluded that the available evidence suggests that human health has not been significantly affected by transgenerational effects of radiation [36].

Linear and Nonlinear

The terms linear and nonlinear can cause confusion. Linear on a graph is a straight line where the change in response is directly proportional to the dose, equivalent to the regression coefficient in a linear regression. Nonlinear can refer to a dose–response relationship which when graphed is not a straight line. Such curves are sometimes called sublinear (convex shape) or supralinear (concave). Curves can take many shapes (Fig. 9.1). Sigmoid curves include both sublinear and supralinear components.

Transformations such as logarithms, applied to the dose and/or the response, or probits or logits can convert curvilinear data into a straight line. (In practice, many of the transformations used in bioassays such as the probit are an attempt to transform curved data

---

1 A recent report by Leuraud et al. (2015) has been interpreted in Nature (Jun. 2015) as providing support to the low-dose linearity theory of radiation risk http://www.nature.com/news/researchers-pin-down-risks-of-low-dose-radiation-1.17876. This work, based upon records of radiation exposure amongst 300,000 nuclear-industry workers, suggests that it is possible to detect an increased (but very small even miniscule) increase in the risk of leukemia from very low doses of radiation. Leuraud K, Richardson DB, Cardis E, Daniels RD, Gillies M, O'Hagan JA, et al. Ionising radiation and risk of death from leukaemia and lymphoma in radiation-monitored workers (INWORKS): an international cohort study. Lancet Haematol 2015;2:e276–81.

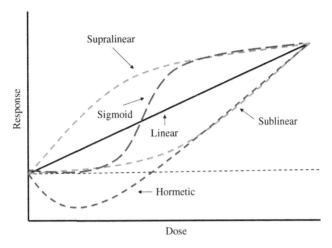

Figure 9.1

Illustration of linear, sublinear, supralinear, and hormetic dose–response
curves. Horizontal dotted line represents background level.

into a straight line to make the analysis more tractable using methods such as least squares
linear regression.) Jeffrey illustrated how the same dataset can have different shaped curves
depending upon the scale used for the axes of the graph [37]. *An important point is that
nonlinear is not synonymous with threshold although there has been a tendency to use the
terms, incorrectly, as interchangeable.*

There is, though, a difference between linear and nonlinear statistical models. In the context
of statistics a linear model does not necessarily imply a straight line but rather that the
parameters in the model are additive. The estimates are derived using a "closed-form"
solution where there is an algebraic procedure. In contrast, the parameters in a nonlinear
model can only be estimated by procedures based upon the use of initial estimates of the
parameters in the model, an iterative approach to fitting a curve though the data and some test
of whether further improvement in fit is unlikely (ie, a goodness of fit test).

Nonlinear regression provides a very flexible approach to curve-fitting [38]. There are many
types of nonlinear shape/curves including: convex, concave, asymptotic, exponential growth
or decay, and sigmoid curves. In all cases the specific function needs to be formulated. This
flexibility comes with a responsibility to identify the model which has the optimal fit to the
data. Expert knowledge in the biological field of interest is an important requirement as the
interpretation of the parameters may not be simple.

Experimental Designs for Dose–Response Modeling

Finney in his book *Probit Analysis* [39] discussed many of the issues related to experimental
designs for bioassays with long sections on the planning of experiments (p. 81–85).

He argued strongly that design was critical. Fisher had earlier developed the important components of randomization, replication, and blocking (or, as it sometimes referred to, local control) during the 1920s and 1930s [40,41]. These concepts remain as relevant today and Fisher's ideas have extended into the fields of design of experiments (DOE) and optimal design [42,43]. The factorial design developed by Fisher is appreciably more efficient than the "one factor at a time" (OFAT) approach often used in biological experiments. It is a design which can be used, for instance, to investigate the responses in both sexes identified by National Institute of Health (USA) (US NIH) as an essential requirement of modern studies [44,45]. Factorial designs/DOE approaches can also provide efficient methods for dose–response experimentation of both individual chemicals and combinations of agents [46]. Holland-Letz and Kopp-Schneider describe identifying optimal experimental designs for dose–response studies with continuous endpoints [47].

There is increasing interest in the development of quantitative methods for the investigation of in vitro experiments and the potential to apply similar methods such as a BMD approaches to these results [15]. Good experimental design is critical to the successful interpretation of such studies. Biomarkers (such as those in genetic toxicology) are sensitive to artefacts and it is potentially easy to carry out studies which are able to detect apparent effects as a consequence of flaws in the experimental design. Considerable care is needed to avoid introducing biases into the design. Statistical tests make a set of assumptions which are not always taken into account in the interpretation of results. Software used for the analyses will not flag up when these have not been met [48].

Identification of the experimental unit and the avoidance of pseudoreplication are key design features [49]. The experimental unit is the smallest unit that can be randomly assigned to the treatments [50] while the observational unit is the smallest unit, such as a cell, which can be measured. Cells from the same culture of animal cannot usually be randomly assigned to the treatment but rather experience the same conditions and their responses are likely to be correlated to some extent. Misspecification of the experimental unit can lead to serious misinterpretation of statistical analyses [49].

A failure to appreciate this in the design and subsequent analysis can lead to serious errors in interpretation. Independence of the experimental unit is an important assumption of many statistical tests such as the *t*-test, ANOVA, chi-square, and Fisher's exact test [51]. Designs with different levels of variability—animals (or cultures), samples from the same animal/cultures, cells from the same sample—can be wrongly analyzed because of a failure to recognize pseudoreplication resulting in an increased risk of false-positive results. For example, if a large number of cells is scored from single cultures each of which is treated with a different concentration of a chemical then apparent differences between the doses may be a consequence of differences between the cultures rather than a dose effect. Increasing the number of cells scored increases the precision of the effect detected. It is now possible to score over a million cells from an animal or a culture for micronuclei using flow cytometry. Torous et al. suggest that if up to 3 million cells are scored from a single sample then it is possible to detect a difference of 0.10% and 0.11% [52]. Large samples can make the estimate from a particular animal or sample very precise but care is needed to ensure that artefactual results do not arise.

There is considerable concern at the perceived lack of reproducibility of studies in the biomedical sciences [53,54]. Nature has been "campaigning" on this issues [55] relating it to and linked into Ioannidis' explanation of "why most published findings are false" [56]. A useful but not universally used framework is to consider another set of 3R's: replication, repeatability, and reproducibility. Replication is variability within an experiment; repeatability is a measure of the variability between experiments within the same laboratory, while reproducibility is a measure of variability between laboratories. More formal definitions of these terms have been developed by the International Standards Organisation in their ISO 5725 guidelines for studies aimed at assessing interlaboratory comparisons [57,58]. Replication and repeatability can be considered as a form of internal validity which reproducibility provides some evidence of external validity.

Bias can be reduced by randomization (at all stages) of an experiment and blinding of scoring/measurement of endpoints. Churchill and coworkers, for instance, have demonstrated the value of randomization in the reproducibility of microarray data [59,60].

The potential of blocking, effectively carrying out mini-experiments, is important in those large experiments where longitudinal effects may be present. An example is the study of micronuclei in male mice treated with 10 logarithmically spaced doses of acrylamide together with a negative control [61]. The group size was 10 so the experiment was split into two to make the work more manageable. This, in practice, created two blocks separated in time. There was no evidence of a dose × block interaction (in other words the dose–response identified was consistent across the two blocks) [61].

Gocke and Muller investigated a potential threshold in the induction of micronuclei by ethylmethanesulfonate (EMS) an accidental contaminant of tablets of Viracept, an HIV medication [62]. The initial experiment with doses between 0 and 80 mg/kg per day showed no strong evidence of a positive dose-response. Consequently, a second experiment was carried out with three higher doses ranging from 140 to 260 mg/kg per day where there was a significant dose-response. The results of the two were combined to provide evidence for a nonlinear response and a threshold for EMS. However, dose effects could be confounded with any uncontrolled differences between the experiments. An interesting aspect of this design was that the lower doses showed a significant negative regression line. The original data for these experiments are provided by Gocke et al. [63] and application of graphical methods such as splines show a marked curved response below the negative control incidence. Gocke and Wall noted this and commented on a possible hormetic dose-response [64]. Calabrese has reviewed the mechanisms and experimental evidence around the concept of hormesis [65].

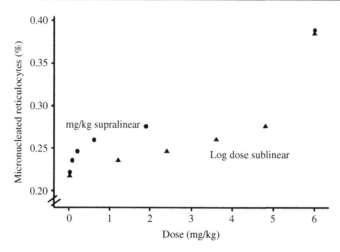

Figure 9.2
Data from Table I of Asano et al. [66] of frequencies of micronucleated reticulocytes
of various doses of 1-β-D-arabinofuranosylcytosine. Statistical comparisons using
the cell as the statistical unit carried out using Fisher's exact test, comparison
using the animal as the statistical unit carried out using Student's t-test.

Asano et al. [66] explored practical thresholds in a study of micronuclei produced by
exposure to 1-β-D-arabinofuranosylcytosine and scored using both manual and automatic
methods. Plots of the group means show different shaped dose–response curves depending
upon whether the dose is expressed on the untransformed dose (supralinear) or on the log
dose (sublinear) illustrating that visual inspection of graphs needs care (Fig. 9.2). Statistical
analysis (Table 9.1) showed significant linear components using both dose metrics but the
quadratic component was only significant with the log dose. Pairwise comparisons without
multiple comparison approaches showed significant differences with the animal as the
experimental unit only at the highest dose. Using the cell (incorrectly) as the experimental unit
showed lower doses becoming significantly different as more cells were scored (Table 9.2).

Experimental design involves the choice of an appropriate number of experimental groups.
The designs used for hazard identification studies often have three or four groups plus
a negative control. This limits the number of parameters than can be fitted in a model
as many of the "standard" models, for instance, use three or four parameters. Including
more experimental dose groups provides a more precise description of the dose–response
relationship. Ideally more doses are required, especially around the dose range of interest
[67]. The Environmental Protection Agency (USA) (US EPA) notes that studies with more
groups and a graded monotonic response will be more useful while studies with single doses
will, in general, not be suitable for BMD derivations and that the number of groups should be
at least one more than the number of parameters planned to be fitted in the models.

Table 9.1 Analysis of variance table of orthogonal breakdown of individual animal scores from raw data provided in Table II of Asano et al. [66].

(a) Using Original Dose Metric (mg/kg)				
Source	**df**	**MS (×100)**	**F**	**P**
Between groups	5	1.856	5.58	0.002
Linear	1	9.102	27.36	<0.001
Quadratic	1	0.001	0.01	0.97
Cubic	1	0.138	0.41	0.91
Deviations	2	0.019	0.06	0.95
Within groups	24	0.333		
Total	29			

(b) Using Log Dose				
Source	**df**	**MS (×100)**	**F**	**P**
Between groups	5	1.856	5.58	0.002
Linear	1	6.776	20.37	<0.001
Quadratic	1	1.634	4.91	0.036
Cubic	1	0.706	2.12	0.16
Deviations	2	0.081	0.24	0.79
Within groups	24	0.333		
Total	29			

Table 9.2 Summary of comparisons between negative control and dose groups from Asano et al. [54].

Dose (mg/kg BW)	Cells				Mice
	2K	**20K**	**200K**	**1M**	**1M**
0.06					
0.19			*	*	
0.60			**	**	
1.89		**	**	**	
6.00		**	**	**	**

*$P<0.05$; **$P<0.01$.

Piegorsch et al. note that greater information could be obtained about the shape of a dose–response relationship by increasing the number of doses [68].

Slob et al. used simulations to show that designs with more than four groups avoided problems with wrongly spaced dose levels and that high dose groups should be included in the modeling [69]. These high doses, they argued, help define the shape of the fitted curve and to identify an appropriate model. A further advantage is being able to obtain a more favorable signal:noise ratio in the region of the BMD. They found that the choice of a specific model was often not critical.

They also argued that more doses with a smaller numbers of experimental units (animals) at each dose level (in contrast to the designs needed for NOEL determination) performed adequately. They also found that the four group design often used for NOEL determination could be satisfactory for obtaining the BMD. However, highly variable responses can affect whether a dose-response is detected. Rhomberg provides a helpful commentary on this paper [70].

Kavlock et al. studied the effect of study design on the calculation of BMDs [71]. A design with six or more dose groups, but with fewer animals per group, can enhance the precision with which the overall dose–response curve can be estimated. The shift from a small number of doses with a number of units per dose to a larger number of doses with fewer replicates at each dose level is equivalent to the move from an analysis of variance to a regression analysis. Replicates in a design are a measure of the "pure error" or the random variation seen between otherwise identical observational units.

Gaylor et al. suggested designs for investigating nonmonotonic dose–response relationships, particularly J-shaped curves [72]. They suggest combining two designs if there is no duplication of doses in order to have six doses plus controls to provide a test for a J-shaped dose-response; with the design also providing a test for reductions below the negative control and the estimation of the zero equivalent dose (ZED). If there are seven doses in the design, there is the possibility of fitting the chosen model and being able to perform a "goodness of fit" test.

Some of the high-throughput in vitro screens associated with the Tox21 program use a large number of concentrations. Tice et al. describe the Tox21 program where over 12,000 chemical are being tested at 15 different concentrations of various toxicological endpoints [73]. Shukla et al. describe the assays used to investigate dose–response relationships in their part of the Tox21 collaboration where their qHTS-based screening assays using 1536-well format plates have generated over 6 million data points and over 400,000 concentration–response curves in specific assays. EC_{50} values are, in general, being derived based upon curve-fitting using a Hill model [74].

No-Observed Genotoxic Effect Level

The NOGEL has been proposed by Pottenger and Gollapudi [75]. It is similar in concept to the traditional NOEL/NOAEL approach used in other areas of toxicology. It defines a RP or a POD to use for deriving estimates of effects at low doses. It is based upon identifying the highest dose where the responses are not statistically significantly different from the negative control level. The lowest dose which is statistically significant is defined as the lowest observed genotoxic effect level (LOGEL). Alternative approaches are taken if no nonsignificant dose level is identified.

The NOGEL suffers, however, from the limitations identified for the NOEL approach in general. The NOGEL is determined by a hypothesis test depending upon factors such as the sample size, the dose spacing, and the specific statistical test used. The limitations of this approach are well known and these to some extent spurred the development of the BMD approach [76].

These limitations can complicate its application to in vitro endpoints where sample sizes may be artificially inflated by the lack of an appreciation of the implication of using the cell as the experimental unit in the statistical analysis (pseudoreplication). Attempts are sometimes made to "dampen down" the significance levels by the use of multiple comparison methods. Dunnett's test is one commonly used but has limitations because it compares each treatment group against the negative control. It is based upon a family-wide error rate: with the critical values dependent upon the number of groups and is set so that there is only an $\alpha = 0.05$ chance that a set of combinations will contain a comparison which is falsely declared significant [77]. The implication is that some real effects will fail to be detected and that the true NOGEL may be lower than the one detected. (Similar problems apply to the use of the more conservative Bonferroni approach.) The design is also vulnerable to biases resulting from artefactual results because of effects occurring at just one concentration.

Ideally the power of and sample sizes for designs should be considered, particularly if the objective is to identify NOGELs. Power is the probability of detecting an effect of a given size, if it exists, with a specific design and using a defined statistical test. Power calculations are easy to obtain for a simple comparison between two groups because there is much commercial and free software available.

One approach is to consider the size of effect in standard deviation (SD) terms. Sample sizes of approximately 16 (calculations give $n = 17$) to detect a 1 SD difference if power of 80% is required using a two-sided test. Sample sizes increase fourfold with each halving of the effect size to be detected: an effect size of 0.5 SD needs group sizes of about 64. Table 9.3 shows the sample sizes needed for 80% and 90% power for various effect sizes. The main problems with such calculations are determining an appropriate biologically important effect and the consequences of the estimates of the SD used in the calculations being highly variable. Power calculations are more complex with more complex designs or for those where identifying trends or shapes of curves is required [78].

Dose–Response Modeling

The BMD methodology in contrast to the NOGEL approach uses modeling techniques. Many of the common statistical methods—*t*-test, analysis of variance, linear and multiple regression—are also forms of a modeling approach called the general linear model (GLM) which in turn is a special case of the generalized linear model (GZM) [79]. The relationship between the different statistical modeling approaches is an active area of research [80].

Table 9.3 Sample sizes to detect various effect sizes with
80% and 90% power.

SD units	Power	
	80%	90%
0.0625	4020	5381
0.1	1571	2103
0.125	1006	1346
0.2	394	527
0.25	253	338
0.3	176	235
0.4	100	133
0.5	64	86
0.6	45	60
0.8	26	34
1.0	17	23
1.25	12	15
1.5	9	11
2.0	6	7
2.5	4	5
3.0	4	4
4.0	3	3

Sample sizes needed in each group to have 80% or 90% power to detect a
difference in means in standard deviation units using a two-sided two group
unpaired t-test with a 0.050 two-sided significance level and assuming
a common standard deviation. Sample sizes were calculated using the
software package, nQuery Advisor but other software gives similar values.
Numbers in bold show the approximate fourfold increase in sample sizes
needed to identify each halving in the effect size.

Toxicology is just one of many fields of science that fits models to data. It is not unusual or special in this respect. The statistical modeling methods used are similar to those widely used in many independent fields. Both the basic software/algorithms and conceptual underpinning are common across these different disciplines. There are a large number of ways of fitting data. The fit may be a predefined standard function (a mathematical model) or a statistical model, a simple example being a least squares linear regression.

There is an important distinction between mathematical and statistical models. The former are created with variables which are directly related to the biological events, while the latter are based upon parameters which link into the underlying distributions of the experimental data. Waller discusses the two concepts as applied in ecology [81].

Modeling of biological data (such as a dose–response relationship) consists of two parts: firstly, the fitting of some type of mathematical function to the data; secondly, the use of this function to make a prediction either within (interpolation) the observed data or beyond the observed data "extrapolation" (see below). These predictions allow the model to be tested and if necessary refined.

In this paradigm models are built, refined, tested, and modified. A model is a simplification but a useful representation of a process. George Box (R.A. Fisher's son-in-law) in a review of Fisher's contribution to statistics pointed out that "All models are wrong." He later modified this to the widely cited quotation: "All models are wrong (but) some are useful" [82].

Most statistical packages have procedures such as multiple regression where models can be built to describe a dependent variable (the Y term) in terms of its relationship to one or more independent variables (the X terms). These packages have various options for building the model such as forward, backward, stepwise or best-subset procedures [83]. In the forward approach parameters are added to the model until adding an extra parameter does not improve the fit to the data. In the reverse approach all the parameters are included in the initial model and parameters are dropped until the fit deteriorates. The stepwise approach is a combination of the forward and backward approaches. The best-subset procedure is a method which gives the "best" models for different numbers of parameters. However, these "automated" methods have their critics in that the models developed do not reflect biological knowledge. Harrell lays out very clearly the philosophy behind model fitting and provides a very clear set of guidelines [84].

In some cases there may be an underlying biological rationale (eg, a biologically based dose–response model) but often there will be a pragmatic approach with complex curves being drawn through data. It is important to appreciate that while such models may be able to describe many datasets they are only empirical models in the sense that they fit an equation to data. There is, in general, no direct relationship between the models and the molecular or biological system being investigated.

There is much software/algorithms available for curve-fitting. In some cases there is a clearly defined function/equation with parameter values such as for polynomials. In others, there is no specific function rather "local" equations providing a close fit to the data points, such as Lowess regression curves and splines [85].

Bonate provides a detailed but accessible account of various techniques such as smoothers, splines, and locally weighted regression (LOESS) describing how they are derived based upon the use of information in the local neighborhood of the data point rather than modeling based upon the totality of the data [86]. (A spline is a piecewise polynomial function which can have a simple form locally but is also flexible and smooth over a wider range. The name relates to the instrument draftsmen had to draw curves.) Splines are sometimes referred to as a nonparametric model fitting approach.

An important consideration is whether the dose–response relationship is monotonic or not. Monotonic is where the responses at higher dose are always equal to or greater than responses at a lower doses. Some models/software make the assumption that the relationship is monotonic and, if this is not so, will only work if data points showing a downturn are excluded.

In general, the more parameters that are include in the model the better will be the fit. These ensure that more inflection points are possible in the curve and, because it can bend more, the curve comes closer to the data points giving a better fit. Five parameter models can give closer fits that two parameter models.

Models can be either overparameterized or underparameterized. If as many parameters are fitted as there are doses, then a perfect fit (the "full model") is obtained which carries the danger of overfitting. This can result in good explanation of the observed or training dataset but a poor(er) prediction of the new independent (or test) data. If too few parameters are included there may be a poor fit. (In modeling it is generally advisable, for prediction, to have two sets of data: the training and the test sets.)

Models used for fitting dose–response relationships for quantitative endpoints in toxicology include the polynomial, power, exponential and Hill function models [87]. Models such as the Hill and exponential have been favored because they produce sigmoid (S-shaped) and bounded curves which are thought to be compatible with biological data and have parameters which can easily be related to the shapes of the dose-response. Bounded means the curves have specified maximum and minimum responses, such as 0% and 100%. Models can also be extended to accommodate, for instance, different variances within the dose groups.

In some models, some of the parameters—top/maximum, bottom/minimum or slope factors—are fixed (or constrained to standard values); the top and/or bottom could be set as the control values and the values "normalized" to 100 or 0, respectively. The curve is then effectively "forced through these values."

The exponential model, for instance is: $y = a*[c-(c-1)*\exp(-bx^d)]$ where y is the response, and x is the dose. The background/baseline level is a while the maximum level is c. (These are often set at fixed values.) The other two parameters—b, the potency parameter and d, the shape parameter—are allowed to vary. Models with fixed parameters may be preferred because they free up degrees of freedom (df) for model testing.

The so-called "hockey-stick" model (based on the "ice" not "field" hockey-stick!) is an example of a piecewise (or segmented or broken-stick) linear regression. It was developed for applications in genotoxicology by Lutz and Lutz [88]. Such models fit straight lines to the data with the aim of detecting discontinuities in datasets such as time series. Hockey-stick models are considered useful in fields such as finance and ecology and have been highly controversial in the debate on global warming [89].

Transformation of the doses and/or the responses is possible. Transformations have three main purposes: to linearize relationships, to stabilize variances, and to reduce the effect of outliers (*see earlier*). Note, however, the earlier comment that developments in modeling are reducing the importance of transformations.

Slob argues for the presentation of the data using a double log scale as the response then shows a relative change [90]. The default option may differ between software packages. The logarithmic transformation is the default option in PROAST but not in BenchMark Dose Software (BMDS). Similarly GraphPad PRISM expects the X values to be log doses [85]. Ritz, on the other hand, argues against the automatic use of logarithmic transformations both on the practical aspect of how to circumvent the problem of the log of zero and on biological grounds [91].

Interpolation and Extrapolations

Interpolation refers to the estimation of an effect within the range of doses included in the study (ie, the known data points); extrapolation is where a prediction is made outside the range of observed values. Interpolation is usually considered more reliable that extrapolation. Prediction becomes less accurate the further away it is made from the range of observed range and should be carried out with care to avoid the risk of serious error. One example is how extrapolations using polynomials can become negative outside the observed range. Identifying effects at low dose, however, is also often referred to as extrapolation [92,93] implying that there is a difference in the data from the negative control and the treated groups because they are being used to make predictions. Often in graphs the negative control data are separated from the rest of the data and the X axis is "broken." When the doses are expressed as logarithms the zero dose needs to be adjusted by adding a small value before the transformations.

Goodness of Fit Issues: Acceptance and Rejection of Models

Identifying which model is the best fit to the data is not a simple task. The choice of which model is the "best" or optimal fit is often made using a test based on the goodness (or lack) of fit of the predicted values to the observed data.

Parsimony is an important concept in this context. Occam's razor (named after the 14th century logician William of Occam) expressed as a statement such as "simpler is better" or "simple but not too simple" is often cited [51]. Its use in modeling is to try to find a model which gives a satisfactory explanation of the observations while using the minimum number of parameters as well as meeting the assumptions implicit in the methods used.

Many of the procedures use conventional goodness of fit tests such as the chi-squared or log-likelihood to measure the quality of the model fit. The value of the statistic is compared against a theoretical distribution for an appropriate number of dfs (usually the number of parameters fitted in the model). The P value associated with the statistic is often interpreted as a measure of how much the observed values differ from the predicted value. Small P values usually imply that the model is a poor fit to the data. The criteria used vary from modeler to modeler. The "traditional $P = 0.05$ cut-off" is sometimes considered too lenient as a criterion for a good model fit and $P = 0.10$, for instance, may be used as the criterion for deciding between an adequate fit and a poor fit [94]. It is though, important, to note that this does not automatically mean that the model is a good fit or that the "size" of the P value can be used as a metric for comparing and assessing which model is the "best." The assumptions on which the model is based should also be checked using the set of diagnostic tools and graphs produced alongside the statistical tests. Model uncertainty should be assessed. Piegorsch et al. have warned that misspecification of the model can have appreciable effects on the estimates of statistics such as the BMD [68].

The likelihood ratio/chi-square test is not appropriate for comparing models from different families such as, for instance, the probit and logistic models. Instead when two models are not nested an "information theory approach," such as the Akaike information criterion (AIC), should be used. The AIC is a measure for a set of models of the relative quality of a statistical model for the specific dataset.

Nested models are where one model can be transformed into another by the addition or subtraction of a single parameter. Consequently, in nested models one model has one more or one less parameter than the other. A model with two parameters is simpler (more parsimonious) than one with three, that is, the original two plus another. This means that the two models being compared differ by the inclusion or exclusion of just one parameter. A formal test between models can only be carried out if the models being compared are part of a "family" of models and are nested or hierarchical. Such a test is a way to obtain an unambiguous test of the effect of including individual parameters in the model. Ritz has shown the relationship that exists between many of the different function uses in the assessment of dose–response relationship and argues for a more uniform approach to modeling [91].

The improved fit that occurs because more parameters are included in a model should be considered. In multiple regression this is done using the adjusted R^2 value. The statistic AIC is an AIC that has been corrected or "penalized" to take into account the extra parameters in a model and is recommended by some modelers.

There may be a number of different models which fit the data on the basis of the goodness of fit criteria. However, it should be stressed again that goodness of fit tests cannot be used to choose between different models. The US EPA recommend plotting the data and inspecting the fit because, although there may appear to be good fit based upon the test, the predicted value may all be above, or below, the observed values [94]. The US EPA suggest identifying all the models that fit the data satisfactorily and then consider choosing the one with the lowest AIC [94]. An alternative is to use the model averaging approach [95].

This characterizes the uncertainty in the value of the BMDLs resulting from incomplete knowledge of the true dose-response.

In summary, although modeling can appear a precise and formal process there is the opportunity for an appreciable amount of expert but subjective input into, for instance, the choice of options and the inclusion or exclusion of outliers and anomalous curve fits. All imply a certain degree of subjectivity in the hands of the modeler. Full transparency of the methods used (and of the assumptions made) is necessary.

BMD Approach

The BMD methodology was first proposed by Crump in 1984 as an alternative to the NOEL/NOAEL approach [76]. For many years this approach has been criticized and its limitations pointed out (see above). The BMD approach has gradually been accepted in the regulatory arena by organizations such as the EFSA [96] and JECFA [19]. JECFA proposed the BMD as the reference dose (RfD) for the calculation of the MoE of genotoxic carcinogens.

The BMD is defined by the US EPA [67] as "A dose or concentration that produces a predetermined change in response rate of an adverse effect (called the benchmark response or BMR) compared to background."

The main advantages of the BMD approach are: (1) the use of confidence limits provides an estimate of uncertainty and this uncertainty is reduced in larger and better designed studies with lower and more conservative PODs; (2) the POD does not have to be one of the actual dose levels tested and can be calculated even when there is no NOAEL identified in a study; (3) the BMDL is a consistent and explicit response level while the NOAEL cannot be assessed in terms of a biological response (compare with the BMR) and can vary from study to study [97].

The lower 95% confidence bound for the BMD, termed the BMDL, is calculated and is then used as a RP or a POD (in a similar way to the NOEL) for extrapolation to low doses or to set guidance levels: for example, PDE, RfD, TDI, or ADI using safety or UFs or adjustment factors depending upon the regulatory context.

The choice of the BMR is an important aspect of the BMD methodology. The BMR may be defined relative to the critical effect size (CES) [98]. This could, for instance, be some percentage increase in the endpoint over the negative control level such as 10% (for the mean adult body weight [99]), some fold change in an enzyme level of clinical chemistry value or a doubling for GST-P-positive foci [90]. Slob used a CES of 5% change from the negative control mean [87].

The BMR used with qualitative data of, say, a 5% or 10% excess risk or a change from 5% to 10% in the proportion of animals with, say, a tumor cannot be equated with percentage changes in quantitative measures such as body weights. In the case of endpoints such as genotoxicity where qualitative events such as gene mutations are used, they are included in the model as if they are continuous variables.

An alternative approach to the BMR is to use a CES based upon the variability seen in the negative control group or the background level. The US EPA suggested using a change equivalent to 1 SD in the endpoint as the CES and defining the BMR as a change equal to 1 SD above the negative control mean [76,100,101]. A BMR of 1 SD is considered to be equivalent to about a 10% excess risk for individuals below and above the 2nd and 98th percentiles [100]. The US EPA suggest a CES of 0.5 SD under certain circumstances (such as frank effects) [94]. One consideration, however, is that a confidence interval associated with an estimate of an SD based upon small sample sizes can be very wide. The US EPA prefers that individual animal/experimental unit data should be used if possible (because covariates can then be included in the model) [94]. However, if these data are not available, then the mean, SEM or SD and *n* at each dose level can be used for the modeling.

Mathematical Modeling for the BMD

Endpoints where there are "visual" trends and a statistically significant dose-response in the data are investigated to see whether dose–response models can be fitted to the experimental data. The BMD derived by fitting a dose–response model to the experimental data and BMDL are determined for each suitable model. The BMD is the dose estimated to be associated with the BMR. The BMD is usually calculated by interpolation between points within the observed part of the dose–response study. If extrapolation below the observed data is necessary then this should be noted (it is less desirable with the results potentially unreliable if considerably outside the observed range).

The BMDL is the lower (one-sided) 95% confidence bound of the BMD (equivalent to one-side of a 90% confidence interval). A simple interpretation of a confidence interval (there is a more complex statistical, and deeply philosophical interpretation) is that there is 95% confidence that the true value of the parameter will lie within this range of values. There are different methods for calculating the lower bound which can produce different results.

Software

Many software packages can carry out nonlinear regression. GraphPad/PRISM, for instance, which is widely used in the biological sciences, has many options for fitting functions/curves to data. Some of these curves have a biological basis, other less so. Genstat has a directive FITCURVE which is "a convenient way of fitting various standard curves"; SAS, SPSS, and STATA have similar capabilities. The programming language R has a number of packages for nonlinear regression including some with thresholds or break points.

Specialist software, such as BDMS or PROAST, has been developed to model the data and provide estimates of statistics such as the BMD and the BMDL. An important consideration is that the different software packages can make different assumptions which are not always explicit to the user.

BMDS and PROAST have had different methods of development. BMDS has the more traditional mode of package development with periodic releases and updates. As at May 2015 it was at Version 2.6 and includes documentation and tutorials. PROAST, on the other hand, has been developed using the statistical programming language R and is in continual development and upgrading. It is now at version 38.9. PROAST now has a GUI to make it easier to use. Previously it needed to run within the R environment. In this sense it fits into the underlying philosophy of the R programming language of being free at use, of innovation, continual development and limited support to the nonprofessional user. The two packages produce similar outputs although there are differences.

BMDS

The BMDS package has over 60 models which can be used to fit models to quantal and continuous data. Details of the specific models available can be found at the BMDS website. The choice of model depends upon the type of data. For quantal data there are a range of standard "tolerance" functions. For quantitative or continuous data the models include polynomial, power, Hill, and a set of nested exponential models. More complex models are included in BMDS for the multilevel data from studies using developmental or teratology data where intralitter correlations may occur.

PROAST

PROAST is an R-based package developed at the RIVM (http://www.rivm.nl/en/Documents_and_publications/Scientific/Models/PROAST). The version on the RIVM website at May 2015 is v38.9. (Further enhanced versions are likely to be released in the future.) PROAST can carry out nonlinear regression across a wide range of scientific fields as well as in vivo and in vitro toxicology. The latest version has a GUI which allows standard applications to be run. The continual development approach means that the software is more flexible for the analysis of in vitro studies, for combinations across studies, the inclusion of covariates, comparison of different subgroups, and more flexibility in graphical outputs. PROAST, however, is not included in the packages that can be loaded directly from the R software.

Drsmooth

The software package *drsmooth*, maintained at the University of Swansea, consists of statistical tools for investigating dose–response curves. It provides tests for linearity and nonlinearity using user-defined cut-off values. Two methods are available for estimating threshold doses or doses where the dose–response function shows a transition to a significantly increasing bilinearity (R package *segmented*) or are smoothed with splines (R package *mgcv*).

Other R Packages

Ritz and Streibig (2008) provide an overview of the facilities available in R for nonlinear regression including the function *nls* [102]. Other R functions for threshold-related work include *Segmented* and *mgcv* which provide fits of linear, quadratic, and higher-order polynomial models and are used by the *drsmooth* package.

The R version of *drsmooth* "provides tools for assessing the shape of a dose–response curve by testing linearity and nonlinearity at user-defined cut-offs." The package can also be accessed and run independently of the University of Swansea website. There is a vignette/pfd outlining the options available (http://cran.r-project.org/web/packages/drsmooth/drsmooth.pdf).

The R package *drc* provides a wide range of facilities for carrying out dose–response modeling [38,102]. More information can be found at http://www.bioassay.dk/. http://cran.r-project.org/web/packages/drc/drc.pdf.

There is also a package, *bmd*, under development by Ritz and aimed at BMD calculations.

The R package *SiZer* has a number of options for exploring structures in curves [103]. The options include the "bent cable" which is, in effect, "a piecewise linear model with a quadratic curve of length 2γ connecting the two linear pieces," a locally weighted polynomial regression smoother and a piecewise linear model which "Fits a degree 1 spline with 1 knot point where the location of the knot point is unknown." (http://cran.r-project.org/web/packages/SiZer/SiZer.pdf)

The R function developed by Lutz and Lutz [88] for the analysis of possible threshold doses was called *thresholddose08111*. Although referenced in a number of papers this function/program may no longer be available; various laboratories may, however, still have copies of the original R code for it.

GraphPad PRISM

Prism includes the standard symmetrical dose–response curve (or four parameter logistic equation, 4PL). The four parameters relate to the top and bottom (plateaus) of the curve, the EC50 and the slope. An extra parameter, S, is needed if the curve is not symmetrical, resulting in the five parameter logistic equation (5PL). The Hill slope or slope factor is 1.0 for the standard symmetrical curve. Slopes of greater than one indicate a steeper slope and less than one a shallower slope.

Conclusions

Understanding the mechanisms of action of genotoxicity is an important aspect of the risk assessment of potential exposures to the human population. Dose–response modeling has a key part to play in this assessment. A wide range of curves, mathematical functions, and models can be fitted to experimental data but cannot prove that a threshold exists. Attempts to equate a threshold with the identification of a NOEL-like measure based upon statistical hypothesis testing have major limitations. Statistical methods applied to carefully designed and conducted experiments can provide estimates of the size of responses together with confidence intervals associated with them, these can provide insight into dose levels where there may be high confidence of negligible risk.

Modeling can provide RDs or PODs which can be used in various regulatory approaches to low-dose risk assessment such as the BMD or MoE.

Advances in the field of high-throughput in vitro screening, -omics technologies, high-throughput sequencing linked with the use multivariate statistical and bioinformatics approaches and applied in conjunction with mathematical modeling will allow a greater mechanistic understanding of low-dose effects.

Acronyms

ADI acceptable daily intake
AIC Akaike information criterion
ALARA as low as reasonably attainable
ALARP as low as reasonably practical
BMD benchmark dose
BMDL$_{10}$ benchmark dose lower bound
BMDS BenchMark Dose Software
BMR benchmark response
COC Committee on Carcinogenicity of Chemicals in Food, Consumer Products and the Environment (UK)
COM Committee on Mutagenicity of Chemicals in Food, Consumer Products and the Environment (UK)
df degrees of freedom
DOE design of experiments
EFSA European Food Safety Authority
EMS ethylmethanesulfonate
EPA Environmental Protection Agency (USA)
FAO Food and Agriculture Organization of the United Nations
GLM general linear model
GZM generalized linear model
ISO International Standards Organisation
JECFA Joint FAO/WHO Expert Committee on Food Additives
LNT linear nonthreshold
LOESS locally weighted regression
LOGEL lowest observed genotoxic effect level
MoE Margin of Exposure

NIH National Institute of Health (USA)
NOAEL no-observed adverse effect level
NOEL no-observed effect level
NOGEL no-observed genotoxic effect level
NRC National Research Council (USA)
OECD Organisation for Economic Cooperation and Development
OFAT one factor at a time
OSTP Office of Science and Technology Policy (USA)
PDE permitted daily exposure
POD point of departure
QRA quantitative risk assessment
RfD reference dose
RP reference point
SD standard deviation
SF safety factors
STT short-term genotoxicity test
TDI tolerable daily intake
TTC threshold of Toxicological Concern
UF uncertainty factor
US EPA United States Environmental Protection Agency
VSD virtually safe dose
WHO World Health Organization
ZED zero equivalent dose

References

[1] Madle S, von der Hude W, Broschinski L, Janig GR. Threshold effects in genetic toxicity: perspective of chemicals regulation in Germany. Mutat Res 2000;464:117–21.

[2] OSTP (Office of Science and Technology Policy, Executive Office of the President). Chemical carcinogens: a review of the science and its associated principles. Fed Regist 1985;50:10371–442.

[3] NRC (National Research Council). Science and judgment in risk assessment. Washington, DC: The National Academies Press; 1994.

[4] COM (2010). Committee on mutagenicity of chemicals in food, consumer products and the environment. Guidance statement: thresholds for in vivo mutagens, <https://www.gov.uk/government/uploads/system/uploads/attachment_data/file/315698/assessment_of_threshold_for_in_vivo_mutagens.pdf>.

[5] Efron E. The apocalyptics. New York, NY: Simon and Schuster; 1984.

[6] Rodericks JV. Calculated risks, 2nd ed. Cambridge. MA: Cambridge University Press; 2007.

[7] Barlow S, Renwick AG, Kleiner J, Bridges JW, Busk L, Dybing E, et al. Risk assessment of substances that are both genotoxic and carcinogenic: report of an International Conference organized by EFSA and WHO with support of ILSI Europe. Food Chem Toxicol 2006;44:1636–50.

[8] O'Brien J, Renwick AG, Constable A, Dybing E, Muller DJ, Schlatter J, et al. Approaches to the risk assessment of genotoxic carcinogens in food: a critical appraisal. Food Chem Toxicol 2006;44:1613–35.

[9] COM. Committee on mutagenicity of chemicals in food, consumer products and the environment. Guidance on a strategy for genotoxicity testing of chemical substances, <https://www.gov.uk/government/uploads/system/uploads/attachment_data/file/315800/in_vivo_testing_of_genotoxicity_of_chemicals.pdf>; 2010.

[10] Parry JM, Parry EM. The use of the in vitro micronucleus assay to detect and assess the aneugenic activity of chemicals. Mutat Res 2006;607:5–8.

[11] Jenkins GJS, Doak SH, Johnson GE, Quick E, Waters EM, Parry JM. Do dose response thresholds exist for genotoxic alkylating agents? Mutagenesis 2005;20:389–98.

[12] Flamm WG, Valcovic LR, deSerres FJ, D'Aguanno W, Fishbein L, Green S, et al. Approaches to determining the mutagenic properties of chemicals: risk to future generations. J Environ Pathol Toxicol 1977;1:301–52.

[13] White RH, Cote I, Zeise L, Fox M, Dominici F, Burke TA, et al. State-of-the-science workshop report: issues and approaches in low dose–response extrapolation for environmental health risk assessment. Environ Health Perspect 2009;117:283–7.

[14] Piegorsch WW, Hoel DG. Exploring relationships between mutagenic and carcinogenic potencies. Mutat Res 1988;196:161–75.

[15] Gollapudi BB, Johnson GE, Hernandez LG, Pottenger LH, Dearfield KL, Jeffrey AM, et al. Quantitative approaches for assessing dose–response relationships in genetic toxicology studies. Environ Mol Mutagen 2013;54:8–18.

[16] Pottenger LH, Schisler MR, Zhang F, Bartels MJ, Fontaine DD, McFadden LG, et al. Dose–response and operational thresholds/NOAELs for in vitro mutagenic effects from DNA-reactive mutagens, MMS and MNU. Mutat Res 2009;678:138–47.

[17] Benford D, Bolger PM, Carthew P, Coulet M, DiNovi M, Leblanc JC, et al. Application of the Margin of Exposure (MOE) approach to substances in food that are genotoxic and carcinogenic. Food Chem Toxicol 2010;48(Suppl. 1):S2–24.

[18] EFSA (European Food Safety Authority). Scientific Committee; Scientific Opinion on Exploring options for providing advice about possible human health risks based on the concept of Threshold of Toxicological Concern (TTC). EFSA J 2012;10:2750–853.

[19] FAO/WHO. JECFA evaluation of certain food contaminants. In Sixty-fourth report of the Joint FAO/WHO Expert Committee on food additives. WHO Technical report series, No. 930; 2005.

[20] EFSA (European Food Safety Authority). Scientific Committee Scientific opinion on the applicability of the Margin of Exposure approach for the safety assessment of impurities which are both genotoxic and carcinogenic in substances added to food/feed. Guidance of the Scientific Committee. EFSA J 2012;10:2578–82.

[21] COC. Committee on carcinogenicity of chemicals in food, consumer products and the environment. Risk characterisation methods COC/G 06 version 1.0, <https://www.gov.uk/government/uploads/system/uploads/attachment_data/file/315883/Risk_characterisation_methods.pdf>; 2012.

[22] ICH. Guideline M7: assessment and control of DNA reactive (mutagenic) impurities in pharmaceuticals to limit potential carcinogenic risk. In: International conference on harmonization of technical requirement of pharmaceuticals for human use; 2014.

[23] Lovell DP. Dose-response and threshold-mediated mechanisms in mutagenesis: statistical models and study design. Mutat Res 2000;464:87–95.

[24] Lovell DP. Experimental design and statistical analysis of studies to demonstrate a threshold in genetic toxicology: a mini-review. Gene Environ 2008;30:139–49.

[25] Kirsch-Volders M, Gonzalez L, Carmichael P, Kirkland D. Risk assessment of genotoxic mutagens with thresholds: a brief introduction. Mutat Res 2009;678:72–5.

[26] Crump KS. Use of threshold and mode of action in risk assessment. Crit Rev Toxicol 2011;41:637–50.

[27] Boobis AR, Daston GP, Preston RJ, Olin SS. Application of key events analysis to chemical carcinogens and noncarcinogens. Crit Rev Food Sci Nutr 2009;49:690–707.

[28] Crump KS, Hoel DG, Langley CH, Peto R. Fundamental carcinogenic processes and their implications for low dose risk assessment. Cancer Res 1976;36:2973–9.

[29] NRC (National Research Council). Toxicology in the 21st century: a vision and a strategy. Washington, DC: The National Academies Press; 2007.

[30] Zhang Q, Bhattacharya S, Andersen ME, Conolly RB. Computational systems biology and dose-response modeling in relation to new directions in toxicity testing. J Toxicol Environ Health B Crit Rev 2010;13:253–76.

[31] MacGregor JT, Frötschl R, White PA, Crump KS, Eastmond DA, Fukushima S, et al. IWGT report on quantitative approaches to genotoxicity risk assessment I. Methods and metrics for defining exposure-response relationships and points of departure (PoDs). Mutat Res 2015;783:55–65.

[32] MacGregor JT, Frötschl R, White PA, Crump KS, Eastmond DA, Fukushima S, et al. IWGT report on quantitative approaches to genotoxicity risk assessment II. Use of point-of-departure (PoD) metrics in defining acceptable exposure limits and assessing human risk. Mutat Res 2015;783:66–78.

[33] Calabrese EJ. Origin of the linear no threshold (LNT) dose-response concept. Arch Toxicol 2013;87:1621–33.

[34] Salomaa S, Prise KM, Atkinson MJ, Wojcik A, Auvinen A, Grosche B, et al. State of the art in research into the risk of low dose radiation exposure—findings of the fourth MELODI workshop. J Radiol Prot 2013;33:589–603.

[35] Nikjoo H, Sankaranarayanan K. State of the art in research into the risk of low dose radiation exposure. J Radiol Prot 2014;34:253–8.

[36] Bridges BA, Goodhead DT, Little MP, Bouffler SD. Evidence for transgenerational effects following exposure to ionising radiation: a briefing note prepared by a subgroup of the advisory group on ionising radiation. Didcot: Health Protection Agency (Great Britain); 2013.

[37] Jeffrey AM. Thresholds: absolute, practical, pragmatic, apparent and virtual. Toxicol Lett 2009;191:365.

[38] Ritz C, Streibig JC. Bioassay analysis using R. J Stat Softw 2005;12:1–22.

[39] Finney DJ. Probit analysis, 1st ed. Cambridge: Cambridge University Press; 1949.

[40] Fisher RA. Statistical methods for research workers, 1st ed. Edinburgh: Oliver and Boyd; 1925.

[41] Fisher RA. The design of experiments, 1st ed. Edinburgh: Oliver and Boyd; 1935.

[42] Box GEP, Hunter WC, Hunter JS. Statistics for experimenters, 2nd ed. New York, NY: Wiley; 2005.

[43] Montgomery DC. Design and analysis of experiments, 6th ed. New York: Wiley; 2005.

[44] Clayton JA, Collins FS. NIH to balance sex in cell and animal studies. Nature 2014;509:282–3.

[45] OECD. OECD guidelines for the testing of chemicals. Test guideline 474: mammalian erythrocyte micronucleus test. Paris: OECD; 2014.

[46] Meadows SL, Gennings C, Carter Jr WH. Experimental designs for mixtures of chemicals along fixed ratio rays. Environ Health Perspect 2002;110:979–83.

[47] Holland-Letz T, Kopp-Schneider A. Optimal experimental designs for dose–response studies with continuous endpoints. Arch Toxicol 2015;10:2059–68. http://dx.doi.org/10.1007/s00204-014-1335-2.

[48] Lovell DP. Commentary: statistics for biomarkers. Biomarkers 2012;17:193–200.

[49] Hurlbert SH. Pseudo-replication and the design of ecological field experiments. Ecol Monogr 1984;54:187–211.

[50] Brook RJ, Arnold G. Applied regression analysis and experimental design. Boca Raton, FL: CRC Press (Chapman & Hall). Marcel Dekker Inc, New York; 1985.

[51] van Belle G. Statistical rules of thumb, 2nd ed. Hoboken, NJ: Wiley; 2008.

[52] Torous D, Asano N, Tometsko C, Sugunan S, Dertinger S, Morita T, et al. Performance of flow cytometric analysis for the micronucleus assay—a reconstruction model using serial dilutions of malaria-infected cells with normal mouse peripheral blood. Mutagenesis 2006;21:11–13.

[53] Prinz F, Schlange T, Asadullah K. Believe it or not: how much can we rely on published data on potential drug targets? Nat Rev Drug Discov 2011;10:712–3.

[54] Collins FS, Tabak LA. Policy: NIH plans to enhance reproducibility. Nature 2014;505:612–3.

[55] Nature Editorial. Announcement: Reducing our irreproducibility. Nature 2013;496:398.

[56] Ioannidis JPA. Why most published research findings are false. PLoS Med 2005;2:e124. http://dx.doi.org/10.1371/journal.pmed.0020124.

[57] ISO. ISO 5725 accuracy (trueness and precision) of measurement methods and results—part 1 general principals and definitions. ISO (International Standards Organisation), Geneva; 1994.

[58] ISO. ISO 5725 accuracy (trueness and precision) of measurement methods and results—part 2 basic methods for the determination of repeatability and reproducibility of a standard measurement method. ISO (International Standards Organisation), Geneva; 1994.

[59] Churchill GA. Fundamentals of experimental design for cDNA microarrays. Nat Genet 2002;32(Suppl.):490–5.

[60] Verdugo RA, Deschepper CF, Munoz G, Pomp D, Churchill GA. Importance of randomization in microarray experimental designs with Illumina platforms. Nucleic Acids Res 2009;37:5610–8.

[61]   Zeiger E, Recio L, Fennell TR, Haseman JK, Snyder RW, Friedman M. Investigation of the low-dose response in the in vivo induction of micronuclei and adducts by acrylamide. Toxicol Sci 2009;107:247–57.

[62]   Gocke E, Muller L. In vivo studies in the mouse to define a threshold for the genotoxicity of EMS and ENU. Mutat Res 2009;678:101–7.

[63]   Gocke E, Ballatyne M, Whitwell J, Muller L. MNT and MutaMouse studies to define the in vivo dose response relations of the genotoxicity of EMS and ENU. Toxicol Lett 2009;190:286–97.

[64]   Gocke E, Wall M. In vivo genotoxicity of EMS: statistical assessment of the dose response curves. Toxicol Lett 2009;190:298–302.

[65]   Calabrese EJ. Hormetic mechanisms. Crit Rev Toxicol 2013;43:580–606.

[66]   Asano N, Torous DK, Tometsko CR, Dertinger SD, Morita T, Hayashi H. Practical threshold for micronucleated reticulocyte induction observed for low doses of mitomycin C, Ara-C and colchicine. Mutagenesis 2006;21:15–20.

[67]   US EPA (U.S. Environmental Protection Agency) Benchmark dose software (BMDS). U.S. Environmental Protection Agency, Rockville, MD; 2010. <http://www.epa.gov/ncea/bmds/>.

[68]   Piegorsch WW, Xiong H, Bhattacharya RN, Lin L. Nonparametric estimation of benchmark doses in environmental risk assessment. Environmetrics 2012;23:717–28.

[69]   Slob W, Moerbeek M, Rauniomaa E, Piersma AH. A statistical evaluation of toxicity study designs for the estimation of the benchmark dose in continuous endpoints. Toxicol Sci 2005;84:167–85.

[70]   Rhomberg LS. Seeking optimal design for animal bioassay studies. Toxicol Sci 2005;84:1–3.

[71]   Kavlock RJ, Allen BC, Faustman EM, Kimmel CA. Dose–response assessments for developmental toxicity. IV. Benchmark doses for fetal weight changes. Fundam Appl Toxicol 1995;26:211–22.

[72]   Gaylor DW, Lutz WK, Conolly RB. Statistical analysis of nonmonotonic dose-response relationships: research design and analysis of nasal cell proliferation in rats exposed to formaldehyde. Toxicol Sci 2004;77:158–64.

[73]   Tice RR, Austin CP, Kavlock RJ, Bucher JR. Improving the human hazard characterization of chemicals: a Tox21 update. Environ Health Perspect 2013;121:756–65.

[74]   Shukla SJ, Huang R, Austin CP, Xia M. The future of toxicity testing: a focus on in vitro methods using a quantitative high-throughput screening platform. Drug Discov Today 2010;15:997–1007.

[75]   Pottenger LH, Gollapudi BB. Genotoxicity testing: Moving beyond qualitative "screen and bin" approach towards characterization of dose–response and thresholds. Environ Mol Mutagen 2010;51:792–9.

[76]   Crump KS. A new method for determining allowable daily intakes. Fundam Appl Toxicol 1984;4:854–71.

[77]   Dunnett CW. New tables for multiple comparisons with a control. Biometrics 1964;20:482–91.

[78]   Ryan TP. Sample size determination and power. John Wiley and Sons Inc, Hoboken, NJ 2013.

[79]   McCullagh P, Nelder J. Generalized linear models Monographs on statistics & applied probability, 2nd ed. Boca Raton, FL: Chapman & Hall/CRC; 1989.

[80]   Dobson AJ, Barnett AG. Introduction to generalized linear models, 3rd ed. Boca Raton, FL: Chapman and Hall/CRC; 2008.

[81]   Waller LA. Bridging gaps between statistical and mathematical modeling in ecology. Ecology 2010;91:3500–14.

[82]   Box GEP. Science and statistics. J Am Stat Assoc 1976;7:791–9.

[83]   Draper NR, Smith H. Applied regression analysis, 3rd ed. Wiley Series in Probability and Statistics John Wiley and Sons Inc, New York; 1998.

[84]   Harrell FE. Regression modeling strategies with applications to linear models, logistic regression, and survival analysis: Springer Series in Statistics New York; 2001.

[85]   Motulsky H, Christopoulos A. Fitting models to biological data using linear and non-linear regression: a practical guide to curve fitting. Oxford: Oxford University Press; 2004.

[86]   Bonate PL. Pharmacokinetic-pharmacodynamic modeling and simulation: Springer New York; 2011.

[87]   Slob W. Dose–response modeling of continuous endpoints. Toxicol Sci 2002;66:298–312.

[88]   Lutz W, Lutz R. Statistical model to estimate a threshold dose and its confidence limits for the analysis of sublinear dose-response relationships, exemplified for mutagenicity data. Mutat Res 2009;678:118–22.

[89]   Khodadadi A, Asgharian M. Change-point problem and egression: an annotated bibliography. Collection of biostatistics research archive (COBRA) preprint series paper 44, <http://biostats.bepress.com/cgi/viewcontent.cgi?article=1075&context=cobra>; 2008.

[90] Slob W. What is a practical threshold? Toxicol Pathol 2007;35:848–9.

[91] Ritz C. Toward a unified approach to dose–response modeling in ecotoxicology. Environ Toxicol Chem 2010;29:220–9.

[92] Morgan BJT. Analysis of quantal response data. London: Chapman & Hall; 1992.

[93] Piegorsch WW. Low-dose extrapolation Encyclopedia of quantitative risk analysis and assessment. John Wiley and Sons Inc, New York; 2008.

[94] US EPA. Benchmark dose technical guidance document (BMD TG). External review draft. EPA/100/R-12/100. Risk assessment forum. Washington, DC: US Environmental Protection Agency; 2012.

[95] Wheeler MW, Bailer AJ. Properties of model-averaged BMDLs: a study of model averaging in dichotomous response risk estimation. Risk Anal 2007;27:659–70.

[96] EFSA (European Food Safety Authority). Use of the benchmark dose approach in risk assessment: guidance of the Scientific Committee EFSA J 2009; 11:1–72.

[97] Sand S, Victorin K, Filipsson AF. The current state of knowledge on the use of the benchmark dose concept in risk. J Appl Toxicol 2008;28:405–21.

[98] Slob W, Pieters MN. A probabilistic approach for deriving acceptable human intake limits and human health risks from toxicological studies: general framework. Risk Anal 1998;18:787–98.

[99] WHO/IPCS. Environmental health criteria 239: principles for modelling dose–response for the risk assessment of chemicals. Geneva: World Health Organization; 2009.

[100] Crump KS. Calculation of benchmark doses from continuous data. Risk Anal 1995;15:79–89.

[101] Kavlock RJ, Schmid JE, Setzer Jr RW. A simulation study of the influence of study design on the estimation of benchmark doses for developmental toxicity Risk Anal 1996;16:399–410

[102] Ritz C, Streibig JC. Nonlinear regression with R. New York, NY: Springer Science; 2008.

[103] Chaudhuri P, Marron JS. SiZer for exploration of structures in curves. J Am Stat Assoc 1999;94:807–23.

CHAPTER 10

Nrf2 as a Possible Determinant of the Threshold for Carcinogenesis

Yasunobu Aoki

Center for Health and Environmental Risk Research, National Institute for Environmental Studies, Tsukuba, Japan

Chapter Outline

Introduction   155
The Regulation of Gene Expression by Nrf2   158
The Susceptibility of Nrf2 Knockout Mice to Xenobiotics   159
The Carcinogenicity and Mutagenicity of Xenobiotics in Nrf2 Knockout Mice   160
Human Carcinogenesis in Regard to Nrf2 Activity   163
Do Nrf2 and Nrf2-Regulating Genes Contribute to the Creation of a Threshold to
   Carcinogenesis?   164
Conclusion   164
Abbreviations   165
References   165

Introduction

Carcinogens are classified into two categories: genotoxic carcinogens, which induce mutations by binding to and modifying DNA nucleotides (also known as direct mutagens; eg, alkylating agents and polycyclic aromatic hydrocarbons), and by modifying without direct binding to DNA (also known as indirect mutagens; eg, agents that generate reactive oxygen species (ROS)) [1–3]. In general, genotoxic carcinogens, especially direct mutagens, are considered to exert their effects even at low dosage, in the absence of a minimal dose required for effect (no-threshold effect). In contrast, nongenotoxic carcinogens, such as dioxins and chemicals that stimulate cell proliferation, are considered to show dose–response mechanics and threshold effects. For assessing the risk of genotoxic carcinogens with no-threshold effect, the excess cancer incidence is estimated by calculating the slope factor ((incidence of cancer)/(dose of carcinogen; eg, mg/kg body weight per day)) by using data from animal experiments or epidemiologic studies in mathematical models. When the carcinogen

Thresholds of Genotoxic Carcinogens.
DOI: http://dx.doi.org/10.1016/B978-0-12-801663-3.00010-0

is assumed to be nongenotoxic, the estimated acceptable daily intake (ADI; that is the no-observed adverse effect level (NOAEL) derived from animal experiments divided by the uncertainty factor) has been used in risk assessment [4–7].

However, some genotoxic carcinogens are considered to show dose–response kinetics that incorporate a so-called "practical" threshold. One example of these carcinogens is those that generate ROS, such as hydroxyl and superoxide radicals, which subsequently modify nucleotides to their oxidized forms [8,9]. These modified nucleotides, known as oxidative DNA adducts (eg, 8-oxo-deoxyguanosine (8-oxo-dG)), cause mutations that induce cancer [10–12]. In this regard, ROS-generating genotoxic carcinogens are sometimes categorized as indirect mutagens. However, the mechanisms that determine whether the dose-response of carcinogenicity includes a threshold for effect are not well characterized, particularly in the case of ROS-generating agents. Because the method used to calculate an agent's risk of carcinogenicity is selected according to the presence (or not) of a threshold, identifying the mechanism that determines this threshold is essential for accurately assessing the carcinogenic risk of various chemicals, especially ROS-generating agents.

As mentioned earlier, not only environmental genotoxic carcinogens, including ROS-generating chemicals, but also endogenous aerobic metabolism and exogenous irradiation modify nucleotides to produce DNA adducts, including oxidative DNA adducts; the formation of DNA adducts induces mutation and is hypothesized to cause aging-related phenomena [13,14]. To prevent these adverse effects, the body mounts various protection mechanisms, including (1) the suppression of metabolic activation catalyzed by phase II drug-metabolizing enzymes and antioxidant enzymes [15,16], (2) DNA excision and repair systems, (3) translesional DNA synthesis by Y family polymerases (eg, Pol eta and Pol kappa) and B family polymerases (eg, Pol zeta) [17,18], and (4) apoptosis (Fig. 10.1). These mechanisms act coordinately to prevent mutagenesis and consequently carcinogenesis. However, environmental carcinogens could overload the capacities of these systems, thus again causing excess DNA

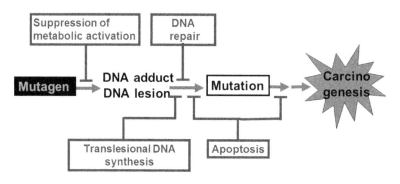

Figure 10.1
Mechanisms for preventing in vivo mutagenesis and carcinogenesis.

adducts and increasing the mutation frequency. The sensitivity of protective mechanisms to overload varies by mechanism and is a possible determinant of the practical threshold.

Among these mechanisms, the suppression of metabolic activation is key in governing the susceptibility to environmental carcinogens. Although some carcinogens, such as alkylating agents, bind to nucleotides to form DNA adducts in the absence of metabolic activation, numerous other environmental carcinogens, especially polycyclic aromatic ring-containing mutagens such as polycyclic aromatic hydrocarbons (eg, benzo[*a*]pyrene) and heterocyclic amines (eg, 2-amino-3-methylimidazo[4,5-*f*]quinolone (IQ)) are transformed to reactive intermediates, for example, their epoxy forms and hydroxylamines, through oxidation that is catalyzed by cytochrome P450 monooxygenases. These reactive intermediates exert various toxicities by binding to biomolecules and modifying their functions (eg, binding to nucleotides to produce DNA adducts; Fig. 10.2). On the other hand, the reactive intermediates are detoxified by conversion to hydrophobic conjugates, such as glutathione conjugates and glucuronic acid conjugates; this process is catalyzed by phase II drug-metabolizing enzymes, such as glutathione *S*-transferase (GST) isoforms (eg, GST-A1, GST-P1, GST-M1, and GST-T1) and UDP-glucuronosyltransferase (UDP-GT), respectively (Fig. 10.2). In addition, the activities of various antioxidant enzymes (eg, superoxide dismutase, peroxiredoxin, and glutathione peroxidase) suppress the formation of oxidative DNA adducts by quenching ROS generated by environmental agents. The suppression of phase II drug-metabolizing and antioxidant enzyme activities is speculated to accelerate the formation of DNA adducts (including oxidative DNA adducts) and increase the susceptibility to carcinogens. Epidemiologic studies of drug-metabolizing enzyme polymorphisms associated with cancer risk support this theory [19,20]. In fact, recent epidemiologic analysis suggests that null polymorphisms in GST (GST-T1, GST-M1, and GST-P1) directly contribute to an increased cancer risk [21–23].

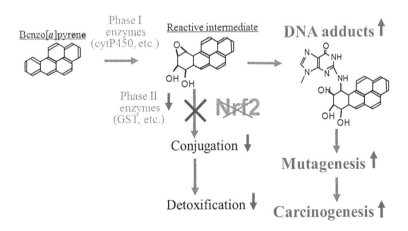

Figure 10.2
Acceleration of DNA adduct formation, mutagenesis, and carcinogenesis in Nrf2 knockout mice.

Phase II drug-metabolizing enzymes (GSTs, UDP-TG, and NADP(H):quinone reductase 1 (NQO1)) and antioxidant enzymes contain the consensus sequence 5′-PuGTGACNNNGC-3′ [24], the antioxidant responsive element (ARE) or electrophile responsive element (EpRE), as a cis element on the 5′ upstream of the structural gene. Various exogenous electrophilic inducers, including metabolites of xenobiotics and ROS-generating agents and phytochemicals, upregulate the transcription of ARE-containing genes by activating Nrf2 (nuclear factor erythroid related 2-related factor 2), a transcription factor binding to ARE [25], which plays a key role in regulating the expression of these genes [26]. In the following section, we review how Nrf2 modulates the susceptibility to genotoxic carcinogens by regulating the levels of phase II drug-metabolizing and antioxidant enzymes. Through this mechanism, the activity of Nrf2 may determine the practical threshold that must be overcome to achieve carcinogenicity.

The Regulation of Gene Expression by Nrf2

Nrf2 is an essential transcription factor that regulates not only the inducible but also the basal expression of phase II drug-metabolizing and antioxidant enzymes whose 5′-flanking sequence contains ARE. Nrf2 binds to ARE as a heterodimer with the small Maf transcription factor, and consequently stimulates the expression of these genes (Fig. 10.3). Under basal

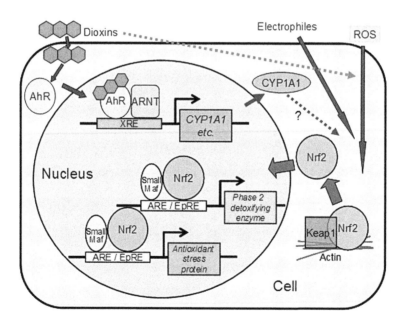

Figure 10.3
Comparison of an Nrf2–ARE signaling system with an AhR–ARNT system. *Source: Reproduced from Aoki Y. Health risk assessment of air pollutants: air pollutant genotoxicity and its enhancement by suppression of phase II drug-metabolizing enzymes. Genes Environ 2012;34(4):186–90 [27].*

conditions, Nrf2 binds to the cytoplasmic repressor named Keap1 (Kelch-like erythroid cell-derived protein with CNC homology-associated protein) and is thus retained in the cytoplasm as a latent form [28]. However, when stimulated by an ARE inducer (an agent that activates ARE-containing genes), Nrf2 translocates to the nucleus. Whereas the transcription of phase I drug-metabolizing enzymes (eg, cytochrome P450-1A1) is regulated by the binding of the well-known ligand-dependent transactivating factor arylhydrocarbon receptor (AhR) as a heterodimer with ARNT (Fig. 10.3, dioxin is used as an example ligand) to the 5′ cis element xenobiotic responsive element (XRE) [29,30], the activation of Nrf2-regulated transcription is controlled through a unique ubiquitin-associated mechanism. Under basal conditions and when bound to Keap1, Nrf2 is polyubiquitinated by the Cul3–Rbx-E3 (ubiquitination complex) [31] that is associated with Keap1 and polyubiquitinated Nrf2 is degraded by a proteasome system. Keap1 is a cysteine-rich protein, and the several thiol residues of cysteine are reactive to ARE inducers [26]. When these reactive thiols on Keap1 are modified due to ARE inducers, the ubiquitination of Nrf2 is inhibited. Consequently, Nrf2 translocates to the nucleus, where it induces ARE-containing genes.

Given that Nrf2 regulates the levels of enzymes that mediate formation of conjugates with various xenobiotics and the cellular redox level, the activity of Nrf2 may modulate DNA adduct formation due to genotoxic carcinogens and thus influence the susceptibility to carcinogens [32,33]. Consequently, the threshold of carcinogenesis may be dependent on the transcriptional activity of Nrf2 and Nrf2-mediated phase II drug-metabolizing enzymes.

The Susceptibility of Nrf2 Knockout Mice to Xenobiotics

Nrf2 knockout mice are an excellent model system for revealing the function of this transcription factor [34,35]. This model has been used extensively to investigate how Nrf2 contributes to protecting against the adverse effects of xenobiotics, including ROS-generating agents, and determines the susceptibility to genotoxic carcinogens.

Histologic studies showed that Nrf2 knockout mice are highly sensitive to hepatotoxicity from acetaminophen, a model chemical that is detoxified through UDP-GT and glutathione [36]. The expression of the ARE-dependent genes *UDP-GT* and *γ-GCS* (glutamylcysteine synthetase) and the level of nonprotein thiols (mainly reduced glutathione) were suppressed in these mice, suggesting that the resulting increased quantities of the reactive metabolite *N*-acetyl-*p*-benzoquinone-imine subsequently bound to intracellular proteins and other macromolecules and induced hepatic necrosis.

The toxicities of various environmental pollutants and model chemicals are enhanced in Nrf2 knockout mice. For example, Nrf2 knockout mice that inhaled diesel exhaust, which contains carcinogenic polycyclic aromatic hydrocarbons, developed severe hyperplasia

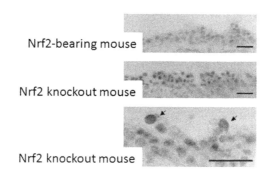

Nrf2-bearing mouse

Nrf2 knockout mouse

Nrf2 knockout mouse

Figure 10.4

Immunostaining of 8-oxo-dG in the lung of an Nrf2 knockout mouse and Nrf2-bearing mouse after their exposure to diesel exhaust. Positive staining (*arrows*) was detected in the bronchial epithelial cells of the Nrf2 knockout mouse. Bar represents 20 μm. *Source: Reproduced from Aoki Y, Sato H, Nishimura N, Takahashi S, Itoh K, Yamamoto M. Accelerated DNA adduct formation in the lung of the Nrf2 knockout mouse exposed to diesel exhaust. Toxicol Appl Pharmacol 2001;173(3):154–60. Epub 2001/07/05. http://dx.doi.org/10.1006/taap.2001.9176. PubMed PMID: 11437637.*

of and produced 8-oxo-dG in the bronchial epidermis [37] (Fig. 10.4). Benzoquinones contained in diesel exhaust may induce the generation of ROS, and subsequently 8-oxo-dG [38]. As expected, the formation of bulky DNA adducts, which are produced in response to polycyclic aromatic hydrocarbons, was accelerated in the lungs of Nrf2 knockout mice, in which the DNA adduct level was approximately 2.3-fold higher than that in Nrf2-bearing mice [37]. In addition, Nrf2 knockout mice were shown to be susceptible to pulmonary injury induced by butylated hydroxytoluene, an ROS-generating chemical [39]. Furthermore, Nrf2 helps to protect against hydroquinone- and benzoquinone-induced cytotoxicity [39]. These observations demonstrate the increased susceptibility of the Nrf2-deficient condition to environmental mutagens and carcinogens, such as diesel exhaust.

The Carcinogenicity and Mutagenicity of Xenobiotics in Nrf2 Knockout Mice

Investigation into the mechanism of chemoprotective agents yielded the first insights into the preventive function of Nrf2 against carcinogenesis induced by xenobiotics. The inducer of ARE-containing gene, oltipraz, a substituted 1,2-dithiole-3-thione developed as an antischistosomal agent, prevented benzo[a]pyrene-induced neoplasia in the forestomach of wild-type mice but had no protective effect in Nrf2 knockout mice [40]. Oltipraz subsequently was shown to induce the expression of the *GST* and *NQO1* genes in wild-type mice. However, the activities of *GST* and *NQO1* were suppressed in Nrf2 knockout mice, even when oltipraz was administered, and the number of benzo[a]pyrene-induced tumors was significantly greater (ie, 1.5 times higher) in nontreated knockout mice than in nontreated wild-type mice.

The administration of oltipraz prevented the urinary bladder carcinoma induced by *N*-nitrosobutyl (4-hydroxybutyl)-amine (BBN), an alkylating agent that binds to nucleotides without subsequent metabolic activation, in wild-type but not Nrf2 knockout mice. Specifically, the incidence of carcinoma was significantly (ie, 1.9 times) higher in Nrf2 knockout mice, in which multiple UDP-GT isoforms were expressed, than in wild-type mice [41], in which Nrf2 protected against the carcinogenesis induced through cooperation between BBN and p53 [42]. Interestingly, although the alkylating agent cyclophosphamide induced oxidative stress, DNA damage, and GST-P-positive foci (an early biomarker of hepatocarcinogenesis) in rats, treatment with astaxanthin, an antioxidant agent, enhanced the expression of the Nrf2-mediated genes *NQO1* and *heme oxygenase-1* and prevented these adverse effects of cyclophosphamide [43]. These combined results suggest that Nrf2 acts to detoxify carcinogens even when a carcinogen does not require metabolic activation to exert its carcinogenicity.

Similarly designed studies have shown the susceptibility of Nrf2 knockout mice to other carcinogens. For example, the number of tumors induced by IQ, a heterocyclic amine, was greater in Nrf2 knockout mice (2.8 times in male and 1.7 times in female mice) than in wild-type mice [44]. A protocol involving combined treatment with the cancer initiator 7,12-dimethylbenzo[*a*]anthracene (DMBA) and the promotor agent 12-*O*-tetradecanoylphorbol-13-acetate led to increased skin tumorigenicity in Nrf2 knockout compared with wild-type mice [45]. The administration of DMBA alone induced the progression of aggressive mammary carcinoma in Nrf2 knockout mice [46].

An increased frequency of mutation was suggested as the mechanism underlying the increased carcinogenicity in Nrf2 knockout mice. In this regard, intratracheal instillation of benzo[*a*]pyrene increased the mutation frequency in the lungs of Nrf2 knockout mice to twice that in Nrf2-bearing mice; in addition, the mutation frequency in vehicle-control Nrf2 knockout mice was higher than that in vehicle-control wild-type mice (Fig. 10.5) [47]. The expression of GST-A3 is essential for preventing the genotoxicity of aflatoxin; DNA adduct formation in the liver was accelerated in knockout mice lacking the GST-A3 isoform as well as in Nrf2-activated mice by knockout of Keap1 (GST-A3/Keap1 double-knockout mice) [48]. Similarly, aerodigestive tract carcinogenesis induced by the administration of 4-nitroquinoline-1-oxide (4-NQO) was enhanced in Nrf2 knockout mice, as expected, but suppressed in Keap1-knockdown mice, in which Nrf2 was activated [49]. Furthermore, Nrf2 knockout mice were susceptible to colitis induced by administration of dextran sulfate sodium, an inducer of colonic inflammation [50], and the incidence of colonic tumors after treatment with azoxymethane and dextran sulfate sodium was 1.7 times higher in Nrf2 knockout mice than in wild-type mice [51]. In comparison, the inflammation and tumor multiplicity induced by azoxymethane–dextran sulfate sodium were enhanced in mice that lacked the gene for glutathione peroxidase 2, an Nrf2-mediated antioxidant enzyme [52]. Together, these observations suggest that Nrf2 acts to prevent the mutagenesis that results from inflammation due to ROS production.

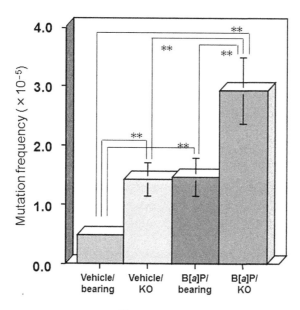

Figure 10.5

Mutation frequency in benzo[*a*]pyrene-treated Nrf2 knockout (KO) and Nrf2-bearing *gpt* delta mice. Columns, mean; Bar, 1 SD. **$P<0.01$. *Source: Reproduced from Aoki Y, Hashimoto AH, Amanuma K, Matsumoto M, Hiyoshi K, Takano H, et al. Enhanced spontaneous and benzo(a)pyrene-induced mutations in the lung of Nrf2-deficient gpt delta mice. Cancer Res 2007;67(12):5643–8. Epub 2007/06/19. http://dx.doi.org/10.1158/0008-5472.can-06-3355. PubMed PMID: 17575130.*

Regarding inflammation, Nrf2 knockout mice had greater steatohepatitis than wild-type mice when fed a high-fat diet [53]. The authors suggested that Nrf2 protected against steatohepatitis in part by increasing the threshold for inflammation. Overall, experimental data seem to indicate that the activity of Nrf2 determines the susceptibility to environmental carcinogens; in Nrf2 knockout mice, this susceptibility is about twice that in wild-type mice. Furthermore, transcriptional suppression of phase II drug-metabolizing and antioxidant enzymes appears to underlie the susceptibility of Nrf2 knockout mice to carcinogens; the metastasis-preventing function of Nrf2 may contribute to this phenotype as well [54].

The idea that susceptibility to carcinogens is increased in Nrf2-deficient conditions is consistent with its function as a transcription factor of detoxifying enzymes. However, urethane (ethyl carbamate)-induced lung tumorigenesis in Nrf2 knockout mice was about half that in wild-type mice [55]. Urethane is metabolized to vinyl carbamate, and the epoxide of this metabolite forms DNA adducts. Genotoxicity testing of urethane in transgenic mice revealed the induction of A-to-G transition in lung [56,57]. Although A-to-G transition in the K-ras gene (CAA to CGA) was frequent in the urethane-induced lung tumors of wild-type mice [58,59], it occurred only rarely in the tumors of Nrf2 knockout mice [59], suggesting that the decreased K-ras mutation in the lung tumors of Nrf2 knockout mice contributed to the decreased carcinogenicity of urethane. The authors then suggested that Nrf2 accelerates tumor progression through K-ras signaling [59]. Similarly, the administration of potassium bromate, a typical ROS generator that induces the formation of 8-oxo-dG, failed to accelerate oxidative DNA damage in the kidneys of Nrf2–Ogg (8-oxoguanine glycosylase, an excision DNA repair enzyme) double-knockout mice but caused severe kidney damage in the double-knockout mice [60]. Given that Nrf2 successfully prevented the renal oxidative stress induced by ferric nitrilotriacetate [61], Nrf2 may be unable to protect against the oxidative stress generated by a specific type of ROS.

Human Carcinogenesis in Regard to Nrf2 Activity

The contribution of Nrf2 to the susceptibility to carcinogens has mainly been shown through experimental data from knockout mice. Does Nrf2 similarly regulate the gene expression of phase II drug-metabolizing enzymes and protect against carcinogenesis in humans? In an attempt to answer this question, several molecular epidemiologic studies have been performed, and numerous genetic polymorphisms have been analyzed.

As mentioned earlier, experiments in mice revealed that the chemopreventive effects of oltipraz, an ARE inducer, are mediated through the activation of Nrf2. A chemoprevention trial of oltipraz was conducted in Qidong, China, where hepatocellular carcinoma is a leading cause of cancer death and where exposure to aflatoxin, a genotoxic carcinogen, may contribute to its high risk. Qidong residents who received 125 mg oltipraz daily for 8 weeks demonstrated increased urinary excretion of aflatoxin mercapturic acid, a phase II metabolite [62]. This result suggests that oltipraz increases the activity of phase II drug-metabolizing enzymes and subsequent excretion of aflatoxin and that the NRF2 activity that governs the expression of these enzymes may influence the susceptibility to carcinogens in humans.

Regarding an NRF2 activity-determining mechanism in humans, somatic mutations in the *NRF2* and *KEAP1* genes have been analyzed intensively. Somatic mutations in *KEAP1* occurred at a frequency of 50% in lung cancer cell lines and of 12% in nonsmall-cell lung cancer samples; these mutations were located in the DGR, an NRF2-binding region [28], and IVR domains [63], respectively. As expected, the activities of NQO1 and GST were higher in the *KEAP1*-mutated lung tumors compared with the corresponding normal tissue, suggesting that *KEAP1* mutation enhanced Nrf2 activity. Somatic mutations within DGR and IVR domains of *KEAP1* in the lung cancer tissue of Japanese patients occurred at the frequency of 8% [64]. Due to conformational changes, the mutated KEAP1 had reduced affinity to NRF2 and thus failed to suppress its activity [65]. In lung cancer cell lines bearing mutated *KEAP1*, NRF2 was constitutively activated, leading to the cell's resistance to various anticancer drugs. Furthermore, mutated *KEAP1* genes have been identified in gall bladder cancer; functional analysis revealed NRF2 activation and subsequent resistance to anticancer drugs that generate oxidative stress [66].

Similar to mutations in *KEAP1*, mutations in *NRF2* reportedly constitutively activate phase II drug-metabolizing enzymes in human cancers. Studies of the cell lines derived from the cancers revealed that these mutations occur in the DLG and ETGE motifs of the KEAP1-binding domain of the *NRF2* gene. The failure of the mutated NRF2 to bind to KEAP1 may escape NRF2 from the ubiquitination, suggesting to provide resistance to chemoprevention [67]. In addition, NRF2 activity is regulated through transcriptional control. DNA sequence analysis identified a single-nucleotide polymorphism in the 5′-upstream promotor region of *NRF2*; the A/A homozygote in this promotor region showed lower *NRF2* expression and greater cancer risk than did the C/C homozygote [68]. Higher activity of NRF2 assumes to tend to be associated with resistance to genotoxic carcinogens. The factors that regulate *NRF2* transcription via this 5′ upstream region have not yet been identified, but in vitro experiments have shown that K-Ras and other oncogenes stimulate *NRF2* transcription [69].

The effects of the *NRF2* and *KEAP1* mutants in human cancer cells provide evidence that the level of NRF2 activity may function as a determinant of the susceptibility to cancer-inducing environmental agents even in humans.

Do Nrf2 and Nrf2-Regulating Genes Contribute to the Creation of a Threshold to Carcinogenesis?

In an experiment addressing the contribution of Nrf2 to the existence of a threshold to carcinogenesis induced by a genotoxic carcinogen, rats fed aflatoxin B_1 for 4 weeks developed GST-P-positive hepatic foci, but those treated with a triterpenoid that has potent ARE-inducing activity, 1-[2-cyano-3,12-dioxooleana-1,9 (11)-dien-28-oyl]imidazole (CDDO-Im), were completely protected against this lesion [70]. In addition, CDDO-Im was shown to elevate the expression of Nrf2-dependent genes and to accelerate the urinary excretion of aflatoxin metabolites in these rats. Furthermore, cotreatment of rats with CDDO-Im and aflatoxin B_1 suppressed the amount of a major aflatoxin B_1–DNA adduct to one-fourth that after treatment with aflatoxin B_1 only. This finding indicates that phase II drug-metabolizing and antioxidant enzymes, whose gene expression is regulated by Nrf2, cooperatively decreased the quantity of aflatoxin–DNA adducts to a level insufficient for the induction of cancer in these animals. This idea is supported by toxicogenomic analysis of gene expression profiling in TK6 human cells treated with potassium bromate and hydrogen peroxide [71]. In that study, the genes of Nrf2-regulating antioxidant enzymes were identified as key players in the threshold responses for genotoxicity.

Conclusion

Nrf2-regulating genes restrict the amount of DNA adducts to below that necessary (the threshold) for inducing carcinogenesis, suggesting that Nrf2 is a determinant of the threshold for genotoxic carcinogenesis. Precisely how Nrf2 activity establishes the level of DNA adducts necessary for carcinogenesis remains unclear. Perhaps the "practical threshold" of carcinogenesis is a dose of carcinogen that provides a particular level of DNA adduct, of which formation was not prevented by drug-metabolizing and antioxidant enzymes but can be repaired completely by an excision repair, a translesional DNA synthesis and related DNA repair systems. To reveal the underlying mechanism for emerging a practical threshold in the carcinogenesis of genotoxic carcinogens indirect mutagen, such as ROS-generating agents, we need to analyze quantitatively how DNA adducts are fixed as in vivo mutations, resulting in initiating carcinogenesis.

Abbreviations

8-oxo-dG 8-oxo-deoxyguanosine
ADI acceptable daily intake
AhR arylhydrocarbon receptor
ARE antioxidant responsive element
BBN *N*-nitrosobutyl (4-bydroxybutyl)-amine
CDDO-Im 1-[2-cyano-3,12-dioxooleana-1,9(11)-dien-28-oyl]imidazole
DMBA 7,12-dimethylbenzo[*a*]anthracene
DSS dextran sulfate sodium
EpRE electrophile responsive element
GCS glutamylcysteine synthetase
GST glutathione *S*-transferase
IQ 2-amino-3-methylimidazo[4,5-f]quinolone
Keap1 Kelch-like erythroid cell-derived protein with CNC homology-associated protein 1
NOAEL no-observed adverse effect level
NQO1 NADP(H):quinone reductase 1
Nrf2 nuclear factor erythroid related 2-related factor 2
Ogg 8-oxoguanine glycosylase
ROS reactive oxygen species
UDP-GT UDP-glucuronosyltransferase
XRE xenobiotic responsive element

References

[1] Kirsch-Volders M, Vanhauwaert A, Eichenlaub-Ritter U, Decordier I. Indirect mechanisms of genotoxicity. Toxicol Lett 2003;140–141:63–74. Epub 2003/04/05. PubMed PMID: 12676452.
[2] Pratt IS, Barron T. Regulatory recognition of indirect genotoxicity mechanisms in the European Union. Toxicol Lett 2003;140–141:53–62. Epub 2003/04/05. PubMed PMID: 12676451.
[3] Eastmond DA. Evaluating genotoxicity data to identify a mode of action and its application in estimating cancer risk at low doses: a case study involving carbon tetrachloride. Environ Mol Mutagen 2008;49(2):132–41. Epub 2008/01/24. http://dx.doi.org/10.1002/em.20368. PubMed PMID: 18213651.
[4] Risk assessment of carcinogenic chemicals in The Netherlands. Health Council of The Netherlands: Committee on the Evaluation of the Carcinogenicity of Chemical Substances. Regul Toxicol Pharmacol 1994;19(1):14–30. Epub 1994/02/01. PubMed PMID: 8159812.
[5] Hengstler JG, Bogdanffy MS, Bolt HM, Oesch F. Challenging dogma: thresholds for genotoxic carcinogens? The case of vinyl acetate. Annu Rev Pharmacol Toxicol 2003;43:485–520. Epub 2002/11/05. http://dx.doi.org/10.1146/annurev.pharmtox.43.100901.140219. PubMed PMID: 12415124.

[6]   Bolt HM, Huici-Montagud A. Strategy of the scientific committee on occupational exposure limits (SCOEL) in the derivation of occupational exposure limits for carcinogens and mutagens. Arch Toxicol 2008;82(1):61–4. Epub 2007/11/17. http://dx.doi.org/10.1007/s00204-007-0260-z. PubMed PMID: 18008062.

[7]   Neumann HG. Risk assessment of chemical carcinogens and thresholds. Criti Rev Toxicol 2009;39(6): 449–61. Epub 2009/06/24. http://dx.doi.org/10.1080/10408440902810329. PubMed PMID: 19545196.

[8]   Kasai H, Chung MH, Yamamoto F, Ohtsuka E, Laval J, Grollman AP, et al. Formation, inhibition of formation, and repair of oxidative 8-hydroxyguanine DNA damage. Basic Life Sci 1993;61:257–62. Epub 1993/01/01. PubMed PMID: 8304936.

[9]   Sekiguchi M, Tsuzuki T. Oxidative nucleotide damage: consequences and prevention. Oncogene 2002;21(58):8895–904. Epub 2002/12/17. http://dx.doi.org/10.1038/sj.onc.1206023. PubMed PMID: 12483507.

[10] Amoroso A, Crespan E, Wimmer U, Hubscher U, Maga G. DNA polymerases and oxidative damage: friends or foes? Curr Mol Pharmacol 2008;1(2):162–70. Epub 2008/06/01. PubMed PMID: 20021430.

[11] Ventura I, Russo MT, De Luca G, Bignami M. Oxidized purine nucleotides, genome instability and neurodegeneration. Mutat Res 2010;703(1):59–65. Epub 2010/07/06. http://dx.doi.org/10.1016/j.mrgentox.2010.06.008. PubMed PMID: 20601098.

[12] Vijg J, Suh Y. Genome instability and aging. Annu Rev Physiol 2013;75:645–68. Epub 2013/02/13. http://dx.doi.org/10.1146/annurev-physiol-030212-183715. PubMed PMID: 23398157.

[13] Moller P, Lohr M, Folkmann JK, Mikkelsen L, Loft S. Aging and oxidatively damaged nuclear DNA in animal organs. Free Radic Biol Med 2010;48(10):1275–85. Epub 2010/02/13. http://dx.doi.org/10.1016/j.freeradbiomed.2010.02.003. PubMed PMID: 20149865.

[14] Jacob KD, Noren Hooten N, Trzeciak AR, Evans MK. Markers of oxidant stress that are clinically relevant in aging and age-related disease. Mech Ageing Dev 2013;134(3–4):139–57. Epub 2013/02/23. http://dx.doi.org/10.1016/j.mad.2013.02.008. PubMed PMID: 23428415; PubMed Central PMCID: PMCPmc3664937.

[15] Kwak MK, Egner PA, Dolan PM, Ramos-Gomez M, Groopman JD, Itoh K, et al. Role of phase 2 enzyme induction in chemoprotection by dithiolethiones. Mutat Res 2001;480-481:305–15. Epub 2001/08/17. PubMed PMID: 11506823.

[16] Motohashi H, Yamamoto M. Nrf2-Keap1 defines a physiologically important stress response mechanism. Trends Mol Med 2004;10(11):549–57. Epub 2004/11/03. http://dx.doi.org/10.1016/j.molmed.2004.09.003. PubMed PMID: 15519281.

[17] Masutani C, Kusumoto R, Yamada A, Yuasa M, Araki M, Nogimori T, et al. Xeroderma pigmentosum variant: from a human genetic disorder to a novel DNA polymerase. Cold Spring Harb Symp Quant Biol 2000;65:71–80. Epub 2003/05/23. PubMed PMID: 12760022.

[18] Katafuchi A, Nohmi T. DNA polymerases involved in the incorporation of oxidized nucleotides into DNA: their efficiency and template base preference. Mutat Res 2010;703(1):24–31. Epub 2010/06/15. http://dx.doi.org/10.1016/j.mrgentox.2010.06.004. PubMed PMID: 20542140.

[19] Nebert DW, Ingelman-Sundberg M, Daly AK. Genetic epidemiology of environmental toxicity and cancer susceptibility: human allelic polymorphisms in drug-metabolizing enzyme genes, their functional importance, and nomenclature issues. Drug Metab Rev 1999;31(2):467–87. Epub 1999/05/21. http://dx.doi.org/10.1081/dmr-100101931. PubMed PMID: 10335448.

[20] Neber DW, Roe AL. Ethnic and genetic differences in metabolism genes and risk of toxicity and cancer. Sci Total Environ 2001;274(1–3):93–102. Epub 2001/07/17. PubMed PMID: 11453308.

[21] Li J, Long J, Hu Y, Tan A, Guo X, Zhang S. Glutathione *S*-transferase M1, T1, and P1 polymorphisms and thyroid cancer risk: a meta-analysis. Cancer Epidemiol 2012;36(6):e333–40. Epub 2012/07/07. http://dx.doi.org/10.1016/j.canep.2012.06.002. PubMed PMID: 22765906.

[22] Wu K, Wang X, Xie Z, Liu Z, Lu Y. Glutathione *S*-transferase P1 gene polymorphism and bladder cancer susceptibility: an updated analysis. Mol Biol Rep 2013;40(1):687–95. Epub 2012/10/12. http://dx.doi.org/10.1007/s11033-012-2109-7. PubMed PMID: 23054023.

[23] Yang H, Yang S, Liu J, Shao F, Wang H, Wang Y. The association of GSTM1 deletion polymorphism with lung cancer risk in Chinese population: evidence from an updated meta-analysis. Sci Rep 2015;5:9392.

Epub 2015/03/24. http://dx.doi.org/10.1038/srep09392. PubMed PMID: 25797617; PubMed Central PMCID: PMCPmc4369748.

[24] Rushmore TH, Morton MR, Pickett CB. The antioxidant responsive element. Activation by oxidative stress and identification of the DNA consensus sequence required for functional activity. J Biol Chem 1991;266(18):11632–9. Epub 1991/06/25. PubMed PMID: 1646813.

[25] Itoh K, Igarashi K, Hayashi N, Nishizawa M, Yamamoto M. Cloning and characterization of a novel erythroid cell-derived CNC family transcription factor heterodimerizing with the small Maf family proteins. Mol Cell Biol 1995;15(8):4184–93. Epub 1995/08/01. PubMed PMID: 7623813; PubMed Central PMCID: PMCPmc230657.

[26] Ma Q, He X. Molecular basis of electrophilic and oxidative defense: promises and perils of Nrf2. Pharmacol Rev 2012;64(4):1055–81. Epub 2012/09/12. http://dx.doi.org/10.1124/pr.110.004333. PubMed PMID: 22966037.

[27] Aoki Y. Health risk assessment of air pollutants: air pollutant genotoxicity and its enhancement by suppression of phase II drug-metabolizing enzymes. Genes Environ 2012;34(4):186–90.

[28] Itoh K, Wakabayashi N, Katoh Y, Ishii T, Igarashi K, Engel JD, et al. Keap1 represses nuclear activation of antioxidant responsive elements by Nrf2 through binding to the amino-terminal Neh2 domain. Genes Dev 1999;13(1):76–86. Epub 1999/01/14. PubMed PMID: 9887101; PubMed Central PMCID: PMCPmc316370.

[29] Gu YZ, Hogenesch JB, Bradfield CA. The PAS superfamily: sensors of environmental and developmental signals. Annu Rev Pharmacol Toxicol 2000;40:519–61. Epub 2000/06/03. http://dx.doi.org/10.1146/annurev. pharmtox.40.1.519. PubMed PMID: 10836146.

[30] Fujii-Kuriyama Y, Kawajiri K. Molecular mechanisms of the physiological functions of the aryl hydrocarbon (dioxin) receptor, a multifunctional regulator that senses and responds to environmental stimuli. Proc Jpn Acad Ser B Phys Biol Sci 2010;86(1):40–53. Epub 2010/01/16. PubMed PMID: 20075607; PubMed Central PMCID: PMCPmc3417568.

[31] Taguchi K, Motohashi H, Yamamoto M. Molecular mechanisms of the Keap1-Nrf2 pathway in stress response and cancer evolution. Genes Cells 2011;16(2):123–40. Epub 2011/01/22. http://dx.doi.org/10.1111/ j.1365-2443.2010.01473.x. PubMed PMID: 21251164.

[32] Higgins LG, Hayes JD. The cap'n'collar transcription factor Nrf2 mediates both intrinsic resistance to environmental stressors and an adaptive response elicited by chemopreventive agents that determines susceptibility to electrophilic xenobiotics. Chem Biol Interact 2011;192(1–2):37–45. Epub 2010/10/12. http://dx.doi.org/10.1016/j.cbi.2010.09.025. PubMed PMID: 20932822.

[33] Slocum SL, Kensler TW. Nrf2: control of sensitivity to carcinogens. Arch Toxicol 2011;85(4):273–84. Epub 2011/03/04. http://dx.doi.org/10.1007/s00204-011-0675-4. PubMed PMID: 21369766.

[34] Itoh K, Chiba T, Takahashi S, Ishii T, Igarashi K, Katoh Y, et al. An Nrf2/small Maf heterodimer mediates the induction of phase II detoxifying enzyme genes through antioxidant response elements. Biochem Biophys Res Commun 1997;236(2):313–22. Epub 1997/07/18. PubMed PMID: 9240432.

[35] Chan K, Kan YW. Nrf2 is essential for protection against acute pulmonary injury in mice. Proce Natl Acad Sci USA 1999;96(22):12731–6. Epub 1999/10/27. PubMed PMID: 10535991; PubMed Central PMCID: PMCPmc23072.

[36] Enomoto A, Itoh K, Nagayoshi E, Haruta J, Kimura T, O'Connor T, et al. High sensitivity of Nrf2 knockout mice to acetaminophen hepatotoxicity associated with decreased expression of ARE-regulated drug metabolizing enzymes and antioxidant genes. Toxicol Sci 2001;59(1):169–77. Epub 2001/01/03. PubMed PMID: 11134556.

[37] Aoki Y, Sato H, Nishimura N, Takahashi S, Itoh K, Yamamoto M. Accelerated DNA adduct formation in the lung of the Nrf2 knockout mouse exposed to diesel exhaust. Toxicol Appl Pharmacol 2001;173(3):154–60. Epub 2001/07/05. http://dx.doi.org/10.1006/taap.2001.9176. PubMed PMID: 11437637.

[38] Kumagai Y, Arimoto T, Shinyashiki M, Shimojo N, Nakai Y, Yoshikawa T, et al. Generation of reactive oxygen species during interaction of diesel exhaust particle components with NADPH-cytochrome P450 reductase and involvement of the bioactivation in the DNA damage. Free Radic Biol Med 1997;22(3): 479–87. Epub 1997/01/01. PubMed PMID: 8981040.

[39]   Rubio V, Zhang J, Valverde M, Rojas E, Shi ZZ. Essential role of Nrf2 in protection against hydroquinone- and benzoquinone-induced cytotoxicity. Toxicol In Vitro 2011;25(2):521–9. Epub 2010/11/10. http://dx.doi.org/10.1016/j.tiv.2010.10.021. PubMed PMID: 21059386.

[40]   Ramos-Gomez M, Kwak MK, Dolan PM, Itoh K, Yamamoto M, Talalay P, et al. Sensitivity to carcinogenesis is increased and chemoprotective efficacy of enzyme inducers is lost in nrf2 transcription factor-deficient mice. Proce Natl Acad Sci USA 2001;98(6):3410–5. Epub 2001/03/15. http://dx.doi.org/10.1073/pnas.051618798. PubMed PMID: 11248092; PubMed Central PMCID: PMCPmc30667.

[41]   Iida K, Itoh K, Kumagai Y, Oyasu R, Hattori K, Kawai K, et al. Nrf2 is essential for the chemopreventive efficacy of oltipraz against urinary bladder carcinogenesis. Cancer Res 2004;64(18):6424–31. Epub 2004/09/18. http://dx.doi.org/10.1158/0008-5472.can-04-1906. PubMed PMID: 15374950.

[42]   Iida K, Itoh K, Maher JM, Kumagai Y, Oyasu R, Mori Y, et al. Nrf2 and p53 cooperatively protect against BBN-induced urinary bladder carcinogenesis. Carcinogenesis 2007;28(11):2398–403. Epub 2007/07/03. http://dx.doi.org/10.1093/carcin/bgm146. PubMed PMID: 17602169.

[43]   Tripathi DN, Jena GB. Astaxanthin intervention ameliorates cyclophosphamide-induced oxidative stress, DNA damage and early hepatocarcinogenesis in rat: role of Nrf2, p53, p38 and phase-II enzymes. Mutat Res 2010;696(1):69–80. Epub 2009/12/30. http://dx.doi.org/10.1016/j.mrgentox.2009.12.014. PubMed PMID: 20038455.

[44]   Kitamura Y, Umemura T, Kanki K, Kodama Y, Kitamoto S, Saito K, et al. Increased susceptibility to hepatocarcinogenicity of Nrf2-deficient mice exposed to 2-amino-3-methylimidazo[4,5-*f*]quinoline. Cancer Sci 2007;98(1):19–24. Epub 2006/11/07. http://dx.doi.org/10.1111/j.1349-7006.2006.00352.x. PubMed PMID: 17083568.

[45]   Xu C, Huang MT, Shen G, Yuan X, Lin W, Khor TO, et al. Inhibition of 7,12-dimethylbenz(*a*)anthracene-induced skin tumorigenesis in C57BL/6 mice by sulforaphane is mediated by nuclear factor E2-related factor 2. Cancer Res 2006;66(16):8293–6. Epub 2006/08/17. http://dx.doi.org/10.1158/0008-5472.can-06-0300. PubMed PMID: 16912211.

[46]   Becks L, Prince M, Burson H, Christophe C, Broadway M, Itoh K, et al. Aggressive mammary carcinoma progression in Nrf2 knockout mice treated with 7,12-dimethylbenz[*a*]anthracene. BMC Cancer 2010;10:540. Epub 2010/10/12. http://dx.doi.org/10.1186/1471-2407-10-540. PubMed PMID: 20932318; PubMed Central PMCID: PMCPmc2964634.

[47]   Aoki Y, Hashimoto AH, Amanuma K, Matsumoto M, Hiyoshi K, Takano H, et al. Enhanced spontaneous and benzo(*a*)pyrene-induced mutations in the lung of Nrf2-deficient gpt delta mice. Cancer Res 2007;67(12):5643–8. Epub 2007/06/19. http://dx.doi.org/10.1158/0008-5472.can-06-3355. PubMed PMID: 17575130.

[48]   Kensler KH, Slocum SL, Chartoumpekis DV, Dolan PM, Johnson NM, Ilic Z, et al. Genetic or pharmacologic activation of Nrf2 signaling fails to protect against aflatoxin genotoxicity in hypersensitive GSTA3 knockout mice. Toxicol Sci 2014;139(2):293–300. Epub 2014/03/29. http://dx.doi.org/10.1093/toxsci/kfu056. PubMed PMID: 24675090; PubMed Central PMCID: PMCPmc4064015.

[49]   Ohkoshi A, Suzuki T, Ono M, Kobayashi T, Yamamoto M. Roles of Keap1-Nrf2 system in upper aerodigestive tract carcinogenesis. Cancer Prev Res (Phila) 2013;6(2):149–59. Epub 2012/12/20. http://dx.doi.org/10.1158/1940-6207.capr-12-0401-t. PubMed PMID: 23250896.

[50]   Khor TO, Huang MT, Kwon KH, Chan JY, Reddy BS, Kong AN. Nrf2-deficient mice have an increased susceptibility to dextran sulfate sodium-induced colitis. Cancer Res 2006;66(24):11580–4. Epub 2006/12/21. http://dx.doi.org/10.1158/0008-5472.can-06-3562. PubMed PMID: 17178849.

[51]   Khor TO, Huang MT, Prawan A, Liu Y, Hao X, Yu S, et al. Increased susceptibility of Nrf2 knockout mice to colitis-associated colorectal cancer. Cancer Prev Res (Phila) 2008;1(3):187–91. Epub 2009/01/14. http://dx.doi.org/10.1158/1940-6207.capr-08-0028. PubMed PMID: 19138955; PubMed Central PMCID: PMCPmc3580177.

[52]   Krehl S, Loewinger M, Florian S, Kipp AP, Banning A, Wessjohann LA, et al. Glutathione peroxidase-2 and selenium decreased inflammation and tumors in a mouse model of inflammation-associated carcinogenesis whereas sulforaphane effects differed with selenium supply. Carcinogenesis 2012;33(3):620–8.

Epub 2011/12/20. http://dx.doi.org/10.1093/carcin/bgr288. PubMed PMID: 22180572; PubMed Central PMCID: PMCPmc3291858.

[53] Meakin PJ, Chowdhry S, Sharma RS, Ashford FB, Walsh SV, McCrimmon RJ, et al. Susceptibility of Nrf2-null mice to steatohepatitis and cirrhosis upon consumption of a high-fat diet is associated with oxidative stress, perturbation of the unfolded protein response, and disturbance in the expression of metabolic enzymes but not with insulin resistance. Mol Cell Biol 2014;34(17):3305–20. Epub 2014/06/25. http://dx.doi.org/10.1128/mcb.00677-14. PubMed PMID: 24958099; PubMed Central PMCID: PMCPmc4135558.

[54] Satoh H, Moriguchi T, Taguchi K, Takai J, Maher JM, Suzuki T, et al. Nrf2-deficiency creates a responsive microenvironment for metastasis to the lung. Carcinogenesis 2010;31(10):1833–43. Epub 2010/06/02. http://dx.doi.org/10.1093/carcin/bgq105. PubMed PMID: 20513672.

[55] Bauer AK, Cho HY, Miller-Degraff L, Walker C, Helms K, Fostel J, et al. Targeted deletion of Nrf2 reduces urethane-induced lung tumor development in mice. PloS one 2011;6(10):e26590. Epub 2011/11/01. http://dx.doi.org/10.1371/journal.pone.0026590. PubMed PMID: 22039513; PubMed Central PMCID: PMCPmc3198791.

[56] Hernandez LG, Forkert PG. Inhibition of vinyl carbamate-induced mutagenicity and clastogenicity by the garlic constituent diallyl sulfone in F1 (Big Bluex A/J) transgenic mice. Carcinogenesis 2007;28(8): 1824–30. Epub 2007/03/08. http://dx.doi.org/10.1093/carcin/bgm051. PubMed PMID: 17341656.

[57] Forkert PG. Mechanisms of lung tumorigenesis by ethyl carbamate and vinyl carbamate. Drug Metab Rev 2010;42(2):355–78. Epub 2010/03/09. http://dx.doi.org/10.3109/03602531003611915. PubMed PMID: 20205516.

[58] Hernandez LG, Forkert PG. Inhibition of vinyl carbamate-induced lung tumors and Kras2 mutations by the garlic derivative diallyl sulfone. Mutat Res 2009;662(1–2):16–21. Epub 2008/12/23. http://dx.doi.org/10.1016/j.mrfmmm.2008.11.013. PubMed PMID: 19101575.

[59] Satoh H, Moriguchi T, Takai J, Ebina M, Yamamoto M. Nrf2 prevents initiation but accelerates progression through the Kras signaling pathway during lung carcinogenesis. Cancer Res 2013;73(13):4158–68. Epub 2013/04/24. http://dx.doi.org/10.1158/0008-5472.can-12-4499. PubMed PMID: 23610445.

[60] Jaloszynski P, Murata S, Shinkai Y, Takahashi S, Kumagai Y, Nishimura S, et al. Dysfunction of Nrf2 decreases $KBrO_3$-induced oxidative DNA damage in Ogg1-null mice. Biochem Biophys Res Commun 2007;364(4):966–71. Epub 2007/11/01. http://dx.doi.org/10.1016/j.bbrc.2007.10.123. PubMed PMID: 17971305.

[61] Kanki K, Umemura T, Kitamura Y, Ishii Y, Kuroiwa Y, Kodama Y, et al. A possible role of nrf2 in prevention of renal oxidative damage by ferric nitrilotriacetate. Toxicol Pathol 2008;36(2):353–61. Epub 2008/03/28. http://dx.doi.org/10.1177/0192623307311401. PubMed PMID: 18364461.

[62] Wang JS, Shen X, He X, Zhu YR, Zhang BC, Wang JB, et al. Protective alterations in phase 1 and 2 metabolism of aflatoxin B1 by oltipraz in residents of Qidong, People's Republic of China. J Natl Cancer Inst 1999;91(4):347–54. Epub 1999/03/02. PubMed PMID: 10050868.

[63] Singh A, Misra V, Thimmulappa RK, Lee H, Ames S, Hoque MO, et al. Dysfunctional KEAP1-NRF2 interaction in non-small-cell lung cancer. PLoS Med 2006;3(10):e420. Epub 2006/10/06. http://dx.doi.org/10.1371/journal.pmed.0030420. PubMed PMID: 17020408; PubMed Central PMCID: PMCPmc1584412.

[64] Ohta T, Iijima K, Miyamoto M, Nakahara I, Tanaka H, Ohtsuji M, et al. Loss of Keap1 function activates Nrf2 and provides advantages for lung cancer cell growth. Cancer Res 2008;68(5):1303–9. Epub 2008/03/05. http://dx.doi.org/10.1158/0008-5472.can-07-5003. PubMed PMID: 18316592.

[65] Padmanabhan B, Tong KI, Ohta T, Nakamura Y, Scharlock M, Ohtsuji M, et al. Structural basis for defects of Keap1 activity provoked by its point mutations in lung cancer. Mol Cell 2006;21(5):689–700. Epub 2006/03/02. http://dx.doi.org/10.1016/j.molcel.2006.01.013. PubMed PMID: 16507366.

[66] Shibata T, Kokubu A, Gotoh M, Ojima H, Ohta T, Yamamoto M, et al. Genetic alteration of Keap1 confers constitutive Nrf2 activation and resistance to chemotherapy in gallbladder cancer. Gastroenterology 2008;135(4):1358–68. 68.e1-4. Epub 2008/08/12. http://dx.doi.org/10.1053/j.gastro.2008.06.082. PubMed PMID: 18692501.

[67] Shibata T, Ohta T, Tong KI, Kokubu A, Odogawa R, Tsuta K, et al. Cancer related mutations in NRF2 impair its recognition by Keap1-Cul3 E3 ligase and promote malignancy. Proce Natl Acad Sci USA 2008;105(36):13568–73. Epub 2008/09/02. http://dx.doi.org/10.1073/pnas.0806268105. PubMed PMID: 18757741; PubMed Central PMCID: PMCPmc2533230.

[68] Suzuki T, Shibata T, Takaya K, Shiraishi K, Kohno T, Kunitoh H, et al. Regulatory nexus of synthesis and degradation deciphers cellular Nrf2 expression levels. Mol Cell Biol 2013;33(12):2402–12. Epub 2013/04/11. http://dx.doi.org/10.1128/mcb.00065-13. PubMed PMID: 23572560; PubMed Central PMCID: PMCPmc3700104.

[69] DeNicola GM, Karreth FA, Humpton TJ, Gopinathan A, Wei C, Frese K, et al. Oncogene-induced Nrf2 transcription promotes ROS detoxification and tumorigenesis. Nature 2011;475(7354):106–9. Epub 2011/07/08. http://dx.doi.org/10.1038/nature10189. PubMed PMID: 21734707; PubMed Central PMCID: PMCPmc3404470.

[70] Johnson NM, Egner PA, Baxter VK, Sporn MB, Wible RS, Sutter TR, et al. Complete protection against aflatoxin B(1)-induced liver cancer with a triterpenoid: DNA adduct dosimetry, molecular signature, and genotoxicity threshold. Cancer Prev Res (Phila) 2014;7(7):658–65. Epub 2014/03/26. http://dx.doi.org/10.1158/1940-6207.capr-13-0430. PubMed PMID: 24662598; PubMed Central PMCID: PMCPmc4082474.

[71] Platel A, Gervais V, Sajot N, Nesslany F, Marzin D, Claude N. Study of gene expression profiles in TK6 human cells exposed to DNA-oxidizing agents. Mutat Res 2010;689(1–2):21–49. Epub 2010/05/15. http://dx.doi.org/10.1016/j.mrfmmm.2010.04.004. PubMed PMID: 20466008.

Assessment of Nongenotoxic Mechanisms in Carcinogenicity Test of Chemicals; Quinone, Quinone Imine, and Quinone Methide as Examples

Yasushi Yamazoe and Kunitoshi Mitsumori

Food Safety Commission, Government of Japan, Akasaka Minato-ku, Tokyo, Japan

Chapter Outline
Quercetin   172
    Genotoxicity   173
    Pharmacokinetics   173
    Carcinogenicity   174
    Toxicology   175
Eugenol and Methyleugenol   175
    Genotoxicity   175
    Pharmacokinetics   176
    Carcinogenicity   177
Phenacetin and Acetaminophen   178
    Genotoxicity   178
    Pharmacokinetics   179
    Carcinogenicity   180
Menadione   180
    Genotoxicity   181
    Pharmacokinetics   181
    Carcinogenicity   182
    Toxicology   182
Ethoxyquin   183
    Genotoxicity   183
    Pharmacokinetics   184
    Carcinogenicity   184
    Mechanism of Carcinogenicity of Ethoxyquin   185
General Discussion for All the Chemicals Shown   185
References   188

Thresholds of Genotoxic Carcinogens.
DOI. http://dx.doi.org/10.1016/B978-0-12-801663-3.00011-X

Chemicals show carcinogenicity in rodent assays through genotoxic and nongenotoxic mechanisms. No threshold levels are defined for genotoxic carcinogens, and thus genotoxic carcinogens are tightly restricted. Nongenotoxic carcinogens often evoke tumorigenicity after chronic administration of high doses and show a threshold when testing multiple doses. However, verification of genotoxic and nongenotoxic carcinogens is not readily achievable in most cases. This is mainly because of overlapping of biological effects. Therefore, mechanistic support is of importance in the assessment of chemicals with tumorigenic potentials.

Formation of quinone, quinone imine, and quinone methide (EQM) metabolites leads to typical classes of adverse outcome pathways. The significance of these adverse outcome pathways is discussed in this chapter, regarding genotoxicity, tumor pathology, and metabolism. Five different types of chemicals are chosen as examples, which include the natural flavonoid quercetin, the flavor components, eugenol and methyleugenol, the medicinal drug, acetaminophen (phenacetin), the vitamin, menadione, and the food additive, ethoxyquin.

Quercetin

Quercetin is a natural occurring component of daily diet in fruits and vegetables, which contains quercetin as glucosides at the 3- and 4'-positions (Fig. 11.1). Quercetin exhibits a wide range of biological activities, including inhibition of tyrosine kinases, protein kinase C,

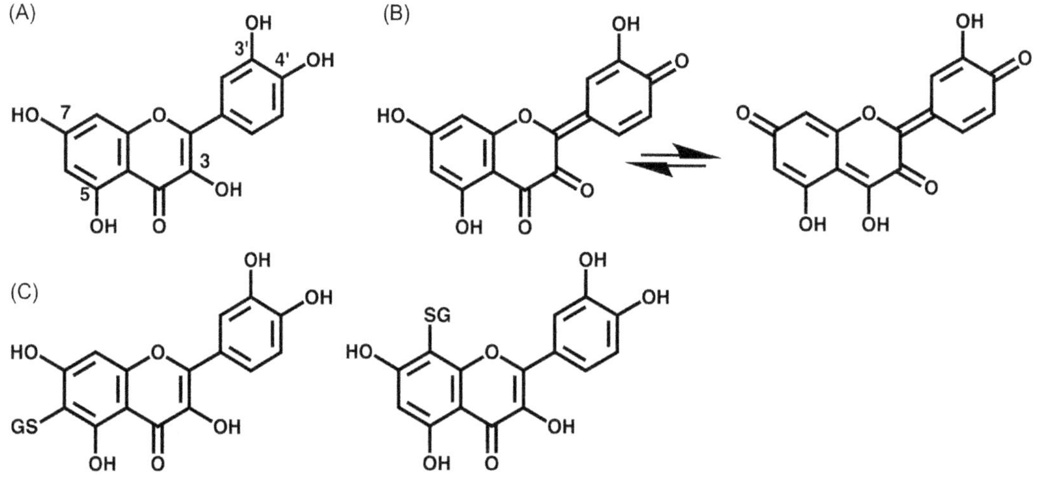

Figure 11.1
Chemical structures of quercetin (A), quinone imine as tautomers (B), and glutathione adducts at 6 and 8 positions (C). *SG*, glutathionyl.

and phosphatidyl inositol-3 kinase [1,2]. The estimated daily average intake of quercetin in the United States is 25 mg [3], although there are variations among different reports [4].

Genotoxicity

In the early 1980s, genotoxic substances in natural products and in the environment were extensively surveyed using mutagen-detecting systems based on *Salmonella* and other bacteria. Flavonoids, which are contained in various edible plants, have been shown to be mutagenic in the Ames test [5]. Quercetin induces mutations in *Salmonella* with and without exogenous metabolic activation, mutations in *Drosophila*, and chromosomal aberrations and sister chromatid exchanges in mammalian cell cultures [3,6,7]. In an experiment using ^{14}C-quercetin in Hep G2 cells, the radioactivity was associated mainly with cellular proteins, but also, to lesser extents, with the DNA [8].

Pharmacokinetics

Due to the low or undetectable plasma levels of quercetin, the bioavailability after oral intake has been questionable in the past. Using recent sensitive methods, unchanged quercetin is not or barely detectable in the plasma of humans, but it mostly appears as 3′-sulfates and 3-glucuronides. After ingestion of 270 g fried onions, in which total 275 μmol of quercetin 3,4′-diglucoside, quercetin 4′-glucoside or isorhamnetin (3′-*O*-methylquercetin)-4′-glucoside are contained, about 4% of the total intake appears in plasma and urine. Under these conditions, two main metabolites in plasma, quercetin 3′-sulfate, and quercetin 3-glucuronide, showed their C_{max} of 665 and 351 nM, respectively, within 1 h after ingestion. More than 90% of the metabolites were excreted within the first 8 h. The main urinary metabolite was quercetin diglucuronide, followed by quercetin 3′-glucuronide, isorhamnetin-3-glucuronide, and quercetin glucuronide sulfate [9].

Quercetin is taken up in the body as aglycon and/or as monoglucoside through the SGLT transporter in the intestine [10]. The glucoside is hydrolyzed prior to its entry into the portal vein, followed by metabolism in the liver to glucuronide and sulfate to be delivered to the bile [11].

In a phase I clinical trial, quercetin aglycon was administrated by short i.v. infusion (60–1700 mg/m²). Quercetin showed a plasma half-life of 43 min and a volume of distribution of 3.7 L/m², indicating rapid clearance from the systemic circulation [1].

Efficient excretion into the bile of the glucuronides of quercetin and of the methylated derivative tamarixetin has also been demonstrated in rats [11].

In another rat study 50 μmol of quercetin-3-*O*-glucoside mixture (glucose $n = 1–7$) was instilled into the duodenum, and higher levels of quercetin conjugate were detected in bile corresponding to 10–30% of the instilled amounts [12].

Carcinogenicity

The carcinogenicity of quercetin has been investigated using rodents. Pamukcu et al. [13] reported that Norwegian rats, having received quercetin at 0.1% in the diet for 58 weeks, showed an increase in the incidence of intestinal and urinary bladder tumors. Other long-term carcinogenicity studies in rats, however, have not confirmed this carcinogenic effect [14,15]. In a 2-year long-term toxicology and carcinogenicity study of quercetin in rats, conducted by the US National Toxicology Program (NTP), there was "some evidence of carcinogenic activity in male F344 rats" based on an increased incidence of renal tubular cell adenomas with increased severity of chronic nephropathy and hyperplasia of the renal tubular epithelium in the highest dose group (40,000 ppm), but not in lower dose groups males or in female rats having received diets containing 1000, 10,000, or 40,000 ppm [16]. In mice, long-term studies of quercetin did not show any carcinogenic effect [17].

As mentioned above, the results of Pamukcu et al. [13] on the intestinal and urinary bladder tumors induced by the treatment of quercetin in rats, were not confirmed by others [15,18]. Carcinogenicity-modifying effects of quercetin were also examined but not detected in two-stage urinary bladder carcinogenesis studies in male rats [19]. In the NTP bioassay of quercetin [3], a treatment-related increase in the severity of nephropathy was seen only in male rats treated with quercetin. Male-specific appearance of quercetin toxicity is apparently due to a greater susceptibility of male rats to spontaneous nephropathy during aging and the exacerbation of this disease by quercetin administration. The possibility of α2u-globulin nephropathy in the male-dominant renal carcinogenicity of quercetin in rats has been discussed by NTP. If this is the case, the renal tumors are unlikely to occur in humans due to low amounts of α2u-globulin excretion in human urine. However, no experimental evidence has been provided on the involvement of α2u-globulin nephropathy in the NTP carcinogenicity study. It is therefore unclear whether the renal tumor induction in male rats treated with quercetin is attributable to α2u-globulin nephropathy. A reevaluation of the histopathology on the kidney in the 2-year carcinogenicity study of quercetin in rats [3] has been performed to determine whether a mode of action underlying the development of renal tumors could be identified [20]. The reevaluation used a semiquantitative method for assessment of chronic progressive nephropathy (CPN) in rats. The exact etiology of the CPN is not clearly defined, but this nephropathy is regarded as an age-related, spontaneously occurring, rodent-specific disease with no relevance for human risk assessment [21]. The CPN leading to hyperplasia has been identified as a factor for a marginal increase in the background incidence of renal tumors in rats. An association between advanced CPN and the exacerbating effect of a test chemical resulting in an increase in renal tubular tumors has been demonstrated for hydroquinone [22] and ethyl benzene [23]. The results of the quercetin reevaluation confirmed that the renal proliferative lesions in the NTP study occurred only at dose levels associated with severe chronic nephropathy, and there were no cellular alterations in the kidney indicative of chemical toxicity at 6, 15 months, or 2 years. These findings supported a mode of action involving quercetin interaction with CPN. The authors pointed out that this mode of action represents a secondary mechanism for renal tumor development, with no relevance for extrapolation to humans [20]. Therefore, the renal tumors observed in the NTP study of male rats can be regarded as being unlikely to occur in humans.

Toxicology

In a clinical trial, renal toxicity has been a dose-limiting factor at over $1700 \, mg/m^2$. Reversible elevation of serum creatinine was observed in patients [1].

Concerning active oxygen and free-radical production, quercetin is oxidized by peroxidase (eg, tyrosinase) to *O*-quinone mono-anion, subsequently to *p*-quinone methides [24]. Two glutathione adducts, 6- and 8-glutathionylquercetin, are formed during the oxidation in the presence of glutathione. The reversible nature of the adduct formation has been shown in vitro. Although a glutathione adduct has been detected in hepatocytes [25], no apparent excretion of a glutathione-derived metabolite of quercetin is observed in experimental animals and humans.

Various factors may lead to the negligible carcinogenicity and toxicity, in spite of a clear genotoxic potential. Low bioavailability upon oral intake, efficient first-pass metabolism prior to the systemic circulation, and low oxygen tension in the body might prevent the oxidation to form the EQM.

Eugenol and Methyleugenol

Eugenol (3-hydroxy-4-methoxyphenyl-3'-propene) is a flavoring component of herbs and a registered food additive (Fig. 11.2). Eugenol is also used as an analgesic and antiseptic agent in dentistry [27]. This chemical interacts with the Ca^{2+} channel [28], cyclooxygenese 2 [29], and chloride ion channel [30]. Methyleugenol (3,4-dimethoxyphenyl-3'-propene), an *O*-methylated derivative of eugenol, is also present in several herbs including basil, clove, and nutmeg as a bitter taste principle. Methyleugenol has an anesthetic action in rodents [31].

Genotoxicity

Eugenol is not mutagenic in Ames test with and without S9 mix [32,33] and in bone marrow micronucleus test [34]. Methyleugenol is also not genotoxic in conventional tests, although methyleugenol forms the DNA adduct in livers of rats [35] and humans [36]. However, in F344 *gpt* delta rats [37] given methyleugenol, significant increases in gpt and Spi-mutant frequencies (MFs) are observed, together with enhanced GST-P-positive foci and PCNA-positive cells in the liver.

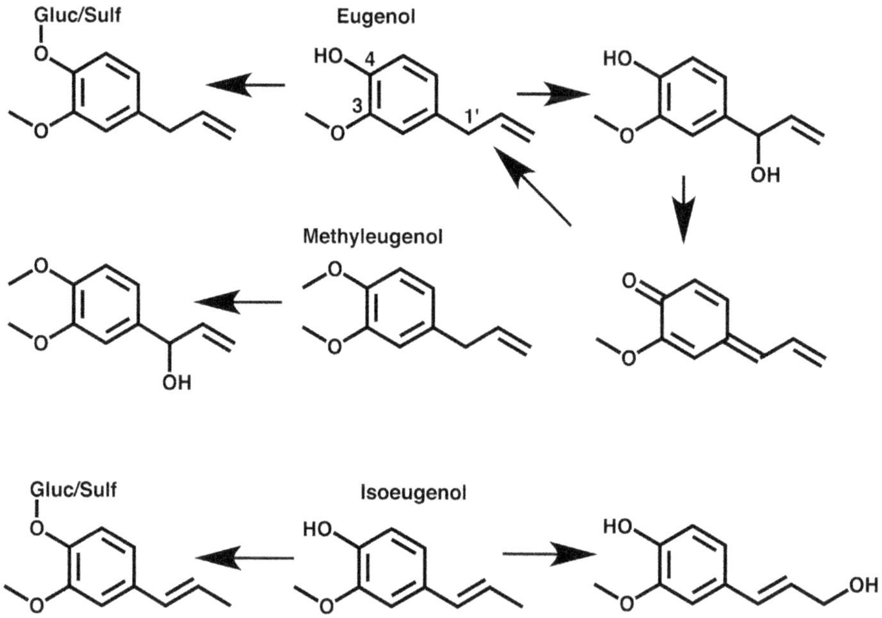

Figure 11.2
Metabolic pathways of eugenol (top), methyleugenol (middle), and isoeugenol (bottom).
Gluc, glucuronide; *Sulf*, sulfate. Metabolic formation of benzylic carbonium ion results
in the rapid quenching to the quinone with eugenol, but offers higher chances to
interact with DNA with methyleugenol due to the possible lack of rapid quenching
system. Isoeugenol exists as a mixture of trans and cis isomers with 7:1 ratio [26].

Pharmacokinetics

In humans [38], ^{14}C-eugenol is absorbed quantitatively and excreted exclusively in urine
after oral administration (150 mg). The metabolism is extensive, and less than 1% of the
dose is detected unchanged. Among the metabolites, more than half of the administered
amount is detected as ^{14}C-eugenol 4-*O*-glucuronide. Glucuronidase-hydrolyzable conjugates
of ^{14}C-1'-hydroxyeugenol are detectable, but at less than 1% of the total excretion. Both
isoeugenol and a 6-thio metabolite, possibly derived from the EQM (4-allyldene-2-methoxy-
2,5-cyclohexadiene-1-one), are isolated in rat and human hepatocyte systems [39], suggesting
similarities of metabolic profiles between rats and humans. Eugenol is thus metabolized in
liver mainly to eugenol-4-*O*-glucuronide, followed by 1'-hydroxyeugenol and an EQM [40].
Glutathione reacts with the eugenol phenoxy radical to reduce it to eugenol. Glutathione
reacts directly with EQM to yield eugenol-glutathione conjugate.

In volunteers, peak levels of methyleugenol in serum are observed 15 min after intake of
gingersnaps containing 216 μg of methyleugenol [41]. The serum level is increased to 53.9

from 16.2 pg/g at fasting level. The elimination half-life is about 90 min. In liver microsomes of rat and human [39,40], methyleugenol is metabolized mainly to 1'-hydroxy-methyleugenol and 3'-hydroxy-methylisoeugenol, followed by eugenol, 3'-oxo-methylisoeugenol and 2',3'-dihydroxy-2',3'-dihydromethyleugenol. Formation of the EQM is detectable, but limited due to the facile *O*-demethylation. Both the formations of 1'-hydroxyeugenol and EQM from eugerol are markedly reduced upon addition of UDPGA to the microsomal reaction mixture, while it has little influence on the metabolic profile of methyleugenol, due to the low efficacy of 4-*O*-glucuronide formation.

Carcinogenicity

Eugenol did not show carcinogenic activity in newborn mice assays when given by stomach tube during the preweaning period at doses of 2.5 μmol/g twice weekly for 5 weeks to CD-1 mice, or given by i.p. injection during the preweaning period at total doses of up to 9.45 μmol/ mouse to male B6C3F1 mice [42]. Just "equivocal evidence" was obtained in male mice, based on an increased incidence of liver tumors [43]. In this NTP study, where eugenol was given in the diets to female F344/N rats (0%, 0.6%, or 1.25%) and to male F344/N rats and male and female B6C3F mice (0%, 0.3%, or 0.6%) for 103 weeks, there was no evidence of carcinogenicity in male or female rats. On the contrary, eugenol caused increased incidences of both carcinomas and adenomas of the liver in male mice of the 0.3% group, but not in the 0.6% group. In fact, the lack of a dose-response in male mice speaks in favor of less than "unequivocal evidence of carcinogenicity." This is in agreement with the lack of DNA adduct formation of eugenol, when male B6C3F1 mice were injected with eugenol on days 1, 8, 15, and 22 after birth and killed on days 23, 29, and 43 for measuring DNA adduct formation using a modified ^{32}P-postlabeling procedure [35].

Regarding methyleugenol, Miller et al. [42] reported that methyleugenol and its 1-hydroxy metabolite induced hepatocellular neoplasms in male B6C3F1 mice treated prior to weaning. Furthermore, methyleugenol showed clear evidence of carcinogenicity in rats and mice [44]. In the NTP study, where rats and mice of both sexes received methyleugenol in 0.5% methylcellulose by gavage at doses of 0, 37, 75, or 150 mg/kg for 105 weeks, liver neoplasms (including hepatocellular adenomas/carcinomas, hepatocholangiomas, and hepatocholangiocarcinomas) occurred in all dosed groups of rats, and neoplasms of the glandular stomach (including benign and malignant neuroendocrine tumors) occurred in the 150-mg/kg groups and in the 75-mg/kg female group. Methyleugenol also induced tumors of the bile duct, kidney, mesothelium, mammary gland, and skin in treated rats. In the NTP study on mice, increases in the incidences of liver neoplasms (including hepatocellular adenomas/carcinomas, hepatoblastomas, and hepatocholangiocarcinomas) were observed in higher-dosed groups of both sexes. Positive results on DNA adduct formation in the liver of rats [35] and humans [36], as well as in in vivo genotoxicity testing using *gpt* delta rats [37], suggest that genotoxicity is an important mechanism in the carcinogenicity of methyleugenol.

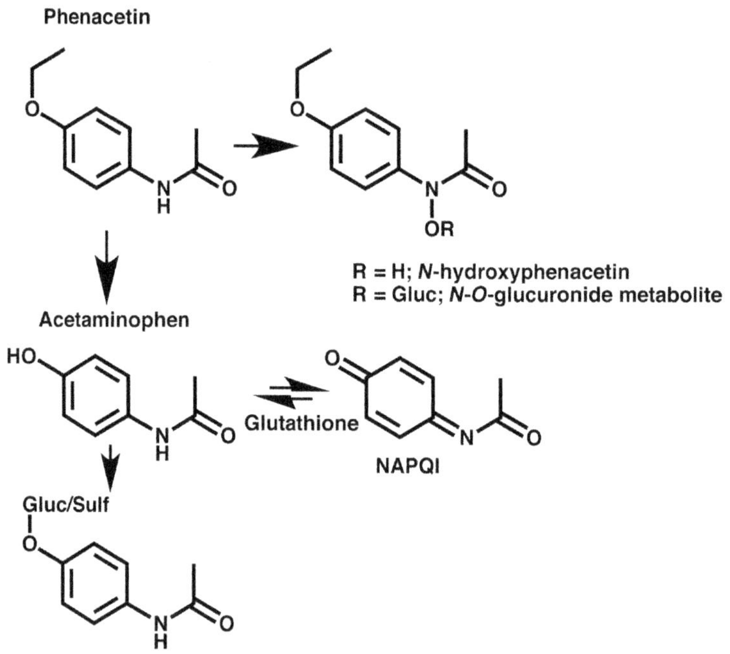

Figure 11.3

Metabolisms of phenacetin (top) and acetaminophen (bottom) in the body. *N*-oxidation of phenacetin leads to the production of *N*-hydroxy metabolite. Oxidation of acetaminophen results in the formation of quinone imine intermediate, which is quenched back to acetaminophen in therapeutic doses. *NAPQI*, *N*-acetylaminophenol quinone imine; *Gluc*, glucuronide; *Sulf*, sulfate.

Phenacetin and Acetaminophen

Both phenacetin and acetaminophen (paracetamol) were introduced in the late 19th century as analgesics. Clinical and epidemiologic studies indicate an increased incidence of renal dysfunction in people who abuse analgesics, particularly phenacetin [45,46]. Phenacetin had been used until the 1980s, but was then mainly replaced by acetaminophen (paracetamol; Fig. 11.3). Acetaminophen is fairly safe in normal use, but overdose may sometimes cause centrilobular hepatic necrosis, which may be fatal [47].

Genotoxicity

Phenacetin is mutagenic in *Salmonella typhimurium* TA100, in plate assays in the presence of liver fractions from aroclor-pretreated hamsters, but not rats. Deacetylated products of the *N*-oxidized metabolite, *N*-hydroxyphenetidine, and 4-nitrosophenetole, were directly mutagenic in *Salmonella* TA100 and TA100 NR (nitroreductase-deficient) strains [48] and bound covalently to nucleic acids [49]. *N*-hydroxyphenacetin and *N*-acetoxyphenacetin are mutagenic, but still require metabolic activation by liver fractions [50]. Phenacetin is positive in micronucleus tests using CD-1 mice [51]. Phenacetin, administered by feeding a 0.5% containing diet for 52 weeks to male Sprague–Dawley *gpt* delta rats, significantly increased *gpt* (point mutations) MFs in the target organ of carcinogenesis, kidney [52]. In this test, both *gpt* MFs and Spi-deletions MF were significantly elevated also in the liver in phenacetin-treated groups of both genders.

Acetaminophen does not induce gene mutations in either bacterial or mammalian cells. It does, however, cause chromosomal damage in cells at high concentrations and in vivo at high doses [53]. In a GPG46 animal model, *gpt* delta rats were exposed to acetaminophen at a dose of 6000 ppm in the diet, and partial hepatectomy was performed to collect liver samples for an in vivo mutation assay. The rats were subsequently administered a single i.p. injection of diethylnitrosamine, and the tumor-promoting activity of the chemical was evaluated based on the development of GST-P-positive foci. No increase was observed in *gpt* MF, and the development of GST-P-positive foci was inhibited [54].

Pharmacokinetics

In rabbit, guinea pig, and rat, 64–88% of an oral dose of acetyl-^{14}C-phenacetin was excreted in urine, and a small percentage appeared in the feces within 3 days. 4-(*N*-acetylamino) phenol represents the major portion of urinary metabolites, both as glucuronide and sulfate [55–57]. Excretion of the 3-cysteine conjugate of 4-(*N*-acetylamino)phenol and an increased proportion of deacetylated metabolites are also detected in higher doses [58]. The bioavailability of phenacetin is very low in human volunteers after oral intake of 0.25 g, and increased with higher dosing (1.0 g) [59].

Following an oral dose of phenacetin (10 mg/kg) to humans, acetaminophen-3-cysteine, -3-mercaturate, and -3-thiomethyl, together with *N*-hydroxyphenacetin, were detected in the urine [60]. Futile metabolic deacetylation and reacetylation of phenacetin are suggested in humans as a possible cause of the sustained presence in the body [61].

Acetaminophen is rapidly absorbed and shows 63% and 89% bioavailability after oral administration of 1000 and 2000 mg, respectively. The drug is extensively metabolized at a plasma half-life of 1.5–2.5 h. About 55% and 30% of a therapeutic dose is excreted in the urine as glucuronide and sulfate conjugates, respectively, whereas mercapturic acid and cysteine conjugates (indicating an intermediate conversion to potentially toxic intermediate metabolites) each account for some 4% of the dose. With hepatotoxic doses, acetaminophen metabolism is impaired and the half-life prolonged. Sulfate conjugation is saturated and the proportion excreted as mercapturic acid and cysteine conjugates is increased [62,63].

Carcinogenicity

Phenacetin is a human carcinogen based on sufficient evidence of carcinogenicity studies in experimental animals. In an 18-month carcinogenicity study, dietary administration of 2.5% phenacetin induced renal cell carcinomas of the renal pelvis and transitional cell carcinomas of the urinary bladder in rats, the tumor incidence in males being greater than in females [64]. In another long-term carcinogenicity study, dietary administration of 0.535% phenacetin for 117 weeks induced renal pelvic tumors in male rats [65]. In B6C3F1 mice of each sex maintained on a diet containing 1.25% or 0.6% phenacetin for 96 weeks, a dose-related induction of renal tumors was observed in male mice, and urinary bladder proliferative lesions developed in mice of either sex fed 1.25% phenacetin [66].

Acetaminophen is a major biotransformation product of phenacetin. In a carcinogenicity study of acetaminophen, where F344 rats of each sex were given diets containing 0.45% or 0.9% acetaminophen in males and 0.65% or 1.3% acetaminophen in females for 104 weeks, no evidence of carcinogenicity was found [67]. On the contrary, an increased incidence of liver tumors was seen in male mice given 1% dietary acetaminophen for 78 weeks [68]. Acetaminophen was demonstrated to exhibit a tumor-promoting activity in the kidneys of rats, but not in the livers of rats [69]. In order to elucidate the tumor-promoting effect of acetaminophen in mice, Hagiwara and Ward [70] conducted a two-stage hepatocarcinogenesis study. Male B6C3F1 mice received an intraperitoneal injection of N-nitrosodiethylamine (DEN) and were fed diets containing 5000 or 10,000 ppm acetaminophen 2 weeks after the DEN treatment, up to 24 weeks. In addition, male B6C3F1 mice were fed diets containing 5000 or 10,000 ppm acetaminophen for 72 weeks (without DEN treatment), to elucidate the potential carcinogenesis of acetaminophen. At 24 weeks, the incidence and number of focal hepatocellular proliferative lesions were significantly increased only in the DEN-treated mice receiving 10,000 ppm acetaminophen. At 72 weeks, 10,000 ppm acetaminophen alone had no effect on the incidence or number of naturally occurring liver tumors, despite severe chronic hepatotoxicity. These findings suggested that acetaminophen has a liver-tumor-promoting effect in mice, but the carcinogenic potential of acetaminophen to the liver in mice is very weak. Similarly to phenacetin, a N-2-hydroxybutyryl, instead of N-ethyl, derivative of 4-phenetidine (bucetin) is genotoxic and carcinogenic in mice [71]. Kidney is a common target for their carcinogenicity. Reduced extents of N-deacylation of phenacetin and bucetin are suggested to contribute to the increased activation through N-hydroxylation of these 4-phenetidine derivatives [72].

Menadione

Menadione (2-methyl-l,4-naphthoquinone) or vitamin K_3 is a lipid-soluble substance that promotes the hepatic biosynthesis of blood clotting factors (Fig. 11.4). This chemical is often used as a model reagent to generate the active oxygen in cell cultures. Menadione, however, has been addressed as being safe as a vitamin K supplement in livestock.

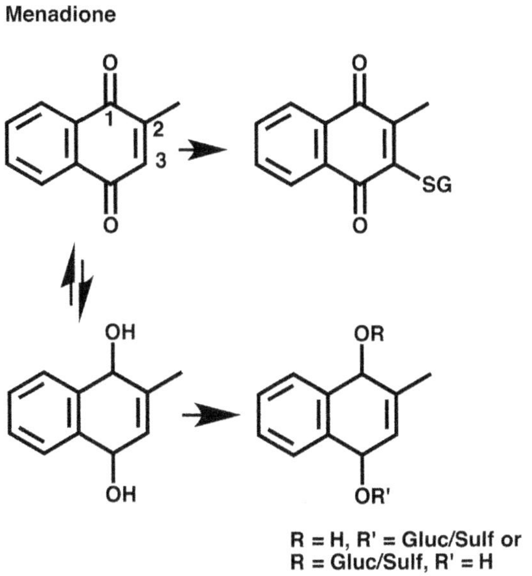

Menadione

R = H, R' = Gluc/Sulf or
R = Gluc/Sulf, R' = H

Figure 11.4

Metabolic pathways of menadione. Rapid reduction into the reduced form (bottom left) and productions of hydrophilic conjugates (bottom right) occur in vivo. SG, glutathionyl.

Genotoxicity

Menadione is mutagenic to *Salmonella* strain TA2637 with metabolic activation, containing plasmid pKM101 [73], and in TA104 [74]. In the presence of metabolic activation, the menadione-induced DNA damage and repair are greatly reduced. Treatment of A549 lung cells with menadione caused formation of single-stranded DNA breaks in the absence of S9 mix. Menadione caused no significant formation of DNA strand breaks in the presence of metabolic activation. Menadione-induced DNA repair was concentration-, time-, and temperature-dependent in A549 cells. Measurement of unscheduled DNA synthesis (UDS) in menadione-treated A549 cells yielded strong UDS responses in the absence of S9 mix [75].

Pharmacokinetics

In a rat liver perfusion system, more than 90% of 2-^{14}C-menadione (^{14}C-VK$_3$) was metabolized within 5 h and 53%, 33%, and 15% was detected in the blood, bile, and liver, respectively [76]. DT-diaphorase (NAD(P)H:quinone oxidoreductase) is at first involved in the metabolism of menadione, to reduce this to 1,4-dihydroxy-2-methyldihydronaphthalene (DHM) [77]. The reduced metabolite is conjugated, mainly in the liver, to *O*-glucuronide and *O*-sulfate [78]. These conjugates are excreted efficiently in the bile. Menadione is conjugated with glutathione, but this is minimal as judged from the analysis of urine and bile.

Efficient reduction of menadione and subsequent conjugation in the liver is likely to limit the systemic availability. In addition, interaction with ABCG2 transporter may have physiological importance on the distribution in the body [79]. Consistent with this idea, menadione shows rather limited distribution in peripheral tissues compared to a methoxy derivative, 2,3-dimethoxy-1,4-naphthoquinone [78]. DHM is susceptible to biological oxidation and undergoes one-electron oxidation to form the radical intermediates [80]. Glutathione interacts with the radical intermediates and is oxidized to the dimer GSSG [81].

Carcinogenicity

No carcinogenicity studies in experimental animals are available for menadione. However, mechanistic studies to clarify the mutagenic and genotoxic potential of menadione have been performed [75]. Measurements of superoxide anion formation, UDS, and alkaline elution assays showed that menadione induces superoxide production and DNA damage and repair. It appears that reactive oxygen species derived from menadione are likely to react with DNA causing DNA damage and repair without leading to apparent carcinogenic effects. Therefore, it is unlikely that menadione has carcinogenic potential.

Toxicology

From experiments in cell culture and rat kidney-perfusion systems, menadione is suggested to cause renal tubule damage. Thiodione (2-methyl-3-S-glutathionyl-1,4-naphthoquinone)-mediated toxicity in the isolated perfused rat kidney can be linked to cellular uptake by anionic transport systems and metabolism by gamma-glutamyltranspeptidase [82,83]. Acute and cumulative toxic effects of menadione were evaluated by intravenous injection in Wistar rats [84]. Menadione, at a dose of 25 mg/kg, produced minimal granular degeneration in the tubular cells of the kidney. At doses of 100 and 150 mg/kg it produced lesions in the kidney, heart, liver, and lung of rats. The characteristic lesions in the kidney included tubular dilatation and formation of protein casts in the lumen of renal tubules, Ca^{2+} mineralization, and vacuolization in proximal and distal tubules, and granular degeneration and necrosis in the cortex. Apoptosis was remarkable in kidneys of rats treated with 100 or 150 mg/kg menadione. Also, mitochondria were swollen in the kidney. Hepatic changes included inflammation, degeneration, vacuolization, and necrosis. Structural damage was more severe in kidney than in other organs [84].

No obvious toxicity is observed in vivo upon feeding menadione to experimental animals. The apparent lack of adverse effect may, at least partly, be due to the efficient elimination system of the liver. Different to quercetin and acetaminophen, glutathione conjugation is not the major detoxification pathway. DT-diaphorase, along with AKR7 (aldoketoreductase), exerts detoxification through reduction. The pharmacokinetic profile of menadione suggests a substantial systemic accumulation only after oral administration of excess amounts.

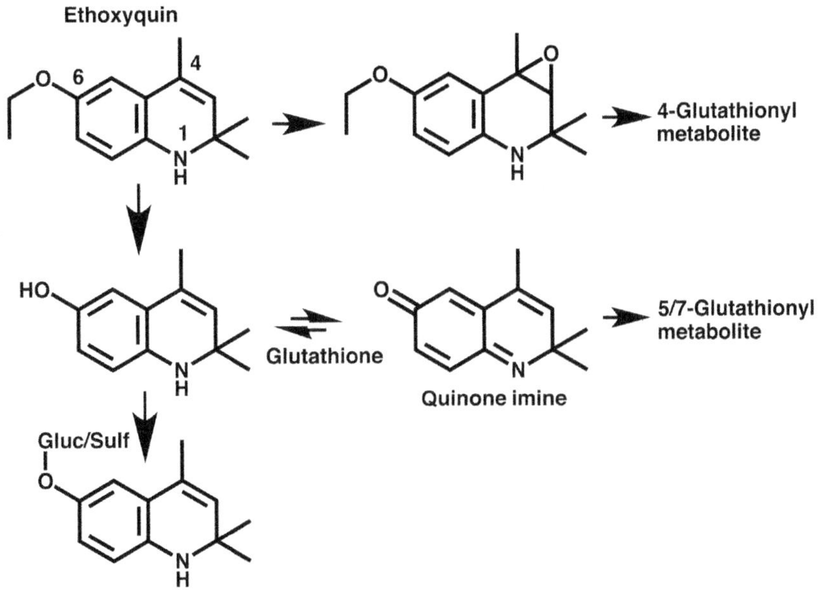

Figure 11.5

Metabolism of ethoxyquin in the body. Quinone imine formed from the major metabolite 6-hydroxyethoxyquin is reduced back in the presence of glutathione. Trace amounts of glutathione conjugates are detected in urine of ethoxyquin-treated rats. *Gluc*, glucuronide; *Sulf*, sulfate.

Ethoxyquin

Ethoxyquin (1,2-dihydro-6-ethoxy-2,2,4-trimethylquinoline) is a dihydroquinoline compound with the ability to scavenge lipid peroxide radicals and thus to terminate the spontaneous oxidation of unsaturated lipids (Fig. 11.5). According to the national surveillance program, ethoxyquin is the most widely used preservative in fish feed.

Genotoxicity

Ethoxyquin is not mutagenic to *Salmonella* TA100 and TA98 [85]. Ethoxyquin induced DNA damage in human lymphocytes in a dose-dependent manner; the observed DNA fragmentation induced by ethoxyquin in the presence of the metabolic activation system was always significantly lower, as compared to cells treated with the same doses of ethoxyquin alone [86]. Ethoxyquin-induced DNA damage is caused by the free radical generated [87]. In vivo, ethoxyquin gave a weak positive response in the liver micronucleus test in juvenile rats, but negative responses in the mouse bone marrow micronucleus test and in the UDS test using rat liver [88]. Although ethoxyquin and/or its metabolite(s) induce chromosomal aberration, the influence on the chromosomal aberration is likely to be associated with ethoxyquin's action on the functional protein component rather than the direct DNA damage.

Pharmacokinetics

After oral administration of ring-^{14}C-ethoxyquin (100 mg/kg), 67–80% of the dose was recovered in 24 h urine and feces of rats. The excretion was slightly higher in urine than in feces, and the total recoveries reached 95% within 6 days. The major metabolite in urine was the *O*-sulfate of the *O*-deethylated product, 6-hydroxy-2,2,4-trimethyl-1,2-dihydroquinoline, followed by the quinone imine, 2,2,4-trimethyl-quinolone, and the sulfates of 3,6-dihydroxylated metabolites [89]. Glutathione conjugates were isolated from bile. These conjugates are expected to be formed from ethoxyquin 3,4-oxide and quinone imine [90]. Ethoxyquin dimers originating during storage [91] are found in fish meat and have only a slow rate of decay compared to the monomer metabolites [92].

Carcinogenicity

A chronic toxicity/carcinogenicity test of ethoxyquin was performed in male and female F344 rats [88]. The animals received ethoxyquin in the diet at 0, 160, 400, 1000, or 2500 ppm for 30 months.

Increases or increasing trends in the absolute and relative kidney weights were seen in males and females of the groups treated with 1000 ppm or more. Histopathologically, epithelial hyperplasia in the mucosa of the urinary bladder was observed in females of the groups given 400 ppm or more and in males of the groups given 1000 ppm or more. Males of the group given 2500 ppm and females of the group given 1000 ppm or more showed papillary hyperplasia of the mucosa. Regarding neoplastic lesions, the incidence of urinary bladder tumors was 16% (12 out of 77 rats) in females of the 2500 ppm group. The value was significantly higher than the background incidence (less than 1–2.5%) of this tumor in F344 rats. These findings suggest that ethoxyquin has carcinogenic potential in the urinary bladder of rats.

A two-stage urinary bladder carcinogenesis study initiated with *N*-butyl-*N*-(4-hydroxybutyl) nitrosamine (BBN) was performed in F344 rats [93]. F344 rats receiving drinking water containing 500 ppm BBN for 4 weeks and subsequently diets containing 8000 ppm ethoxyquin for 32 weeks. The group treated with BBN followed by ethoxyquin showed simple hyperplasia, papillary or nodular hyperplasia, papillomas and carcinomas, and the incidences of papillary or nodular hyperplasia and papillomas were significantly increased compared to those in the BBN-alone group. Moreover, ethoxyquin alone without BBN for 32 weeks induced papillary or nodular hyperplasia but not tumors. In another experiment, F344 rats received drinking water containing 500 ppm BBN for 2 weeks and subsequently diets containing 1250, 2500, or 5000 ppm ethoxyquin for 22 weeks [94]. In the group treated with BBN followed by ethoxyquin, papillomas were observed in the 5000 ppm, and papillary or nodular hyperplasia and papillomas were observed in the 1250 and 2500 ppm groups, but their incidences were not significantly different from those in the BBN-alone group. In the group treated with 5000 ppm ethoxyquin alone without BBN treatment for 22 weeks, proliferative lesions such as hyperplasia were not observed.

In these two studies, the 8000 ppm group treated only with ethoxyquin for 32 weeks showed simple hyperplasia and papillary or nodular hyperplasia, but the 5000 ppm group treated only with ethoxyquin for 22 weeks did not show any proliferative lesion such as hyperplasia. A question arises as to whether ethoxyquin may have an initiating activity to the urinary bladder in rats. Simple hyperplasia and papillary or nodular hyperplasia detected in the group without BBN initiation were also observed in a study of animals treated with sodium L-ascorbate, an antioxidant, which acts as a tumor promoter [95,96]. Therefore, the hyperplasia observed in the urinary bladder of the ethoxyquin-alone group in the two-stage urinary bladder carcinogenesis model suggests that the ethoxyquin is a tumor promoter, but not a tumor initiator.

Mechanism of Carcinogenicity of Ethoxyquin

The metabolic pathway leading to the major urinary and fecal metabolites of ethoxyquin observed in rats is *O*-deethylation yielding a phenol and also the conjugation (conjugates a glucuronide acid or sulfate). Some of these metabolites (eg, quinone imine, a metabolite formed during peroxidase reactions) may have the potential of inducing prooxidative effects.

Vitamin E derivatives and tea extracts with antioxidant properties are known to exert prooxidant effects at high doses [97,98]. The proliferative lesions observed in the mucosa of the urinary bladder in the ethoxyquin-treated animals, thus, may be enhanced by continuous prooxidant stimuli derived from ethoxyquin metabolites, not from the parent compound [99].

Based on these findings, the carcinogenicity in the urinary bladder observed in the 30-month chronic toxicity/carcinogenicity test in rats was judged as being mediated through a nongenotoxic mechanism [88]. FSCJ thus recognized it as feasible to set a threshold value.

Other substances known to exert carcinogenicity in the urinary bladder in rats through nongenotoxic mechanisms include allyl isothiocyanate [100] found in cruciferous plants, such as Wasabi, and OPP (2-phenylphenol) [101] used as an agricultural chemical, food additive, or disinfectant.

General Discussion for All the Chemicals Shown

In this context, carcinogenicities of five chemicals were assessed based on their mechanisms of carcinogenicity and metabolism. Chemicals like quercetin show genotoxic properties in bacterial reverse mutation assays and chromosome aberration tests at high dose levels.

Chronic oral administration of such a chemical in experimental animals results in no or only weak carcinogenicity, even at high dose levels. Eugenol and methyleugenol are not mutagenic to *Salmonella* strains. In vivo, methyleugenol, but not eugenol, forms hepatic DNA-adducts, detected by ^{32}P-postlabeling. A popular analgesic, acetaminophen, is a major metabolite of phenacetin. Phenacetin, but not acetaminophen, induces renal tumor in rodents, and an overdose is associated with renal dysfunction in humans. Plausible links of pharmacokinetics and carcinogenicity are observed between phenacetin and acetaminophen, and between eugenol and methyleugenol.

No obvious differences between rodents and human exist in the pharmacokinetics of phenacetin and acetaminophen. Acetaminophen, once absorbed, is efficiently metabolized to the sulfate and glucuronide during the first pass. Parts of the drug enter the systemic circulation. Most of acetaminophen metabolites including 4-aminophenol is, without enterohepatic circulation, excreted in urine. Both the sulfation and glucuronidation processes have high capacities for detoxification, but are saturated after the intakes of very high and therefore toxic doses. Hepatic cytochrome P450 species, mainly CYP2E1, mediate the oxidation of acetaminophen to the quinone imine (*N*-acetylaminophenol quinone imine, NAPQI). In the presence of high levels of cellular glutathione, NAPQI is reduced back to acetaminophen, and also the glutathione adduct is formed. This adduct is excreted in bile and partly through the kidney after conversion to the cysteine adduct. Phenacetin is extensively oxidized during the first pass after the oral intakes. Its *O*-deethylated metabolite, acetaminophen, is further metabolized as described above. Formation of *N*-hydroxyphenacetin is increased in the liver after intakes of the high doses. Parts of semistable *N*-hydroxyphenacetin and the *N-O*-glucuronide are delivered through the bloodstream to the kidney. Unlike NAPQI, *N*-hydroxyphenacetin is a poor substrate of the glutathione transferase system, and has a higher chance to interact with DNA. Clear differences thus exist in pharmacokinetics between the noncarcinogenic acetaminophen and the carcinogenic phenacetin. (1) High-capacity conjugation pathways (glucuronidation and sulfation) exist for parent drug acetaminophen, while a relatively slow metabolic process, oxidation, is necessary prior to undergoing the conjugation for phenacetin in vivo. (2) Oxidized metabolites of phenacetin are poor substrates of the glutathione transferase system, and thus enter the systemic circulation and possibly reach the kidney [102]. Pharmacokinetic differences are also observed in the case of the flavor components, eugenol and methyleugenol. High-capacity detoxification pathways, glucuronidation and sulfation of the phenol part, are operative for eugenol, but not for methyleugenol. Oxidation of the benzylic position (1′-oxidation) may lead to the quinone imine formation of eugenol, but this reactive intermediate is eliminated efficiently through reduction to the parent compound with glutathione transferase system. For methyleugenol, the 1′-oxidation is a main route of the metabolism, followed by the semistable sulfate formation. The 1′-*O*-sulfate and resultant 1′-carbonium ion react poorly with glutathione and thus are prone to interaction with DNA.

Methyleugenol *O*-demethylation does occur to eugenol, but not extensively. Eugenol is partly metabolized to 3′-hydroxyisoeugenol. The formation is possible through 1′-hydroxylation of eugenol and migration of carbonium ion from the 1′ position to 3′. No significant DNA adduct in the liver is, however, detected with ^{32}P-postlabeling analysis after the treatment with eugenol in mice [35], suggesting the nonsubstantial role of the 1″-hydroxylation pathway.

Similar to eugenol, isoeugenol (1-(3-methoxy-4-hydroxyphenyl)-1-propene) has a phenol moiety in its molecule and thus possibly undergoes conjugation to form a hydrophilic metabolite. In fact, the phenolic sulfate and glucuronide of isoeugenol are detected in urine after oral administration in rats [103]. In addition, considerable amounts of side chain oxidized metabolites (3′-hydroxylated isoeugenol) are detected as the sulfate. The 3′-position of isoeugenol is not prone to form the EQM after side chain oxidation. Thus, inactivation through the EQM formation is not expected to occur for isoeugenol at an extent similar to eugenol. In fact, isoeugenol is hepatocarcinogenic in mice [26].

Highly efficient detoxification pathways exist for quercetin and menadione. Hepatic conjugation of quercetin and of a metabolite reduced by DT-diaphorase of menadione leads to efficient bile excretion prior to their systemic circulation. Glutathione adducts were detected as trace metabolites for both chemicals in vivo. These data suggest an efficient quenching action against radical intermediates from quercetin and menadione and for the EQM of quercetin.

An antioxidant, ethoxyquin, is oxidized mainly to the *O*-deethylated metabolite, 6-hydroxy-2,2,4-trimethyl-1,2-dihydroquinoline, and then excreted as conjugates in the urine of rats and mice. The phenolic metabolite is further oxidized in the liver to a reactive quinone imine, 2,6-dihydro-2,2,4-trimethyl-6-quinolone. A glutathione adduct, expected to be formed from the quinone imine, is present in the bile of rat and mice. Another glutathione adduct, 6-ethoxy-3-hydroxy-4-(S-glutathionyl)-1,2,3,4-tetrahydro-2,2,4-trimethylquinoline, was also isolated in the bile. Although no direct data are available on the covalent binding to DNA of ethoxyquin in experimental animals, negative results obtained in all bacterial reverse mutation tests support the notion that the genotoxicity observed is not elicited through a direct interaction of ethoxyquin (or its metabolite) with DNA. The presence of 2,2,4-trimethyl group of ethoxyquin may hamper the reactivity of the metabolically generated 3,4-epoxide to DNA. Observed influences of ethoxyquin, in the 30-month carcinogenicity study with F344 rats (given the 400 ppm (17.7–20.6 mg/kg) and higher amounts (up to 115–139 mg/kg)), on the kidney, thyroid gland, and urinary bladder may be interpreted as the insults triggered through the prooxidant action of ethoxyquin and/or the metabolites, in a manner similar to the tumorigenic action of sodium ascorbate in the urinary bladder in rats [95,104].

Experimental data, as discussed above, suggest a separation of chemical carcinogens into two general categories, those that contain or can form an electrophile to interact directly with DNA, and those that have no mutagenic or no DNA-damaging properties directly or indirectly, but have modulating properties of normal cell functions. Often, radical-generators including quinones, quinone imines, and EQMs are mutagenic through generation of active oxygen. Their biological reactions are often discordant in vitro and in vivo.

From pathological and pharmaco(toxico)kinetic points of view, quinoids and precursors may be a category of genotoxicants different from those acting through a direct electrophilic reaction with DNA. Many food additives are capable of producing free radicals, and many food additives are able to act as free-radical scavengers. Free- and oxygen-radical scavenging mechanisms also function in the body, whereas such mechanisms are generally not present in tests of genotoxicity in vitro. Detailed investigations of in vivo pathological examinations and pharmaco(toxico)kinetic profiles on quinoid-related chemicals offer us clear assessments with regard to human safety.

References

[1]   Ferry DR, Smith A, Malkhandi J, Fyfe DW, deTakats PG, Anderson D, et al. Phase I clinical trial of the flavonoid quercetin: pharmacokinetics and evidence for in vivo tyrosine kinase inhibition. Clin Cancer Res 1996;2:659–68.

[2]   Duarte J, Perez-Vizcaino F, Zarzuelo A, Jimenez J, Tamargo J. Vasodilator effects of quercetin in isolated rat vascular smooth muscle. Eur J Pharmacol 1993;239:1–7.

[3]   National-Toxicology-Program. Toxicology and carcinogenesis studies of quercetin (CAS No. 117-39-5) in F344 rats (FEED studies). Natl Toxicol Program Tech Rep Ser 1992;409:1–171.

[4]   Crozier A, Lean MEJ, McDonald MS, Black C. Quantitative analysis of the flavonoid content of commercial tomatoes, onions, lettuce, and celery. J Agric Food Chem 1997;45:590–5.

[5]   Bjeldanes LF, Chang GW. Mutagenic activity of quercetin and related compounds. Science 1977;197:577–8.

[6]   IARC. Quercetin. IARC Monogr Eval Carcinog Risks Hum 1983;31:213–30.

[7]   Brown JP. A review of the genetic effects of naturally occurring flavonoids, anthraquinones and related compounds. Mutat Res 1980;75:243–77.

[8]   Maruta A, Enaka K, Umeda M. Mutagenicity of quercetin and kaempferol on cultured mammalian cells. Gann 1979;70:273–6.

[9]   Mullen W, Edwards CA, Crozier A. Absorption, excretion and metabolite profiling of methyl-, glucuronyl-, glucosyl- and sulpho-conjugates of quercetin in human plasma and urine after ingestion of onions. Br J Nutr 2006;96:107–16.

[10] Walle T. Absorption and metabolism of flavonoids. Free Radic Biol Med 2004;36:829–37.

[11] Arts IC, Sesink AL, Faassen-Peters M, Hollman PC. The type of sugar moiety is a major determinant of the small intestinal uptake and subsequent biliary excretion of dietary quercetin glycosides. Br J Nutr 2004;91:841–7.

[12] Matsukawa N, Matsumoto M, Hara H. High biliary excretion levels of quercetin metabolites after administration of a quercetin glycoside in conscious bile duct cannulated rats. Biosci Biotechnol Biochem 2009;73:1863–5.

[13] Pamukcu AM, Yalciner S, Hatcher JF, Bryan GT. Quercetin, a rat intestinal and bladder carcinogen present in bracken fern (*Pteridium aquilinum*). Cancer Res 1980;40:3468–72.

[14] Ito N, Hagiwara A, Tamano S, Kagawa M, Shibata M, Kurata Y, et al. Lack of carcinogenicity of quercetin in F344/DuCrj rats. Jpn J Cancer Res 1989;80:317–25.

[15] Hirono I, Ueno I, Hosaka S, Takanashi H, Matsushima T, Sugimura T, et al. Carcinogenicity examination of quercetin and rutin in ACI rats. Cancer Lett 1981;13:15–21.

[16] Dunnick JK, Hailey JR. Toxicity and carcinogenicity studies of quercetin, a natural component of foods. Fundam Appl Toxicol 1992;19:423–31.

[17] Saito D, Shirai A, Matsushima T, Sugimura T, Hirono I. Test of carcinogenicity of quercetin, a widely distributed mutagen in food. Teratog Carcinog Mutagen 1980;1:213–21.

[18] Ito N. Is quercetin carcinogenic? Jpn J Cancer Res 1992;83:312–3.

[19] Hirose M, Fukushima S, Sakata T, Inui M, Ito N. Effect of quercetin on two-stage carcinogenesis of the rat urinary bladder. Cancer Lett 1983;21:23–7.

[20] Hard GC, Seely JC, Betz LJ, Hayashi SM. Reevaluation of the kidney tumors and renal histopathology occurring in a 2-year rat carcinogenicity bioassay of quercetin. Food Chem Toxicol 2007;45:600–8.

[21] Hard GC, Khan KN. A contemporary overview of chronic progressive nephropathy in the laboratory rat, and its significance for human risk assessment. Toxicol Pathol 2004;32:171–80.

[22] Hard GC, Whysner J, English JC, Zang E, Williams GM. Relationship of hydroquinone-associated rat renal tumors with spontaneous chronic progressive nephropathy. Toxicol Pathol 1997;25:132–43.

[23] Hard GC. Significance of the renal effects of ethyl benzene in rodents for assessing human carcinogenic risk. Toxicol Sci 2002;69:30–41.

[24] Awad HM, Boersma MG, Boeren S, Van Bladeren PJ, Vervoort J, Rietjens IM. Quenching of quercetin quinone/quinone methides by different thiolate scavengers: stability and reversibility of conjugate formation. Chem Res Toxicol 2003;16:822–31.

[25] Omar K, Grant MH, Henderson C, Watson DG. The complex degradation and metabolism of quercetin in rat hepatocyte incubations. Xenobiotica 2014;44:1074–82.

[26] National-Toxicology-Program. Toxicology and carcinogenesis studies of isoeugenol (CAS No. 97-54-1) in F344/N rats and B6C3F1 mice (gavage studies). Natl Toxicol Program Tech Rep Ser, 2010, 1–178.

[27] Markowitz K, Moynihan M, Liu M, Kim S. Biologic properties of eugenol and zinc oxide-eugenol. A clinically oriented review. Oral Surg Oral Med Oral Pathol 1992;73:729–37.

[28] Seo H, Li HY, Perez-Reyes E, Lee JH. Effects of eugenol on T-type Ca^{2+} channel isoforms. J Pharmacol Exp Ther 2013;347:310–7.

[29] Okada N, Hirata A, Murakami Y, Shoji M, Sakagami H, Fujisawa S. Induction of cytotoxicity and apoptosis and inhibition of cyclooxygenase-2 gene expression by eugenol-related compounds. Anticancer Res 2005;25:3263–9.

[30] Yao Z, Namkung W, Ko EA, Park J, Tradtrantip L, Verkman AS. Fractionation of a herbal antidiarrheal medicine reveals eugenol as an inhibitor of Ca^{2+} -Activated Cl- channel TMEM16A. PLoS One 2012;7:e38030.

[31] Carlini EA, Dallmeier K, Zelger JL. Methyleugenol as a surgical anesthetic in rodents. Experientia 1981;37:588–9.

[32] Green NR, Savage JR. Screening of safrole, eugenol, their ninhydrin positive metabolites and selected secondary amines for potential mutagenicity. Mutat Res 1978;57:115–21.

[33] Swanson AB, Chambliss DD, Blomquist JC, Miller EC, Miller JA. The mutagenicities of safrole, estragole, eugenol, *trans*-anethole, and some of their known or possible metabolites for *Salmonella typhimurium* mutants. Mutat Res 1979;60:143–53.

[34] Maura A, Pino A, Ricci R. Negative evidence in vivo of DNA-damaging, mutagenic and chromosomal effects of eugenol. Mutat Res 1989;227:125–9.

[35] Phillips DH, Reddy MV, Randerath K. ^{32}P-post-labelling analysis of DNA adducts formed in the livers of animals treated with safrole, estragole and other naturally-occurring alkenylbenzenes. II. Newborn male B6C3F1 mice. Carcinogenesis 1984;5:1623–8.

[36] Herrmann K, Schumacher F, Engst W, Appel KE, Klein K, Zanger UM, et al. Abundance of DNA adducts of methyleugenol, a rodent hepatocarcinogen, in human liver samples. Carcinogenesis 2013;34:1025–30.

[37] Jin M, Kijima A, Hibi D, Ishii Y, Takasu S, Matsushita K, et al. In vivo genotoxicity of methyleugenol in gpt delta transgenic rats following medium-term exposure. Toxicol Sci 2013;131:387–94.

[38] Fischer IU, von Unruh GE, Dengler HJ. The metabolism of eugenol in man. Xenobiotica 1990;20:209–22.

[39] Cartus AT, Merz KH, Schrenk D. Metabolism of methylisoeugenol in liver microsomes of human, rat, and bovine origin. Drug Metab Dispos 2011;39:1727–33.

[40] Minet EF, Daniela G, Meredith C, Massey ED. A comparative in vitro kinetic study of [(14)C]-eugenol and [(14)C]-methyleugenol activation and detoxification in human, mouse, and rat liver and lung fractions. Xenobiotica 2012;42:429–41.

[41]   Schecter A, Lucier GW, Cunningham ML, Abdo KM, Blumenthal G, Silver Jr AG, et al. Human consumption of methyleugenol and its elimination from serum. Environ Health Perspect 2004;112:678–80.

[42]   Miller EC, Swanson AB, Phillips DH, Fletcher TL, Liem A, Miller JA. Structure-activity studies of the carcinogenicities in the mouse and rat of some naturally occurring and synthetic alkenylbenzene derivatives related to safrole and estragole. Cancer Res 1983;43:1124–34.

[43]   National-Toxicology-Program. NTP technical report on the carcinogenesis studies of eugenol (CAS NO, 97-53-0) in F344 rats and B6C3F1 mice (feed studies). Natl Toxicol Program Tech Rep Ser 1983;223:1–159.

[44]   National-Toxicology-Program. NTP toxicology and carcinogenesis studies of methyleugenol (CAS NO. 93-15-2) in F344/N rats and B6C3F1 mice (gavage studies). Natl Toxicol Program Tech Rep Ser 2000;491:1–412.

[45]   Brown AK, Pell-Ilderton R. Phenacetin and the kidney. Lancet 1964;2:121–3.

[46]   De Broe ME, Elseviers MM. Analgesic nephropathy. N Engl J Med 1998;338:446–52.

[47]   Editorial. Paracetamol hepatotoxicity. Lancet 1975; 306:1189–1191.

[48]   Camus AM, Friesen M, Croisy A, Bartsch H. Species-specific activation of phenacetin into bacterial mutagens by hamster liver enzymes and identification of N-hydroxyphenacetin O-glucuronides as a promutagen in the urine. Cancer Res 1982;42:3201–8.

[49]   Vaught JB, McGarvey PB, Lee MS, Garner CD, Wang CY, Linsmaier-Bednar EM, et al. Activation of N-hydroxyphenacetin to mutagenic and nucleic acid-binding metabolites by acyltransfer, deacylation, and sulfate conjugation. Cancer Res 1981;41:3424–9.

[50]   Shudo K, Ohta T, Orihara Y, Okamoto T, Nagao M, Takahashi Y, et al. Mutagenicities of phenacetin and its metabolites. Mutat Res 1978;58:367–70.

[51]   Sutou S, Kondo M, Mitsui Y. Effects of multiple dosing of phenacetin in the micronucleus test. Mutat Res 1990;234:183–6.

[52]   Kawamura Y, Hayashi H, Masumura K, Numazawa S, Nohmi T. Genotoxicity of phenacetin in the kidney and liver of Sprague-Dawley gpt delta transgenic rats in 26-week and 52-week repeated-dose studies. Toxicology 2014;324:10–17.

[53]   Bergman K, Muller L, Teigen SW. Series: current issues in mutagenesis and carcinogenesis, No. 65. The genotoxicity and carcinogenicity of paracetamol: a regulatory (re)view. Mutat Res 1996;349:263–88.

[54]   Matsushita K, Kijima A, Ishii Y, Takasu S, Jin M, Kuroda K, et al. Development of a medium-term animal modelusing *gpt* delta rats to evaluate chemical carcinogenicity and genotoxicity. J Toxicol Pathol 2013;26:19–27.

[55]   Smith RL, Timbrell JA. Metabolism of (acetyl-^{14}C)phenacetin in various species. Biochem J 1972;128:140P–1P.

[56]   Valle GF, Biesterfeld RC, Taintor JF. Phenacetin: an update. J Endod 1979;5:201–7.

[57]   Smith JN, Williams RT. Studies in detoxication. 22. The metabolism of phenacetin (*p*-ethoxyacetanilide) in the rabbit and a further observation on acetanilide metabolism. Biochem J 1949;44:239–42.

[58]   Smith RL, Timbrell JA. Factors affecting the metabolism of Phenacetin I. Influence of dose, chronic dosage, route of administration and species on the metabolism of [1-i4c-acetyl]phenacetin. Xenobiotica 1972;4:489–501.

[59]   Raaflaub J, Dubach UC. On the pharmacokinetics of phenacetin in man. Eur J Clin Pharmacol 1975;8:261–5.

[60]   Veronese ME, McLean S, D'Souza CA, Davies NW. Formation of reactive metabolites of phenacetin in humans and rats. Xenobiotica 1985;15:929–40.

[61]   Nicholls AW, Wilson ID, Godejohann M, Nicholson JK, Shockcor JP. Identification of phenacetin metabolites in human urine after administration of phenacetin-C_2H_3: measurement of futile metabolic deacetylation via HPLC/MS-SPE-NMR and HPLC-ToF MS. Xenobiotica 2006;36:615–29.

[62]   Prescott LF. Kinetics and metabolism of paracetamol and phenacetin. Br J Clin Pharmacol 1980;10(Suppl. 2):291S–8S.

[63]   Rawlins MD, Henderson DB, Hijab AR. Pharmacokinetics of paracetamol (acetaminophen) after intravenous and oral administration. Eur J Clin Pharmacol 1977;11:283–6.

[64] Isaka H, Yoshii H, Otsuji A, Koike M, Nagai Y, Koura M, et al. Tumors of Sprague-Dawley rats induced by long-term feeding of phenacetin. Gan 1979;70:29–36.

[65] Johansson SL. Carcinogenicity of analgesics: long-term treatment of Sprague-Dawley rats with phenacetin, phenazone, caffeine and paracetamol (acetamidophen). Int J Cancer 1981;27:521–9.

[66] Nakanishi K, Kurata Y, Oshima M, Fukushima S, Ito N. Carcinogenicity of phenacetin: long-term feeding study in B6C3F1 mice. Int J Cancer 1982;29:439–44.

[67] Hiraga K, Fujii T. Carcinogenicity testing of acetaminophen in F344 rats. Jpn J Cancer Res 1985;76:79–85.

[68] Flaks A, Flaks B. Induction of liver cell tumours in IF mice by paracetamol. Carcinogenesis 1983;4:363–8.

[69] Tsuda H, Sakata T, Masui T, Imaida K, Ito N. Modifying effects of butylated hydroxyanisole, ethoxyquin and acetaminophen on induction of neoplastic lesions in rat liver and kidney initiated by *N*-ethyl-*N*-hydroxy ethylnitrosamine. Carcinogenesis 1984;5:525–31.

[70] Hagiwara A, Ward JM. The chronic hepatotoxic, tumor-promoting, and carcinogenic effects of acetaminophen in male B6C3F1 mice. Fundam Appl Toxicol 1986;7:376–86.

[71] Togei K, Sano N, Maeda T, Shibata M, Otsuka H. Carcinogenicity of bucetin in (C57BL/6 X C3H)F1 mice. J Natl Cancer Inst 1987;79:1151–8.

[72] Nohmi T, Ishidate Jr M, Hiratsuka A, Watabe T. Mechanism of metabolic activation of the analgetic bucetin to bacterial mutagens by hamster liver microsomes. Chem Pharm Bull (Tokyo) 1985;33:2877–85.

[73] Tikkanen L, Matsushima T, Natori S, Yoshihira K. Mutagenicity of natural naphthoquinones and benzoquinones in the *Salmonella*/microsome test. Mutat Res 1983;124:25–34.

[74] Chesis PL, Levin DE, Smith MT, Ernster L, Ames BN. Mutagenicity of quinones: pathways of metabolic activation and detoxification. Proc Natl Acad Sci USA 1984;81:1696–700.

[75] Cojocel C, Novotny L, Vachalkova A. Mutagenic and carcinogenic potential of menadione. Neoplasma 2006;53:316–23.

[76] Losito R, Owen Jr CA, Flock EV. Metabolism of [^{14}C]menadione. Biochemistry 1967;6:62–8.

[77] Gong X, Gutala R, Jaiswal AK. Quinone oxidoreductases and vitamin K metabolism. Vitam Horm 2008;78:85–101.

[78] Parry JD, Pointon AV, Lutz U, Teichert F, Charlwood JK, Chan PH, et al. Pivotal role for two electron reduction in 2,3-dimethoxy-1,4-naphthoquinone and 2-methyl-1,4-naphthoquinone metabolism and kinetics in vivo that prevents liver redox stress. Chem Res Toxicol 2009;22:717–25.

[79] Shukla S, Wu CP, Nandigama K, Ambudkar SV. The naphthoquinones, vitamin K3 and its structural analogue plumbagin, are substrates of the multidrug resistance linked ATP binding cassette drug transporter ABCG2. Mol Cancer Ther 2007;6:3279–86.

[80] Watanabe N, Dickinson DA, Liu RM, Forman HJ. Quinones and glutathione metabolism. Methods Enzymol 2004;378:319–40.

[81] Bellomo G, Mirabelli F, DiMonte D, Richelmi P, Thor H, Orrenius C, et al. Formation and reduction of glutathione-protein mixed disulfides during oxidative stress. A study with isolated hepatocytes and menadione (2-methyl-1,4-naphthoquinone). Biochem Pharmacol 1987;36:1313–20.

[82] Redegeld FA, Hofman GA, van de Loo PG, Koster AS, Noordhoek J. Nephrotoxicity of the glutathione conjugate of menadione (2-methyl-1, 4-naphthoquinone) in the isolated perfused rat kidney. Role of metabolism by gamma-glutamyltranspeptidase and probenecid-sensitive transport. J Pharmacol Exp Ther 1991;256:665–9.

[83] Haenen HE, Rogmans P, Temmink JH, van Bladeren PJ. Differential detoxification of two thioether conjugates of menadione in confluent monolayers of rat renal proximal tubular cells. Toxicol In Vitro 1994;8:207–14.

[84] Chiou TJ, Zhang J, Ferrans VJ, Tzeng WF. Cardiac and renal toxicity of menadione in rat. Toxicology 1997;124:193–202.

[85] Ohta T, Moriya M, Kaneda Y, Watanabe K, Miyazawa T, Sugiyama F, et al. Mutagenicity screening of feed additives in the microbial system. Mutat Res 1980;77:21–30.

[86] Blaszczyk A. DNA damage induced by ethoxyquin in human peripheral lymphocytes. Toxicol Lett 2006;163:77–83.

[87] Skolimowski JJ, Cieslinska B, Zak M, Osiecka R, Blaszczyk A. Modulation of ethoxyquin genotoxicity by free radical scavengers and DNA damage repair in human lymphocytes. Toxicol Lett 2010;193:194–9.

[88] Food Safety Commission of Japan. Risk assessment report on food additive and agricultural chemical ethoxyquin p1-59. The report is available in Japanese at <http://www.fsc.go.jp/fsciis/evaluationDocument/show/kya20120912002>. An English summary is also available as Food Safety 2013; 2(1) 14–15 (doi:1014252/foodsafetyfscj.2014013s).

[89] Skaare JU, Solheim E. Studies on the metabolism of the antioxidant ethoxyquin, 6-ethoxy-2,2,4-trimethyl-1,2-dihydroquinoline in the rat. Xenobiotica 1979;9:649–57.

[90] Burka LT, Sanders JM, Matthews HB. Comparative metabolism and disposition of ethoxyquin in rat and mouse. II. Metabolism. Xenobiotica 1996;26:597–611.

[91] He P, Ackman RG. Purification of ethoxyquin and its two oxidation products. J Agric Food Chem 2000;48:3069–71.

[92] Bohne VJ, Lundebye AK, Hamre K. Accumulation and depuration of the synthetic antioxidant ethoxyquin in the muscle of Atlantic salmon (*Salmo salar* L.). Food Chem Toxicol 2008;46:1834–43.

[93] Fukushima S, Kurata Y, Shibata M, Ikawa E, Ito N. Promotion by ascorbic acid, sodium erythorbate and ethoxyquin of neoplastic lesions in rats initiated with N-butyl-N-(4-hydroxybutyl) nitrosamine. Cancer Lett 1984;23:29–37.

[94] Fukushima S, Ogiso T, Kurata Y, Hirose M, Ito N. Dose-dependent effects of butylated hydroxyanisole, butylated hydroxytoluene and ethoxyquin for promotion of bladder carcinogenesis in N-butyl-N-(4-hydroxybutyl)nitrosamine-initiated, unilaterally ureter-ligated rats. Cancer Lett 1987;34:83–90.

[95] Cohen SM, Anderson TA, de Oliveira LM, Arnold LL. Tumorigenicity of sodium ascorbate in male rats. Cancer Res 1998;58:2557–61.

[96] Shibata MA, Fukushima S, Asakawa E, Hirose M, Ito N. The modifying effects of indomethacin or ascorbic acid on cell proliferation induced by different types of bladder tumor promoters in rat urinary bladder and forestomach mucosal epithelium. Jpn J Cancer Res 1992;83:31–9.

[97] Tafazoli S, Wright JS, O'Brien PJ. Prooxidant and antioxidant activity of vitamin E analogues and troglitazone. Chem Res Toxicol 2005;18:1567–74.

[98] Lambert JD, Elias RJ. The antioxidant and pro-oxidant activities of green tea polyphenols: a role in cancer prevention. Arch Biochem Biophys 2010;501:65–72.

[99] Manson MM, Green JA, Driver HE. Ethoxyquin alone induces preneoplastic changes in rat kidney whilst preventing induction of such lesions in liver by aflatoxin B1. Carcinogenesis 1987;8:723–8.

[100] National-Toxicology-Program. Carcinogenesis bioassay of allyl isothiocyanate (CAS No. 57-06-7) in F344/N rats and B6C3F1 mice (gavage study). Natl Toxicol Program Tech Rep Ser 1982;234:1–142.

[101] Brusick D. Analysis of genotoxicity and the carcinogenic mode of action for ortho-phenylphenol. Environ Mol Mutagen 2005;45:460–81.

[102] Nery R. The binding of radioactive label from labelled phenacetin and related compounds to rat tissues in vivo and to nucleic acids and bovine plasma albumin in vitro. Biochem J 1971;122:311–5.

[103] Badger DA, Smith RL, Bao J, Kuester RK, Sipes IG. Disposition and metabolism of isoeugenol in the male Fischer 344 rat. Food Chem Toxicol 2002;40:1757–65.

[104] Chen TX, Wanibuchi H, Murai T, Kitano M, Yamamoto S, Fukushima S. Promotion by sodium L-ascorbate in rat two-stage urinary bladder carcinogenesis is dependent on the interval of administration. Jpn J Cancer Res 1999;90:16–22.

Mode of Action and Assessment of Human Relevance for Chemical-Induced Animal Tumors

Masahiko Kushida[1], Tomoya Yamada[1] and Yasuyoshi Okuno[2]

[1]*Environmental Health Science Laboratory, Sumitomo Chemical Co. Ltd., Osaka, Japan*
[2]*Sumika Technical Information Service, Inc., Osaka, Japan*

Chapter Outline

Introduction 193
Importance of Mode of Action (MOA) Analyses for Chemical-Induced Animal Tumors and
    Assessment of Human Relevance Based on MOA 194
Human Relevance of the Constitutive Androstane Receptor (CAR) Activator-Induced Liver
    Tumors in Rodents Based on MOA 195
    Hepatic Tumor Induction by CAR Activators in Rodents 195
    MOA for Rodent Liver Tumor Formation via CAR 195
    Human Relevance of a Rodent CAR-Activator Liver Tumor MOA 196
Human Relevance of the Mutagen-Induced Tumors in Rodents Based on Threshold 197
Future Prospects of the Mechanistic Research in Genotoxic and Nongenotoxic Tumor
    Inducers 199
References 200

Introduction

Cancer is one of the leading causes of death in the world. Since Percival Pott first suggested in 1775 that a cancer was caused by an environmental carcinogen, many epidemiological studies have revealed clear relationships between human cancers and chemical exposures. This evidence has also been experimentally demonstrated in animal carcinogenesis models; therefore, assessment of the carcinogenicity hazard of chemicals in humans has been determined primarily on the basis of long-term testing in animals, particularly rats and mice. In all these experiments in animals, two fundamental assumptions are made: (1) the results are relevant to humans (interspecies extrapolation) and (2) the doses used are relevant

Thresholds of Genotoxic Carcinogens.
DOI: http://dx.doi.org/10.1016/B978-0-12-801663-3.00012-1

for estimating risk at known or expected human exposure levels (dose extrapolation) [1]. Although these assumptions are valid for many chemicals with respect to carcinogenesis, rodents in standard cancer tests are chronically given a near-toxic dose: the maximum tolerated dose. About 50% of the chemicals tested in standard animal carcinogenicity studies using such high doses have been determined to be positive [2]. For a rational assessment of hazard and risk to humans, it is important that the cancers observed in the animal carcinogenicity tests also occur in humans, especially at the low levels to which humans are usually exposed.

Importance of Mode of Action (MOA) Analyses for Chemical-Induced Animal Tumors and Assessment of Human Relevance Based on MOA

The outcome of a mechanistically based cancer risk assessment is critical for a rational assessment of hazard and risk to humans. No totally unified approach is currently available, but a harmonized approach has been developed. The WHO International Programme on Chemical Safety (IPCS), the International Life Science Institute (ILSI), and the US Environmental Protection Agency (US EPA) provide frameworks for cancer risk assessment [3–8]. The human relevance assessment framework for cancer risk is based on a mode of action (MOA) as the means of describing the "necessary but not sufficient" steps required for exposure to a chemical to produce a tumor. In this framework, an empirically observable causal precursor step to the adverse outcome that is itself a necessary element of the MOA is designated as a "key event." Key events are required events for the MOA, but often are not sufficient to induce the adverse outcome in the absence of other events; whereas "associative events" are biological processes that are themselves not causally necessary key events for the MOA, but are reliable indicators or markers for key events. Associative events can often be used as surrogate markers for a key event in an MOA evaluation or as indicators of exposure to a xenobiotic that has stimulated the molecular initiating event or a key event. In addition, there can be modulating factors such as biological responses, or cooperative factors that are not necessary to induce the adverse outcome but that could modulate the dose–response behavior or probability of inducing one or more key events or the adverse outcome [4].

During the past four decades, understanding of MOAs of carcinogenesis has greatly improved our ability to evaluate human relevance of animal tumors induced by specific chemicals [1]. A fundamental breakthrough in understanding MOAs was the recognition of distinction between genotoxic and nongenotoxic MOAs [1]. Threshold approaches traditionally have been used for the assessment of the human risk for carcinogenicity of nongenotoxic carcinogens, and nonthreshold approaches have been used for genotoxic carcinogens. As progress has been made in determining the MOAs of chemicals that produce neoplasia in animal tests, it has become increasingly clear that some kinds of rodent tumor induced by nongenotoxic carcinogens, such as alpha-2u globulin-associated male rat renal tubule tumors, are not relevant to humans. Therefore, it has become increasingly important to evaluate the relevance of MOAs of animal carcinogenicity with respect to humans.

Human Relevance of the Constitutive Androstane Receptor (CAR) Activator-Induced Liver Tumors in Rodents Based on MOA

Hepatic Tumor Induction by CAR Activators in Rodents

Phenobarbital (phenobarbitone, PB) is a prototypical constitutive androstane receptor (CAR) activator. Many studies have shown that PB and/or its sodium salt (sodium phenobarbital; NaPB) can produce liver tumors in rats and mice [9,10]. Other known CAR activators, including 1,4-bis[2-(3,5-dichloropyridyloxy)]benzene (TCPOBOP), chlordane, cyproconazole, dieldrin, α-hexachlorocyclohexane, 2,4,5,2′,4′,5′-hexachlorobipheny, fluopyram, metofluthrin, oxazepam, phenytoin, potassium perfluorooctanesulfonate, pronamide, propiconazole, pyrethrins, sulfoxaflor, and 1,1,1,-trichloro-2,2-bis (4-chlorophenyl)ethane (DDT) have also produced liver tumors in rats and/or mice [11–19].

MOA for Rodent Liver Tumor Formation via CAR

A number of evaluations have identified key and other events in this MOA for rodent liver tumor formation [4]. The MOA for rodent liver tumor formation by PB and related compounds involves activation of CAR leading to a pleiotropic response. In a recent evaluation of the MOA for PB-induced rodent liver tumor formation, the key events in the MOA were considered to be CAR activation, altered gene expression specific to CAR activation, increased cell proliferation, and the development of altered hepatic foci leading to liver tumor formation [4]. In addition, associative events, including the induction of cytochrome P450 (CYP) enzymes (in particular the CYP2B subfamily enzymes), liver hypertrophy (increased liver weight and hepatocellular hypertrophy), and inhibition of apoptosis, were also identified [4]. This evaluation also included consideration of inhibition of gap junctional intercellular communication and oxidative stress as potential associative events or modulating factors [4]. Since the disruption of gap junctional intercellular communication by PB may contribute to the process of tumor development, this process was considered to be an associative event or a modulating factor; however, while oxidative stress can play a role in chemically induced carcinogenesis, this was not considered to constitute such an event or factor [4].

CAR is the molecular target of PB [20], and activation of this receptor is an essential requirement for liver tumor development [21–23]. The pivotal role of CAR in the MOA for PB-induced liver tumor formation has been demonstrated in transgenic mice lacking this nuclear receptor (CAR knockout mice) or both the CAR and pregnane X receptor (PXR) receptors (CAR/PXR knockout mice). In CAR or CAR/PXR knockout mice, PB does not increase liver weight, does not induce CYP2B enzymes, and does not stimulate replicative DNA synthesis [21–23]. Recently, a study with CAR knockout rats revealed similar findings [24]. The treatment of rat hepatocytes with CAR-siRNA significantly reduced CAR mRNA in the presence of PB, resulting in a significant reduction in the magnitude of induction of CYP2B1 mRNA levels by PB [20]. While PB and the more potent CAR activator TCPOBOP promoted liver tumor production in wild-type mice initiated with a single dose of diethylnitrosamine, no liver adenomas or carcinomas were observed in the CAR knockout mice [21]. Thus, there is clear evidence from studies in knockout mice or rats that CAR plays an essential role in PB-induced liver tumor formation.

Human Relevance of a Rodent CAR-Activator Liver Tumor MOA

To assess the human relevance of a proposed rodent tumor MOA, the IPCS human relevance framework requires answers to the following questions: [3]

1. Is the weight of evidence sufficient to establish an MOA in animals?
2. Can human relevance of the MOA be reasonably excluded on the basis of fundamental, qualitative differences in key events between experimental animals and humans?
3. Can human relevance of the MOA be reasonably excluded on the basis of quantitative differences in either kinetic or dynamic factors between experimental animals and humans?

For a CAR-activation MOA by PB and related compounds, since a robust MOA has been established for rodent liver tumor formation, the answer to the first question is "yes." A number of the hepatic effects of PB that have been reported in rodents can also be observed in humans [4]. However, comparisons of effects of some of the key and associative events in the MOA for PB-induced rodent liver tumor production between rodent and human liver could prove that some clear species differences have been reported. For example, while PB produces an increase in replicative DNA synthesis in cultured rodent hepatocytes, as well as after in vivo administration, PB does not appear to increase replicative DNA synthesis in cultured human hepatocytes [6,25,26]. Unlike in rodent liver, PB has also been reported not to inhibit apoptosis in human hepatocytes [27].

Supportive evidence for the conclusion that PB does not stimulate replicative DNA synthesis in human hepatocytes has been provided in our recent study using chimeric mice with human hepatocytes [28]. In the study, NaPB was administered at various dietary levels for 7 days to male Wistar rats, CD-1 mice, and chimeric mice with human hepatocytes. The treatment of chimeric mice with 1000–1500 ppm NaPB resulted in plasma PB levels around threefold to fivefold higher than those observed in human subjects given therapeutic doses of PB. Treatment with NaPB produced liver hypertrophy and induction of CYP2B mRNA levels and enzyme activity in Wistar rats, CD-1 mice, and chimeric mice. However, while NaPB produced dose-dependent increases in hepatocyte replicative DNA synthesis in Wistar rats and CD-1 mice, no increase in replicative DNA synthesis was observed in human hepatocytes of the chimeric mice. In addition, hepatic mRNA levels for some cell proliferation genes, including *Ki-67*, *PCNA*, *GADD45β*, and *MDM2*, were also increased in Wistar rats and/or CD-1 mice, but not in chimeric mice with human hepatocytes. The study thus provides additional strong evidence that, unlike rodent hepatocytes, human hepatocytes are refractory to the mitogenic effects of NaPB [28].

The lack of effect of PB and related compounds on replicative DNA synthesis in human hepatocytes represents a key species difference between rodents and humans [4,14]. Based on such data it can be concluded that the answer to Question 2 is "no"; that is, the MOA for CAR activator-induced rodent liver tumor formation is not plausible for humans [4,14]. This conclusion is supported by data from a number of epidemiological studies conducted in humans chronically exposed to PB, in which there is no clear evidence of increased liver tumor risk [9,29–32]. Thus there is no need to analyze Question 3.

Human Relevance of the Mutagen-Induced Tumors in Rodents Based on Threshold

Much research has demonstrated that the framework of analysis for an MOA and its human relevance is useful for not only nongenotoxic carcinogens, but also genotoxic carcinogen-induced animal tumors, such as aflatoxin B_1, tamoxifen, and vinyl chloride [33,34], formaldehyde and glutaraldehyde [35], cyclophosphamide [36], and 4-aminobihenyl [37]. The human relevance framework consists of three steps: first, to establish an MOA of tumor induction by a chemical in animals and to find key events of the MOA; second, to analyze its qualitative relevance between humans and animals; and third, to analyze its quantitative relevance. Preston and Williams [34] summarized and Jarabek et al. [38] modified the key events in the carcinogenicity of DNA-reactive mutagenic carcinogens (Table 12.1). Basically, a reactive mutagen is capable of forming DNA adducts or inducing interaction of other cellular target structures that result in specific DNA damage. As a consequence of the mutations that can result from these reactions at critical sites of critical oncogenes and/or tumor suppressor genes, neoplastic cells eventually develop.

All of these previous studies that evaluated the human relevancy based on the human relevancy framework demonstrated that the key events of MOA of genotoxic carcinogen-induced tumors are DNA interactions, and the tumors are considered to be produced by this chemical via direct mutagenicity. In addition, these human relevance framework analyses also showed the analyzed MOA of genotoxic carcinogens is qualitatively relevant to humans, because DNA reactivity is observed in both humans and nonhumans. Therefore, this observation has led to the default use of linear extrapolation from the rodent test tumor data to exposure levels consistent with human environmental or occupational exposure. Certainly, linear extrapolation is adequate at high concentration exposures; however, difficulty arises

Table 12.1 Key events for tumor development: DNA-reactive MOAs.

1a. Exposure of target cells (eg, stem cells) to electrophilic species—in some cases this requires metabolism
1b. Reactions with other non-DNA cellular targets that have impact on adduct fate (eg, depletions of detoxication pathways critical to clearance)
2. Reaction with DNA in target cells to produce DNA damage
3. Misreplication on damaged DNA template or misrepair of DNA damage
4. Mutations in critical genes in replicating target cell
5. Mutations in critical genes result in enhanced DNA/cell replication
6. New cell replication leads to clonal expansion of mutant cells
7. DNA replication leads to further mutations in critical genes
8. Imbalanced and uncontrolled clonal growth of mutant cells may lead to preneoplastic lesions
9. Progression of preneoplastic cells results in emergence of overt neoplasms, solid tumors (which require neoangiogenesis), or leukemia
10. Additional mutations in critical genes as a result of uncontrolled cell division results in malignant behavior

Source: Originally by Preston RJ, Williams GM. DNA-reactive carcinogens: mode of action and human cancer hazard. Crit Rev Toxicol 2005;35:673–83 and modified by Jarabek AM, Pottenger LH, Andrews LS, Casciano D, Embry MR, Kim JH, et al. Creating context for the use of DNA adduct data in cancer risk assessment: I. Data organization. Crit Rev Toxicol 2009;39:659–78.

when evaluating in detail the dose–response relationship between a chemical exposure and genotoxic carcinogen-induced cancer formation at low dose, since humans have several tiers of protection against DNA damage [39], including (1) epithelial barriers to genotoxin entry, (2) detoxification processes leading to excretion of water-soluble genotoxins, (3) compartmentalization of tissues leading to reduced access for genotoxins, (4) cellular and nuclear membranes reducing access of genotoxins to the nucleus, (5) DNA repair to remove damaged DNA sequences, (6) DNA redundancy (<1% genes are thought to code for proteins), and (7) apoptosis/autophagy/anoikis to remove damaged cells. In addition, because of the effect of endogenous DNA damage on the mutagenic process and the multistep nature of that process, the dose response for induced mutations does not reflect the dose response for chemical-specific DNA adducts [38–41]. Furthermore, even if this DNA damage becomes stable and inheritable, it is not sufficient to induce a cancer, because carcinogenesis is a complex tissue response that requires multiple steps or key events that include early events of a genetic and/or epigenetic nature, as well as later steps such as cell selection and cell–cell and cell–microenvironment interactions [38]. Indeed, Fukushima's group demonstrated that the genotoxic hepatocarcinogens 2-amino-3,8-dimethylimidazo [4,5-*f*]quinoxaline [42,43] and 2-amino-3-methylimidazo [4,5-*f*]quinoline [44] induced DNA adduct formation and in vivo mutagenicity at low dose, but carcinogenicity was observed only at high dose. Therefore, DNA adduct formation and DNA mutation are informative biomarkers of chemical exposure and suggestive of potential cancer risk; [38,40] however, the dose response for DNA damage is not sufficient for quantitative evaluation for human relevancy.

Future Prospects of the Mechanistic Research in Genotoxic and Nongenotoxic Tumor Inducers

Assessment of the carcinogenicity hazard of chemicals to humans is determined primarily on the basis of long-term animal testing even now. The assessment of human risk requires the application of a series of default options, from laboratory animals to humans, from high dose to low dose, from intermittent to chronic lifetime exposures, and among routes of exposure. There is no available perfect approach, but an MOA/human relevance framework is useful for human risk assessment of carcinogenicity of chemicals. In the human relevance framework, one of the most important steps is to identify key events of adverse outcome pathways (AOPs) [58] and mechanisms of cancer formation. For this purpose, the application of molecular biology techniques has certainly aimed at the pursuit of mechanisms of mutagenicity and carcinogenicity. To evaluate qualitative human relevance of the results observed in animal testing, especially for nongenotoxic carcinogens, direct in vitro and in vivo comparisons between laboratory animals and humans are important as we recently demonstrated using human hepatocytes (in vitro) and chimeric mice with human hepatocytes (in vivo) [25,26,28].

In contrast to qualitative assessment, there are many difficulties in evaluating quantitative human relevance. First of all, correct determination of the shape of the dose–response curve is not easy. Basically, thresholds for carcinogenicity induced by nongenotoxic carcinogens certainly exist. For example, Fukushima's group demonstrated that phenobarbital and DDT have hormesis effects for hepatocarcinogenesis and their dose–response curves are "J-shaped" [45–49]. Their data suggested these chemicals clearly have thresholds for hepatocarcinogenesis, but it is difficult to establish a true "no (adverse) effect" level. For genotoxic carcinogens, a huge number of animals are needed to establish a precise dose–response relationship between genotoxic carcinogen exposure and carcinogenicity in detail at low dose [43,50]. Improved statistical analysis can reduce the number of animals used to accurately define a point of departure (PoD) [51–54]. One of the methods to analyze exposure–response relationships and to drive PoD metrics for human health risk assessment is the benchmark dose (BMD). In general, quantitative BMD approaches are considered to be preferable to the no-observed-effect level (NOEL) approach, and have been used by many agencies for determining PoDs for health-based guidance [54], and have achieved less than half the number of animals being used to define a PoD [52]. However, Fukushima et al. demonstrated that comparison of NOEL and BMD approaches demonstrates that neither approach separately is applicable for all types of carcinogens, and therefore the most appropriate approach must be selected on the basis of scientific judgment [55]. In vitro assays are certainly useful tools, but the extrapolation premise required for the use of an in vitro assay to describe the dose response for humans versus ex vivo or in vivo data in mammalian species is not likely to carry the same weight of evidence [38]. As the German/Swiss/ Austrian Society of Environmental Mutagenesis (GUM) reviewed recently [56], evidence that genotoxins showed a nonlinear dose response is increasing. In the food and feed area, the Threshold of Toxicological Concern (TTC) approach was considered as a tool for providing scientific advice about possible human health risks from low levels of exposure to chemicals. TTC values were published for substances with a structural alert for genotoxicity (0.15 µg/ person per day or 0.0025 µg/kg bw per day) except for high-potency carcinogens (cohort of concern: aflatoxin-like compounds, *N*-nitrosocompounds, azoxy-compounds, benzidines, hydrazines), inorganic substances; metals and organometallics; proteins, steroids; substances known/predicted to bioaccumulate; nanomaterials, radioactive substances; mixture [57]. However, as Fukushima et al. demonstrated, there is a practical threshold for carcinogenicity even for *N*-nitrosocompounds [43]. To determine the human relevance of a genotoxic carcinogen precisely, novel qualitative and quantitative approaches will play essential roles. Humanized animals such as chimeric mice with human hepatocytes may pave the way for future studies to evaluate quantitative as well as qualitative human relevance.

References

[1] Cohen SM, Klaunig J, Meek ME, Hill RN, Pastoor T, Lehman-McKeeman L, et al. Evaluating the human relevance of chemically induced animal tumors. Toxicol Sci 2004;78:181–6.
[2] Ames BN, Gold LS. Paracelsus to parascience: the environmental cancer distraction. Mutat Res 2000;447:3–13.
[3] Boobis AR, Cohen SM, Dellarco V, McGregor D, Meek ME, Vickers C, et al. IPCS framework for analyzing the relevance of a cancer mode of action for humans. Crit Rev Toxicol 2006;36:781–92.
[4] Elcombe CR, Peffer RC, Wolf DC, Bailey J, Bars R, Bell D, et al. Mode of action and human relevance analysis for nuclear receptor-mediated liver toxicity: a case study with phenobarbital as a model constitutive androstane receptor (CAR) activator. Crit Rev Toxicol 2014;44:64–82.
[5] Meek ME, Bucher JR, Cohen SM, Dellarco V, Hill RN, Lehman-McKeeman LD, et al. A framework for human relevance analysis of information on carcinogenic modes of action. Crit Rev Toxicol 2003;33:591–653.
[6] Parzefall W, Erber E, Sedivy R, Schulte-Hermann R. Testing for induction of DNA synthesis in human hepatocyte primary cultures by rat liver tumor promoters. Cancer Res 1991;51:1143–7.
[7] Sonich-Mullin C, Fielder R, Wiltse J, Baetcke K, Dempsey J, Fenner-Crisp P, et al. IPCS conceptual framework for evaluating a mode of action for chemical carcinogenesis. Regul Toxicol Pharmacol 2001;34:146–52.
[8] U.S. Environmental Protection Agency. <http://www.epa.gov/sites/production/files/2013-09/documents/cancer_guidelines_final_3-25-05.pdf> Guidelines for carcinogen risk assessment. EPA/630/P-03/001F2005.
[9] IARC. Some thyrotropic agents: phenobarbital and its sodium salt. IARC Monogr Eval Carcinog Risks Hum 2001;79:161–288.
[10] Whysner J, Ross PM, Williams GM. Phenobarbital mechanistic data and risk assessment: enzyme induction, enhanced cell proliferation, and tumor promotion. Pharmacol Ther 1996;71:153–91.
[11] Currie RA, Peffer RC, Goetz AK, Omiecinski CJ, Goodman JI. Phenobarbital and propiconazole toxicogenomic profiles in mice show major similarities consistent with the key role that constitutive androstane receptor (CAR) activation plays in their mode of action. Toxicology 2014;321:80–8.
[12] Elcombe CR, Elcombe BM, Foster JR, Chang S-C, Ehresman DJ, Butenhoff JL. Hepatocellular hypertrophy and cell proliferation in Sprague-Dawley rats from dietary exposure to potassium perfluorooctanesulfonate results from increased expression of xenosensor nuclear receptors PPARα and CAR/PXR. Toxicology 2012;293:16–29.

[13] Ellis-Hutchings RG, Rasoulpour RJ, Terry C, Carney EW, Billington R. Human relevance framework evaluation of a novel rat developmental toxicity mode of action induced by sulfoxaflor. Crit Rev Toxicol 2014;44(Suppl. 2):45–62.

[14] Lake BG, Price RJ, Osimitz TG. Mode of action analysis for pesticide-induced rodent liver tumours involving activation of the constitutive androstane receptor: relevance to human cancer risk. Pest Manage Sci 2015;71:829–34.

[15] LeBaron MJ, Rasoulpour RJ, Gollapudi BB, Sura R, Kan HL, Schisler MR, et al. Characterization of nuclear receptor-mediated murine hepatocarcinogenesis of the herbicide pronamide and its human relevance. Toxicol Sci 2014;142:74–92.

[16] Osimitz TG, Lake BG. Mode-of-action analysis for induction of rat liver tumors by pyrethrins: relevance to human cancer risk. Crit Rev Toxicol 2009;39:501–11.

[17] Peffer RC, Moggs JG, Pastoor T, Currie RA, Wright J, Milburn G, et al. Mouse liver effects of cyproconazole, a triazole fungicide: role of the constitutive androstane receptor. Toxicol Sci 2007;99:315–25.

[18] Tinwell H, Rouquie D, Schorsch F, Geter D, Wason S, Bars R. Liver tumor formation in female rat induced by fluopyram is mediated by CAR/PXR nuclear receptor activation. Regul Toxicol Pharmacol 2014;70:648–58.

[19] Yamada T, Uwagawa S, Okuno Y, Cohen SM, Kaneko H. Case study: an evaluation of the human relevance of the synthetic pyrethroid metofluthrin-induced liver tumors in rats based on mode of action. Toxicol Sci 2009;108:59–68.

[20] Deguchi Y, Yamada T, Hirose Y, Nagahori H, Kushida M, Sumida K, et al. Mode of action analysis for the synthetic pyrethroid metofluthrin-induced rat liver tumors: evidence for hepatic CYP2B induction and hepatocyte proliferation. Toxicol Sci 2009;108:69–80.

[21] Huang W, Zhang J, Washington M, Liu J, Parant JM, Lozano G, et al. Xenobiotic stress induces hepatomegaly and liver tumors via the nuclear receptor constitutive androstane receptor. Mol Endocrinol 2005;19:1646–53.

[22] Wei P, Zhang J, Egan-Hafley M, Liang S, Moore DD. The nuclear receptor CAR mediates specific xenobiotic induction of drug metabolism. Nature 2000;407:920–3.

[23] Yamamoto Y, Moore R, Goldsworthy TL, Negishi M, Maronpot RR. The orphan nuclear receptor constitutive active/androstane receptor is essential for liver tumor promotion by phenobarbital in mice. Cancer Res 2004;64:7197–200.

[24] Chamberlain M, Haines C, Elcombe CR. Characterisation of the hepatic effects of phenobarbital in constitutive androstane receptor (CAR, NR1I3) knockout rats. Toxicol Sci 2014;138(Suppl. 1):301.

[25] Hirose Y, Nagahori H, Yamada T, Deguchi Y, Tomigahara Y, Nishioka K, et al. Comparison of the effects of the synthetic pyrethroid Metofluthrin and phenobarbital on CYP2B form induction and replicative DNA synthesis in cultured rat and human hepatocytes. Toxicology 2009;258:64–9.

[26] Yamada T, Kikumoto H, Lake BG, Kawamura S. Lack of effect of metofluthrin and sodium phenobarbital on replicative DNA synthesis and Ki-67 mRNA expression in cultured human hepatocytes. Toxicol Res 2015;4:901–13.

[27] Hasmall SC, Roberts RA. The perturbation of apoptosis and mitosis by drugs and xenobiotics. Pharmacol Ther 1999;82:63–70.

[28] Yamada T, Okuda Y, Kushida M, Sumida K, Takeuchi H, Nagahori H, et al. Human hepatocytes support the hypertrophic but not the hyperplastic response to the murine nongenotoxic hepatocarcinogen sodium phenobarbital in an in vivo study using a chimeric mouse with humanized liver. Toxicol Sci 2014;142:137–57.

[29] Friedman GD, Jiang S-F, Udaltsova N, Quesenberry CP, Chan J, Habel LA. Epidemiologic evaluation of pharmaceuticals with limited evidence of carcinogenicity. Int J Cancer 2009;125:2173–8.

[30] La Vecchia C, Negri E. A review of epidemiological data on epilepsy, phenobarbital, and risk of liver cancer. Eur J Cancer Prev 2014;23:1–7.

[31] Olsen JH, Boice Jr JD, Jensen JP, Fraumeni Jr JF. Cancer among epileptic patients exposed to anticonvulsant drugs. J Natl Cancer Inst 1989;81:803–8.

[32] Olsen JH, Schulgen G, Boice Jr JD, Whysner J, Travis LB, Williams GM, et al. Antiepileptic treatment and risk for hepatobiliary cancer and malignant lymphoma. Cancer Res 1995;55:294–7.

[33] Pottenger LH, Andrews LS, Bachman AN, Boogaard PJ, Cadet J, Embry MR, et al. An organizational approach for the assessment of DNA adduct data in risk assessment: case studies for aflatoxin B1, tamoxifen and vinyl chloride. Crit Rev Toxicol 2014;44:348–91.

[34] Preston RJ, Williams GM. DNA-reactive carcinogens: mode of action and human cancer hazard. Crit Rev Toxicol 2005;35:673–83.

[35] McGregor D, Bolt H, Cogliano V, Richter-Reichhelm HB. Formaldehyde and glutaraldehyde and nasal cytotoxicity: case study within the context of the 2006 IPCS Human Framework for the Analysis of a cancer mode of action for humans. Crit Rev Toxicol 2006;36:821–35.

[36] McCarroll N, Keshava N, Cimino M, Chu M, Dearfield K, Keshava C, et al. An evaluation of the mode of action framework for mutagenic carcinogens case study: cyclophosphamide. Environ Mol Mutagen 2008;49:117–31.

[37] Cohen SM, Boobis AR, Meek ME, Preston RJ, McGregor DB. 4-Aminobiphenyl and DNA reactivity: case study within the context of the 2006 IPCS Human Relevance Framework for analysis of a cancer mode of action for humans. Crit Rev Toxicol 2006;36:803–19.

[38] Jarabek AM, Pottenger LH, Andrews LS, Casciano D, Embry MR, Kim JH, et al. Creating context for the use of DNA adduct data in cancer risk assessment: I. Data organization. Crit Rev Toxicol 2009;39:659–78.

[39] Jenkins GJ, Zair Z, Johnson GE, Doak SH. Genotoxic thresholds, DNA repair, and susceptibility in human populations. Toxicology 2010;278:305–10.

[40] Swenberg JA, Fryar-Tita E, Jeong YC, Boysen G, Starr T, Walker VE, et al. Biomarkers in toxicology and risk assessment: informing critical dose-response relationships. Chem Res Toxicol 2008;21:253–65.

[41] Nakamura J, Mutlu E, Sharma V, Collins L, Bodnar W, Yu R, et al. The endogenous exposome. DNA Repair (Amst) 2014;19:3–13.

[42] Hoshi M, Morimura K, Wanibuchi H, Wei M, Okochi E, Ushijima T, et al. No-observed effect levels for carcinogenicity and for in vivo mutagenicity of a genotoxic carcinogen. Toxicol Sci 2004;81:273–9.

[43] Fukushima S, Wanibuchi H, Morimura K, Wei M, Nakae D, Konishi Y, et al. Lack of a dose-response relationship for carcinogenicity in the rat liver with low doses of 2-amino-3,8-dimethylimidazo[4,5-*f*] quinoxaline or *N*-nitrosodiethylamine. Jpn J Cancer Res 2002;93:1076–82.

[44] Wei M, Wanibuchi H, Nakae D, Tsuda H, Takahashi S, Hirose M, et al. Low-dose carcinogenicity of 2-amino-3-methylimidazo[4,5-*f*]quinoline in rats: evidence for the existence of no-effect levels and a mechanism involving p21(Cip/WAF1). Cancer Sci 2011;102:88–94.

[45] Fukushima S, Kinoshita A, Puatanachokchai R, Kushida M, Wanibuchi H, Morimura K. Hormesis and dose-response-mediated mechanisms in carcinogenesis: evidence for a threshold in carcinogenicity of non-genotoxic carcinogens. Carcinogenesis 2005;26:1835–45.

[46] Kinoshita A, Wanibuchi H, Morimura K, Wei M, Shen J, Imaoka S, et al. Phenobarbital at low dose exerts hormesis in rat hepatocarcinogenesis by reducing oxidative DNA damage, altering cell proliferation, apoptosis and gene expression. Carcinogenesis 2003;24:1389–99.

[47] Kitano M, Ichihara T, Matsuda T, Wanibuchi H, Tamano S, Hagiwara A, et al. Presence of a threshold for promoting effects of phenobarbital on diethylnitrosamine-induced hepatic foci in the rat. Carcinogenesis 1998;19:1475–80.

[48] Kushida M, Sukata T, Uwagawa S, Ozaki K, Kinoshita A, Wanibuchi H, et al. Low dose DDT inhibition of hepatocarcinogenesis initiated by diethylnitrosamine in male rats: possible mechanisms. Toxicol Appl Pharmacol 2005;208:285–94.

[49] Sukata T, Uwagawa S, Ozaki K, Ogawa M, Nishikawa T, Iwai S, et al. Detailed low-dose study of 1,1-bis (*p*-chlorophenyl)-2,2,2-trichloroethane carcinogenesis suggests the possibility of a hormetic effect. Int J Cancer 2002;99:112–8.

[50] Eaton DL, Gilvert SG. Principles of toxicology Klaassen CD, editors. Casarett and Doull's toxicology: the basic science of poisons. 8th ed. New York, NY: McGraw-Hill Education; 2013. p. 13–48.

[51] Benford D, Bolger PM, Carthew P, Coulet M, DiNovi M, Leblanc JC, et al. Application of the Margin of Exposure (MOE) approach to substances in food that are genotoxic and carcinogenic. Food Chem Toxicol 2010;48(Suppl. 1)):S2–24.

[52]   Johnson GE, Slob W, Doak SH, Fellows MD, Gollapudi BB, Heflich RH, et al. New approaches to advance the use of genetic toxicology analyses for human health risk assessment. Toxicol Res 2015;4:667–76.

[53]   MacGregor JT, Frotschl R, White PA, Crump KS, Eastmond DA, Fukushima S, et al. IWGT report on quantitative approaches to genotoxicity risk assessment II. Use of point-of-departure (PoD) metrics in defining acceptable exposure limits and assessing human risk. Mutat Res Genet Toxicol Environ Mutagen 2015;783:66–78.

[54]   MacGregor JT, Frotschl R, White PA, Crump KS, Eastmond DA, Fukushima S, et al. IWGT report on quantitative approaches to genotoxicity risk assessment I. Methods and metrics for defining exposure-response relationships and points of departure (PoDs). Mutat Res Genet Toxicol Environ Mutagen 2015;783:55–65.

[55]   Fukushima S, Gi M, Kakehashi A, Wanibuchi H, Matsumoto M. Qualitative and quantitative approaches in the dose-response assessment of genotoxic carcinogens. Mutagenesis 2015 [Epub ahead of print doi:10.1093/mutage/gev049].

[56]   Guerard M, Baum M, Bitsch A, Eisenbrand G, Elhajouji A, Epe B, et al. Assessment of mechanisms driving non-linear dose-response relationships in genotoxicity testing. Mutat Res Rev Mutat Res 2015;763:181–201.

[57]   European Food Safety Authority. Scientific opinion on evaluation of the toxicological relevance of pesticide metabolites for dietary risk assessment. EFSA J 2012;10:2799. <http://www.efsa.europa.eu/sites/default/files/scientific_output/files/main_documents/2799.pdf>.

[58]   Organisation for Economic Co-operation and Development (OECD). Guidance document on developing and assessing adverse outcome pathways. Series Testing and Assessment No.184. ENV/JM/MONO(2013)6, <http://www.oecd.org/officialdocuments/publicdisplaydocumentpdf/?cote=env/jm/mono%282013%296&doclanguage=en>.

Index

Note: Page numbers followed by "*f*" and "*t*" refer to figures and tables, respectively.

A

Aberrant crypt foci (ACF), 10–11
Absolute risk (AR), 38*t*
Acceptable daily intake (ADI),
    50–52, 62, 103, 130,
    155–156
Acetaldehyde
  DNA damage in risk assessment,
    84–88
Acetaminophen, 178–180
  carcinogenicity of, 180
  genotoxicity of, 178–179
  metabolisms of, 178*f*
  pharmacokinetics of, 179,
    186–187
2-Acetylaminofluorene (2-AAF)
  effect on liver carcinogenesis
    initiation, 23*t*, 25–28, 30–31
  nonthreshold theory for, 2
  low-dose carcinogenicity of,
    qualitative and quantitative
    analyses on, 2
  DNA adduct formation, 10–11
Acrylamide, genotoxicity of, 52–54
Aflatoxin B_1 (AFB$_1$), 54, 164
  effect on liver carcinogenesis
    initiation, 23
  genotoxic thresholds, 105
Akaike information criterion (AIC),
    144–145
ALARA (as low as reasonably
    attainable), 130, 132
ALARP (as low as reasonably
    practical), 130, 132
Aldehydes
  DNA damage in risk assessment,
    84–88

Alkylating agents
  DNA damage in risk assessment,
    88–90
  mechanism of action, 70–71
  paradigm shift in response to low
    doses of, 69
Ames test, 52–54, 104
4-Aminobiphenyl (4-ABP), 10–11
2-Amino-3, 8-dimethylimidazo[4,
    5-*f*]quinoxaline (MeIQx)
  effect on liver carcinogenesis
    initiation, 24–25
  low-dose carcinogenicity of,
    qualitative and quantitative
    analyses on, 3–7, 12*f*
  DNA adduct formation, 3, 4*f*,
    5, 10
  dose–response relationship,
    6–7, 6*f*
  GST-P-positive foci, induction
    of, 4–5, 4*f*, 10–13
  lacI gene mutation, 5–6, 5*f*
  8-OHdG DNA damage,
    elevation of, 3–5, 4*f*, 10
2-Amino-3-methylimidazo[4, 5-*f*]
    quinolone (IQ), 157
  low-dose carcinogenicity of,
    qualitative and quantitative
    analyses on, 7–8
  DNA adduct formation, 7, 8*f*
  GST-P-positive foci, induction
    of, 7, 8*f*
  p21$^{Cip1/WAF1}$ expression, 7, 8*f*, 13
  relative mRNA expression, 7, 8*f*
2-Amino-1-methyl-6-
    phenylimidazo [5, 6-*b*]
    pyridine (PhIP)

low-dose carcinogenicity of
    DNA adduct formation,
    10–11
Apurinic endonuclease (APE), 71
1-β-D-Arabinofuranosylcytosine,
    136, 136*f*
Assays
  genotoxicity, 53*t*
  indicator, 52–54
  mutagenicity, 52–54
Ataxia telangiectasia mutated
    (ATM) kinase, 73
ATM and Rad 3-related (ATR)
    kinases, 73

B

Basal cell carcinoma (BCC),
    epidemiological analysis of,
    38–39, 40*f*
Base excision repair (BER)
    pathway, 71–73
BAT (Biologischer Arbeitsstoff-
    Toleranzwert) values
    (BLVs), 118–120
Bayesian belief network (BBN),
    95–98, 96*f*, 97*f*
Benchmark dose (BMD), 67, 131,
    145–146, 199–200
  advantages of, 145
  choice of, 145
  definition of, 68*t*, 145
  mathematical modeling for, 146
Benzo(*a*)pyrene, 157
  genotoxic thresholds, 105
Benzo[*e*]pyrene (B[*e*]P)
  co-carcinogenicity, 31
Blocking (local control), 133–134

Bmd, 148
BMDS, 143, 147
Bonferroni approach, 139
Bottom-up method, 93–94
Breakpoint doses (BPDs), 67
  definition of, 68t
N-Butyl-N-(4-hydroxybutyl)
  nitrosamine (BBN),
  184–185

C

Cadmium, practical threshold of,
  125–126
Cancer risk, low-dose radiation–
  chemicals interaction in, 37
  data from animal experiments,
    42–46
    skin tumors, 42–43
    thymic lymphoma, 43–46,
      43f, 44f
  epidemiological analysis of,
    38–41
    leukemia, 40–41
    solid cancer, 38–40, 39f, 40f
    radiation–carcinogen interaction,
    41–42
Chlorpromazine, genotoxicity of,
  52–54
Chromosomal aberration test,
  52–54, 104
Chronic progressive nephropathy
  (CPN), 174–175
Clean Air Act, 92–93
Co-carcinogenicity, 31
Compound-specific TTC,
  112–113
Constitutive androstane receptor
  (CAR) activator-induced
  liver tumors, based on
  MOA, 195–197
    hepatic tumor induction, by CAR
    activators, 195
    human relevance of, 196–197
    liver tumor formation, via CAR
    activators, 195–196
Critical effect size (CES),
  145–146
1-[2-Cyano-3, 12-dioxooleana-1, 9
  (11)-dien-28-oyl]imidazole
  (CDDO-Im), 164

D

Delaney Clause, 107
Design of experiments (DOE),
  133–134
Deutsche Forschungsgemeinschaft
  (DFG), 118–120
2, 4-Diaminotoluene, genotoxicity
  of, 52–54
Diethylnitrosamine. See
  N-Nitrosodiethylamine
  (DEN)
Diethylstilbesterol (DES), 30
Distributional method, 94–95, 95t
DNA adducts, 52–54
  formation
    in 2-AAF mutagenicity, 10–11
    and aberrant crypt foci,
      correlation between, 10–11
    in IQ mutagenicity, 7, 8f
    in MeIQx mutagenicity, 3, 4f,
      5, 10
    in PhIP mutagenicity, 10–11
DNA damage in risk assessment,
  endogenous versus
  exogenous, 83
    aldehydes, 84–88
    alkylating agents, 88–90
    oxidative stress, 90–91
    ionizing radiation, 92
    complex dose–response
      relationships to support risk
      assessments, quantifying,
      92–98
      threshold models, 93
      bottom-up method, 93–94
      distributional method, 94–95,
        95t
      Bayesian belief network,
        95–98, 96f, 97f
DNA–DNA cross-links, 84
DNA–glutathione adducts, 84
DNA polymerases
  in E. coli, 59–60, 59f
  in humans, 61–62, 61t
  in S. typhimurium, 59–60, 60f
DNA–protein cross-links (DPCs),
  84–86
DNA repair
  of alkyl adducts, influences on
    points of departure, 71–73

mechanisms
  mutagenesis and tumorigenesis
    in mammals, suppression
    of, 55–57
DNA strand breaks, 52–54
Dose–effect studies, of liver
  carcinogenesis initiation,
  22–28, 23t, 26t, 29t
  2-acetylaminofluorene, 23t,
    25–28
  aflatoxin B$_1$, 23
  2-amino-3, 8-dimethylimidazo[4,
    5-f]quinoxaline, 24–25
  in humans, 30–32
  3′-methyl-4-(dimethylamino)
    azobenzene, 22
  N-nitrosodiethylamine, 23t, 25,
    26t
  N-nitrosomorpholine, 24
  phenobarbital, 22, 26, 26t
  vinyl chloride, 25
Dose–response modeling, 139–143
  experimental designs for,
    133–138
  in radiation, 132
Drsmooth, 147–148
Dunnett's test, 139

E

Endogenous versus exogenous
  DNA damage in risk
  assessment, role of, 83
  aldehydes, 84–88
  alkylating agents, 88–90
  complex dose–response
    relationships to support risk
    assessments, quantifying,
    92–98
    Bayesian belief network,
      95–98, 96f, 97f
    bottom-up method, 93–94
    distributional method, 94–95,
      95t
    threshold models, 93
  ionizing radiation, 92
  oxidative stress, 90–91
Escherichia coli (E. coli)
  DNA polymerases in, genetic
    map position of,
    59–60, 59f

Ethoxyquin (1, 2-dihydro-6-ethoxy-2, 2, 4-trimethylquinoline), 183–185, 187
  carcinogenicity of, 184–185
    mechanism of, 185
  genotoxicity of, 183
  pharmacokinetics of, 184
Ethyl carbamate, genotoxicity of, 52–54
Ethylene oxide (EO)
  DNA damage in risk assessment, 89–90
Ethyl methanesulfonate (EMS), 68
  chemistry of, 70*t*
  DNA damage in risk assessment, 88
  genotoxicity of, 54
  mechanism of action, 70
  paradigm shift in response to low doses of, 69
  points of departure for, mechanistic evidence supporting, 74–75
  potential threshold of, 135
N-Ethyl-*N*-nitrosourea (ENU), 68
  chemistry of, 70*t*
  DNA damage in risk assessment, 88–89
  exposure, and T-cell lymphoma, 43–45, 43*f*, 44*f*
  mechanism of action, 70
  paradigm shift in response to low doses of, 69
  points of departure for, mechanistic evidence supporting, 75
Eugenol (3-hydroxy-4-methoxyphenyl-3′-propene), 175–178
  carcinogenicity of, 177
  genotoxicity of, 175
  metabolic pathways of, 176*f*
  pharmacokinetics of, 176–177
European Academy Bad Neuenahr-Ahrweiler, 120
Excess absolute risk (EAR), 38–39, 38*t*
Excess relative risk (ERR), 38–39, 38*t*, 39*f*, 40*f*, 41*f*
Extrapolations, 143

F

Fluoranthene
  co-carcinogenicity, 31
Food and Drug Administration (FDA) "Threshold of Regulation" policy, 107
Food Quality Protection Act of 1996, 107
Food Sanitation Act, 109
Formaldehyde
  DNA damage in risk assessment, 84–88

G

Gene mutation tests, 52–54
General linear model (GLM), 139
Genotoxic carcinogens, 104–105
  characteristics of, 50–52, 51*f*
  dose–response of, 49–50, 50*f*
  risk management for, 107–109, 108*f*
  self-defense mechanisms, 50–52, 51*f*
Genotoxicity. *See also individual entries*
  assays, 53*t*
  challenges in identification of, 52–54
Genstat, 146
Germ cell genotoxicity assay, 53*t*
Glutathione *S*-transferase (GST) isoforms, 157
Glutathione *S*–transferase placental form (GST-P)-positive foci, induction of, 3
  IQ mutagenicity, 7, 8*f*
  in MeIQx mutagenicity, 4–5, 4*f*, 10–13
Goodness of fit, 143–145
GraphPad PRISM, 143, 148

H

Hepatocellular altered foci (HAF) NOAEL for, 22–28
H-ras mutation, in MeIQx mutagenicity, 11–12
Humans
  DNA polymerases in, 61–62, 61*t*
  liver carcinogenesis initiation, dose–effect studies of, 30–32, 31*t*

Hydrogen peroxide (H_2O_2)
  DNA damage in risk assessment, 90
8-Hydroxy-2′-deoxyguanosine (8-OHdG) DNA damage
  in MeIQx mutagenicity, 3–5, 4*f*, 10
  and oxidative stress, 10
Hypoxanthine phosphoribosyl transferase (HPRT), 69, 74, 88

I

Immunohistochemical staining, 22
Indicator assays, 52–54, 53*t*
Interpolation, 143
In vivo mutagenesis and carcinogenesis, mechanisms for preventing, 156*f*
Ionizing radiation, 42
  DNA damage in risk assessment, 92
Isoeugenol (1-(3-methoxy-4-hydroxyphenyl)-1-propene), 187

K

Keap1 (Kelch-like erythroid cell-derived protein with CNC homology-associated protein), 158–159, 163–164

L

lacI gene mutation, in MeIQx mutagenicity, 5–6, 5*f*
Less-than-lifetime (LTL) TTC, 112, 113*f*, 113*t*
Leukemia, epidemiological analysis of, 40–41, 41*f*
Likelihood ratio/chi-square test, 144
Linear, 132–133, 133*f*
Linearized Multistage Model (LMS), 83–84
Linear nonthreshold (LNT) model, 120, 132
Lipid peroxidation (LPO), 87–88, 91
Lowest observed adverse effect level (LOAEL), 123–124
Lowest observed genotoxic effect level (LOGEL), 138

M

MAK (Maximale Arbeitsstoffkonzentration) Commission, 118–120
Margin of exposure (MoE), 131–132
Menadione (2-methyl-l, 4-naphthoquinone), 180–183
  carcinogenicity of, 182
  genotoxicity of, 181
  metabolic pathways of, 181*f*
  pharmacokinetics of, 181–182
  toxicology of, 182
3′-Methyl-4-(dimethylamino) azobenzene (MDAB)
  effect on liver carcinogenesis initiation, 22
Methyleugenol (3, 4-dimethoxyphenyl-3′-propene), 175–178
  carcinogenicity of, 177
  genotoxicity of, 175
  metabolic pathways of, 176*f*
  pharmacokinetics of, 176–177
Methylguanine-DNA methyltransferase (MGMT)
  DNA repair of, 71–73
Methyl methanesulfonate (MMS), 68
  chemistry of, 70*t*
  DNA damage in risk assessment, 88
  mechanism of action, 70
  paradigm shift in response to low doses of, 69
  points of departure for, mechanistic evidence supporting, 76
4-(Methylnitrosoamino)-1-(3-pyridyl)-1-butanone (NNK)
  and thymic lymphoma, 45–46
N-Methyl-*N*-nitrosourea (MNU), 68
  chemistry of, 70*t*
  DNA damage in risk assessment, 88–89
  mechanism of action, 70
  paradigm shift in response to low doses of, 69
  points of departure for, mechanistic evidence supporting, 76–77

N-Methylpurine-DNA glycosylase (MPG), 72–77
Metronidazole, genotoxicity of, 52–54
mgcv, 148
Mismatch repair (MMR), 71
Mode of action (MOA), 19–21
  chemical-induced animal tumors, human relevance assessment for, 193
    genotoxic and nongenotoxic tumor inducers, future prospects of mechanistic research in, 199–200
    hepatic tumor induction, by CAR activators, 195
    importance of, 194–195
    liver tumor formation, via CAR activators, 195–196
    mutagen-induced tumors based on threshold, 197–198, 198*t*
MTH1
  role in avoiding 8-oxoG-related mutagenesis, 55, 56*f*
Mutagenicity assays, 52–54, 53*t*
Mutation, definition of, 62
MUTYH
  -associated familial adenomatous polyposis, 55–57
  role in avoiding 8-oxoG-related mutagenesis, 55, 56*f*
  role in avoiding ROS-induced mutagenesis, 57, 58*f*

N

*N*3-alkyladenine (*N*3alkA), 68–69, 72–73
*N*7-alkylguanine (*N*7alkG), 68–73
*N*7-methylguanine (*N*7MeG), 71
N-acetylaminophenol quinone imine (NAPQI), 186–187
Naphthalene, practical threshold of, 123–124
Nested models, 144
Nickel, practical threshold of, 124–125
4-Nitroquinoline-1-oxide (4-NQO), 161
N-Nitrosobutyl (4-hydroxybutyl)-amine, 161

N-Nitrosodiethylamine (DEN), 180
  effect on liver carcinogenesis initiation, 23*t*, 25, 26*t*, 30–31
  genotoxicity of, 52–54
  quantitative low-dose hepatocarcinogenicity of, 9
  GST-P-positive foci, induction of, 9, 9*f*
N-Nitrosomorpholine (NNM)
  effect on liver carcinogenesis initiation, 24
Nongenotoxic carcinogens, 50–52, 104–105
  characteristics of, 50–52, 51*f*
  dose–response of, 49–50, 50*f*
Nonlinear, 132–133, 133*f*
No observed adverse effect level (NOAEL), 19–22, 50–52, 120, 124, 130, 138, 155–156
  for hepatocellular altered foci (HAF), 22–28
No-observed genotoxic effect level (NOGEL), 67, 131, 138–139
  definition of, 68*t*
No safe dose of radiation concept, 130, 132
Nrf2, 155
  activity, human carcinogenesis in, 163–164
  DNA adduct formation, acceleration of, 157, 157*f*
  gene expression by, regulation of, 158–159, 158*f*
  threshold creation, 164
  xenobiotics
    carcinogenicity and mutagenicity of, 160–163, 162*f*
    susceptibility to, 159–160, 160*f*

O

O^6-alkylguanine (O^6alkG), 68–71
Occam's razor principle, 143
Occupational exposure limits (OELs)
  for carcinogenic substances, derivation of, 118

Ochratoxin A, genotoxicity of, 54
OGG1
  role in avoiding 8-oxoG-related
    mutagenesis, 55, 56*f*
O^6-methylguanine (O^6MeG), 71
One factor at a time (OFAT)
    approach, 133–134
Oxidative stress
  DNA damage in risk assessment,
    90–91
  8-OHdG DNA damage and, 10
Oxidative stress-induced
    tumorigenesis, 55–57, 56*f*
8-*Oxo*-7, 8-dihydroguanosine
    (8-*oxo*-dG), 156
  genotoxic thresholds, 106
  immunostaining of, 159–160, 160*f*
  -related mutagenesis in
    mammalian cells, 55–57

P

p21$^{\text{Cip1/WAF1}}$ expression, in IQ
    mutagenicity, 7, 8*f*, 13
Parsimony, 143
PBPK (physiologically based
    pharmacokinetic) model,
    123–124
Perfect threshold, 121
Permitted daily exposures (PDEs),
    130
Phase II drug-metabolizing
    enzyme, 156–158
Phenacetin, 178–180
  carcinogenicity of, 180
  genotoxicity of, 178–179
  metabolisms of, 178*f*
  pharmacokinetics of, 179, 186–187
Phenobarbital (PB)
  effect on liver carcinogenesis
    initiation, 5–6, 22, 26, 26*t*
Points of departure (PoDs), 67,
    199–200
  mechanistic evidence supporting
    ethyl methanesulfonate
    (EMS), 74–75
  N-ethyl-*N*-nitrosourea (ENU), 75
  methyl methanesulfonate
    (MMS), 76
  N-methyl-*N*-nitrosourea
    (MNU), 76–77
  metrics, 68*t*

Potassium bromate (KBrO$_3$)
  DNA damage in risk assessment,
    90
  genotoxicity of, 55–57
Power, 139
Practical threshold, 19–21, 50–52,
    105, 156
  of cadmium, 125–126
  of naphthalene, 123–124
  of nickel, 124–125
  in occupational exposure limits
    derivation, 117
  of propylene oxide, 122–123
PROAST, 143, 147
Procarbazine, genotoxicity of,
    52–54
Propylene oxide, practical threshold
    of, 122–123
Pseudoreplication, 134–135
Pyrene
  co-carcinogenicity, 31

Q

Quantitative structure–activity
    relationship (QSAR)
    methodology, 110–112
Quercetin, 172–175, 187
  carcinogenicity of, 174–175
  chemical structure of, 172*f*
  genotoxicity of, 173
  pharmacokinetics of, 173
  toxicology of, 175

R

Radon gas
  health risks associated with, 42
  radioactive progeny of,
    inhalation of, 42
Randomization, 133–134
Reactive oxygen species (ROS),
    55, 90
Relative risk (RR), 38*t*
Repeatability, 135
Replication, 133–135
Reproducibility, 135
R packages, 148

S

S-adenosylmethionine (SAM)
  DNA damage in risk assessment,
    88

Safe Drinking Water Act, 92–93
Salmonella typhimurium
    (*S. typhimurium*), 75
  DNA polymerases in,
    59–60, 60*f*
SAS, 146
SCOEL (Scientific Committee on
    Occupational Exposure
    Limits of the European
    Union), 121–126, 122*f*
Segmented, 148
SiZer, 148
Skin tumors, low-dose
    radiation–chemicals
    interaction in, 42–43
Solid cancer risk, epidemiological
    analysis of, 38–40, 39*f*,
    40*f*
SPSS, 146
Squamous cell carcinoma (SCC),
    epidemiological analysis of,
    38–39
STATA, 146
Syncarcinogenesis, 30–31

T

T-cell lymphoma
  exposure to X-irradiation
    followed by *N*-ethyl-*N*-
    nitrosourea treatment,
    43–45, 43*f*, 44*f*
Thioacetamide (TAA), liver damage
    induced by, 6–7, 6*f*
Threshold(s)
  of chemical genotoxicity,
    105–106, 106*f*
  definitions of, 131–132
  for DNA-reactive carcinogens
    hepatocarcinogenicity, 19
    practical, 19–21
  doses. *See* Breakpoint doses
    (BPDs)
  genotoxic, mechanisms
    underlying, 54–55
  models, 93
  perfect, 121
  practical. *See* Practical
    threshold
  studies, experimental design and
    statistical analysis of, 129
  zero-risk, 107

Threshold of toxicological concern
(TTC), 62–63, 131, 199–200
for genotoxic impurities, in
pharmaceuticals, 103
compound-specific TTC,
112–113
less-than-lifetime TTC, 112,
113*f*, 113*t*
risk assessment and control,
principles for, 109–112,
111*f*, 111*t*
Thymic lymphoma (TL)
low-dose radiation–chemicals
interaction in, 43–46, 43*f*, 44*f*
mechanism of combined
exposure, in, 45–46
Tolerable daily intake (TDI),
50–52, 54, 62, 130

Toxicologically insignificant daily
intake (TIDI), 30–31, 31*t*
Translesion DNA synthesis
(TLS), as critical factor for
mutagenesis, 58–62, 59*f*

U
UDP-glucuronosyltransferase
(UDP-GT), 157
Urethane (ethyl carbamate),
genotoxicity of, 52–54

V
Vinyl chloride (VC)
effect on liver carcinogenesis
initiation, 25
Virtually safe doses (VSDs), 19–21,
107, 108*f*, 132

X
Xeroderma pigmentosum variant
(XPV), 61–62

Z
Zero equivalent dose (ZED), 138
Zero-risk thresholds, 107

Printed in the United States
By Bookmasters